The Study of Surgery:
Comprehensive Clinical Tutorials in Problem-Solving
for Anatomic and Specialty Fields of General Surgery

The Study of Surgery:
Comprehensive Clinical Tutorials in Problem-Solving for Anatomic and Specialty Fields of General Surgery

Glenn W. Geelhoed, M.D., M.P.H., F.A.C.S.
Professor of Surgery
Professor of International Medical Education
George Washington University Medical Center
Washington, D.C.

J&S

J&S Publishing Company Inc., Alexandria, Virginia

J&S

Composition and Layout: Ronald C. Bohn, Ph. D.
Cover Design and Editing: Kurt E. Johnson, Ph. D.
Printing Supervisor: Robert Perotti, Jr.
Printing: Goodway Graphics, Springfield, Virginia

Library of Congress Catalog Card Number 94-079793

ISBN 0-9632873-6-2

About the Author

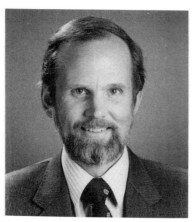

The author is an academic general surgeon with additional subspecialty expertise in endocrine surgery, and background in surgical oncology and transplantation. His undergraduate education was at Calvin College (A.B. cum laude 1964, B.S. 1965) and he attended the University of Michigan Medical School (M.D. cum laude 1968). He was a Harvard surgical resident at the Peter Bent Brigham Hospital and Boston Children's Hospital Medical Center. Following five years in surgical oncology in the Surgery Branch of the National Cancer Institute, Bethesda, M.D., he has been involved full time as Professor of Surgery at George Washington University Medical Center since 1973 developing a transplantation program, trauma service, and interests in surgical physiology in critical illness and sepsis.

Certified and recertified by the American Board of Surgery, he is an active Fellow of the American College of Surgeons, and is past president of the Washington Academy of Surgeons. In 1975 he was awarded an appointment as Clinical Scholar of the Robert Wood Johnson Foundation and in 1986, traveling Surgical Scholar of the James IV Surgical Association. He was inducted in 1990 into the Academie du Chirurgie de Paris. A member of many academic, medical and surgical societies, he is currently vice president of the American Association of Endocrine Surgeons.

He has been continuously active in undergraduate, graduate, and continuing medical education with an interest in evaluating effectiveness of student and resident teaching. He has maintained a strong interest in health and health care education internationally, focusing on the relationship between health and development in the Third World. He has successfully completed additional graduate degrees in International Affairs from George Washington University's Elliot School, as well as an M.P.H. in Epidemiology: Health Promotion/Disease Prevention, the D.T.M.H. from the London School of Tropical Medicine and Hygiene and a Master's degree in Anthropology, investigating the biological anthropology of health and disease in Central Africa. He continues to develop opportunities for international experience for students and physicians interested in pursuing global health issues.

He is an avid outdoorsman, marathon runner, scuba diver, photographer, and enjoys wilderness adventure travel. He assures students of medicine at all levels that writing examination questions is not nearly so exciting as answering them for real.

DEDICATED TO:

PAUL E. SHORB, JR., M.D.
THE "VERY MODEL OF A MAJOR GENERAL SURGEON"
AND A
WONDERFUL FRIEND IN NEED.

CONTENTS

PART VI

PART VII

vii

Preface

This book is a comprehensive review of the clinical applications of the principles of Surgery. The author has used real clinical scenarios from many years of surgical practice in the setting of the treatment potentials and limits of modern medicine. This book emphasizes clinical problem-solving, and taking this test on one's surgical knowledge base is informative, up-to-date, with entertaining flashes of self-deprecating humor along the way. Anyone who clutches up at the prospect of multiple choice test-taking might begin with the very helpful final chapter "How to use _The Study of Surgery_", which gives suggestions on how to approach examination test items.

The book is intended for medical students learning Surgery for the first time, for residents solidifying their knowledge base, and for practicing surgeons who wish to refresh their fundamental principles in applying surgical skills. The study of Surgery calls for knowledge of biologic principles, technical skills, compassion and cautious courage. _The Study of Surgery_ is an appropriate amalgam of these characteristics to form a solid foundation for Surgery examinations.

At a time when Dr. Geelhoed was a highly successful student in the University of Michigan Medical School, the Professor and Chairman of Surgery was C. Gardner Child, who described the prototypical medical students of the era as "addicts for cold dope". We can be grateful for Glenn Geelhoed's provision of a lucid book, _The Study of Surgery_ as a means for ready application of up-to-date "cold dope" in surgical science.

Timothy S. Harrison, M.D.
Professor of Surgery and Physiology, Emeritus
Pennsylvania State University College of Medicine
Hershey, PA, November, 1994

Acknowledgements

The author would like to thank Dr. Ronald C. Bohn for his expertise in formatting these documents for production. The author would also like to thank Diane Downing, R.N., M.P.H. Without her skill and support this typescript would not appear before you. The author is grateful for all this help and acknowledges any errors in this book as his own.

Disclaimer

The clinical information presented in this book is accurate for the purposes of review for licensure examinations but in no way should be used to treat patients or substituted for modern clinical training. Proper diagnosis and treatment of patients requires comprehensive evaluation of all symptoms, careful monitoring for adverse responses to treatment and assessment of the long-term consequences of therapeutic intervention.

Figure Credits

Some of the images used at the beginning of each section in Parts IV, V, and VI were taken from the LifeART Collection, Copyright © 1994, TechPool Studios Corp. USA. The remainder were from CorelDraw! Clipart for CorelDraw 3.0, © 1992, Corel Corporation. The clinical photographs are from the author's personal collection.

PART I
PATIENT MANAGEMENT PROBLEMS

Items 1-3

The 30 year-old woman whose operation, removing a deep mole and the regional nodes, has just been completed as shown below. She has histologic evidence of melanoma in 4 of 34 lymph nodes. Following this treatment:

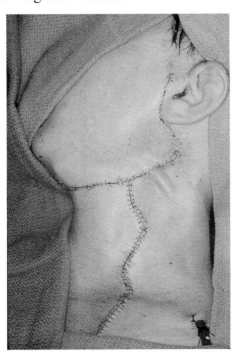

1.   Her five year survival should approximate

(A)   95%
(B)   75%
(C)   60%
(D)   35%
(E)   10%

2.   Her expected recurrence site would be most likely to be

(A)   bone
(B)   wound
(C)   lung
(D)   skin
(E)   opposite neck

3.   Her next line treatment for evidence of recurrence would be

(A)   radiation
(B)   chemotherapy
(C)   immunotherapy
(D)   endocrine therapy
(E)   debulking

ANSWERS AND TUTORIAL ON ITEMS 1-3

The answers are: **1-C; 2-C; 3-C.**

Melanoma on the extremities has better survival than that on the trunk, (including the head and neck) and in women has a generally 10% better overall prognosis than in men for the same site and stage. This is Stage II disease, and the thickness or level of invasion for the primary tumor is only helpful to get to an estimation of the likelihood that it would invade lymph nodes to become Stage II, so that is no longer a very helpful prognostic indicator to determine the nature of the primary lesion and its affect on prognosis when the disease is already present in lymph nodes. The five year survival would be less than 50% in males, and would be around 60% for females. If and when it recurs, the recurrence site would be most likely in lung, since the pulmonary metastases are the most common visceral metastases following primary melanoma treatment.

There is essentially no effective radiotherapy for this disease, and debulking does not increase survival or decrease symptoms generally as it might for some other specific tumors. There is a puzzling unpredictability about melanoma which has led many to postulate some form of immunologic control, and it is for that reason that the most extensive clinical experimentation with immunotherapy has been done with melanoma. Because it is not monotonous in its predictable behavior pattern such as many of the sarcomas, it takes larger numbers of patients to determine whether there is any effectiveness to the immunotherapy. However, it is an option to be tried should the disease recur at pulmonary or other regional sites. It is unlikely that the disease would cross the midline to involve the lymphatics of the opposite side of the neck.

This man has a scalp lesion that has been enlarging for over a year with heaped up edges and occasional ulceration.

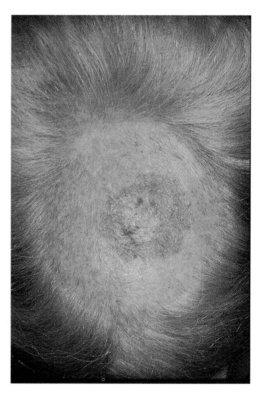

4.   Biopsy would show histologically

    (A)   amelanotic melanoma
    (B)   squamous cell carcinoma
    (C)   basal cell carcinoma
    (D)   actinic keratosis
    (E)   granuloma

5.   Treatment might include all of the following **EXCEPT:**

    (A)   radical neck dissection
    (B)   local excision
    (C)   rotation flap graft
    (D)   chemosurgery
    (E)   free skin graft

6. Recurrence might be expected in the

    (A)   local wound
    (B)   lymph nodes
    (C)   lungs
    (D)   skull
    (E)   liver

ANSWERS AND TUTORIAL ON ITEMS 4-6

The answers are: **4-C; 5-A; 6-A.**

This is the classic "rodent ulcer" recognizable by its heaped-up edges. It is malignant, basal cell carcinoma in origin, and recurs locally, but almost never metastasizes to lymphatics or beyond. It is frequently treated by chemosurgery if it is too extensive for simple excision, and this "Moh's paste" treatment causes destruction of the local tumor back to areas where it will show biopsy negative margins. Simple rotation flaps are sufficient to achieve coverage in most instances, but split thickness skin graft may be employed as well. The one therapy that is inappropriate is radical neck dissection, since it is so rarely metastatic beyond the area of the local wound.

Items 7-9

This pigmented lesion on the neck of a young boy is about to be removed.

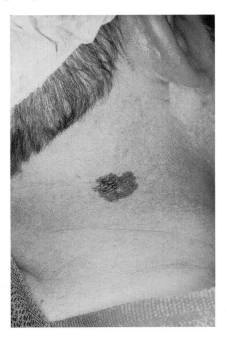

7. Indications for this procedure include each of the following **EXCEPT:**

    (A)   central clearing
    (B)   nodularity
    (C)   irregular border
    (D)   high malignancy rate in this age and sex
    (E)   cosmetic appearance in this position

8. Removal would best be done by

    (A)   laser ablation
    (B)   excisional biopsy
    (C)   in continuity neck dissection
    (D)   hyfrecator
    (E)   incisional biopsy and frozen section

9. The differential diagnosis includes all the following **EXCEPT:**

(A) junctional nevus
(B) Hutchinson's lentigo
(C) compound nevus
(D) nodular melanoma
(E) superficial spreading melanoma

ANSWERS AND TUTORIAL ON ITEMS 7-9

The answers are: **7-D; 8-B; 9-B.**

This is a pigmented nevus histologically unknown but clinically suspected of being either a junctional nevus (worrisome enough for future degeneration that it is by itself an indication for removal) or a compound nevus (for which the indication toward removal is only its cosmetic position and its confusion with the other forms that would be more worrisome, since compound nevus is benign). Simple excisional biopsy is sufficient to treat a compound nevus. This nevus has each of the features described including some of those that pertain to melanoma, such as central clearing and irregular border with some nodularity. However, this is not an age group in which this malignancy is expected at a very high rate. Methods of removal would involve anything that ablates the primary lesion but still gives evidence of its histology for complete and thorough evaluation. For that reason, destruction of it or less than full excision of it is not indicated, and anything more radical than simple excision is certainly inappropriate given the high probability that it is benign.

4

Items 10-12

This 12 year-old boy had noted a neck lump for most of his life, recently enlarging.

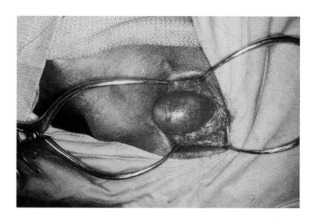

10. It is a derivative of

(A) thyroglossal tract
(B) neuroectoderm
(C) first pharyngeal pouch
(D) second pharyngeal pouch
(E) dental anlage

11. On cut section it would be

(A) a solid tumor
(B) a pseudocyst
(C) hemorrhagic
(D) filled with colloid
(E) containing cystic secretions

12. The most likely complication would be

    (A) malignant degeneration
    (B) infection
    (C) fistula formation
    (D) hypothyroidism
    (E) sialolithiasis

ANSWERS AND TUTORIAL ON ITEMS 10-12

The answers are: **10-D; 11-E; 12-B.**

This clinical photograph is of a second pharyngeal pouch cyst presenting in the classic position. The first pharyngeal pouch is at the level of the external auditory meatus. The boy has had it most of his life, and the "rule of sevens" suggests that this is likely to be congenital (seven days inflammatory, seven months neoplastic and seven years congenital). This one, in fact, was filled with cystic secretion materials with a sebaceous character; many can be purulent when secondarily infected. That secondary infection is the most likely complication, and if there is interior communication and incision and drainage is done, fistula formation may result, but that is less common than infection which is the usual complicating feature to which it is predisposed.

Items 13-15

This adult male is quite worried about the rapidly expanding mass in his neck.

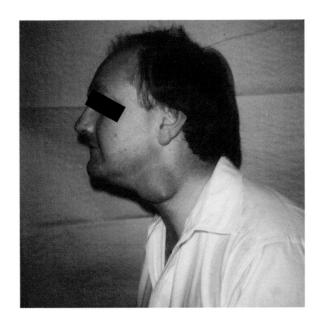

13. The best treatment would be

    (A) reassurance
    (B) incision and drainage
    (C) antibiotics
    (D) immediate excision
    (E) schedule urgent radical neck dissection

14. Tissue biopsy results would reveal

    (A) squamous cell carcinoma
    (B) necrotic melanoma
    (C) purulent inflammation
    (D) papillary thyroid carcinoma
    (E) mixed salivary tumor

15. Definitive treatment would be

    (A)   radiation therapy
    (B)   methotrexate and leucovorin rescue
    (C)   radio-iodine
    (D)   radical neck dissection
    (E)   elective local excision in six weeks

ANSWERS AND TUTORIAL ON ITEMS 13-105

The answers are: **13-B; 14-C; 15-E.**

You may not have thought that a congenital abnormality would wait until adult life for presentation! As many things that may present to the clinic may come in pairs or threes, so may some test questions, and this is an adult with a second pharyngeal pouch cyst. In this instance, the patient has become aware of it because it is secondarily infected. In this form it is an abscess despite the predisposition to the collection of fluid there in the cystic remnant of the second pharyngeal pouch. As almost all abscesses are treated by incision and drainage after some warm compresses to encourage the "pointing" of the abscess, that is the treatment for this one as well; however, note that it is already "pointing" and it would be a simple matter to relieve him of this rapid inflammatory expansion. When this considerable quantity of pus is drained, a period of healing would follow in which the cyst may scar down, but when it is no longer inflamed and primary healing would be likely to take place without the complication of infection, the patient could be scheduled for an elective excision of the pharyngeal pouch cyst that gave rise to this abscess.

Items 16-18

This Kampuchean refugee woman has had this mass for several years and sought an opinion regarding its nature and treatment.

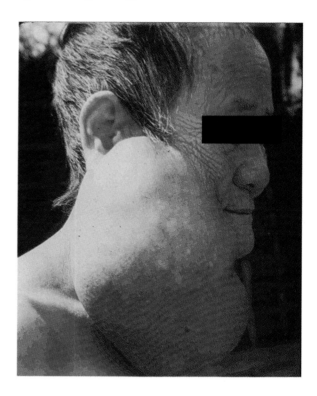

16. It is most probably

    (A)   congenital
    (B)   inflammatory
    (C)   benign
    (D)   malignant
    (E)   metastatic

17. Operation for its removal would carry the biggest risk of

    (A)   hemorrhage
    (B)   facial nerve palsy
    (C)   inadequate closure
    (D)   spreading metastases
    (E)   rapid local recurrence

18. Alternatives to operation would include

   (A) antibiotics
   (B) radiation therapy
   (C) 5-fluorouracil
   (D) corticosteroids
   (E) none

ANSWERS AND TUTORIAL ON ITEMS 16-18

The answers are: **16-C; 17-B; 18-E.**

This patient, isolated from most advanced forms of medical care, patiently awaited my attention and exhibited a massive mixed parotid salivary gland tumor. Parotid tumors are most often benign. Note that she has an intact facial nerve despite the pendulous nature of this enlarged mass. It would be relatively easy to get control of both the bleeding and accomplish skin closure around this with a subtotal parotid excision, but the single biggest hazard would be to the facial nerve, which in fact happened for a period of transient paralysis in this individual. Of the alternatives to operation, the simplest is the true one; there are no alternatives, since this benign tumor does not respond to any of the other treatment modalities listed.

Items 19-21

This wound has been a problem in management so the operation seen here has just been performed.

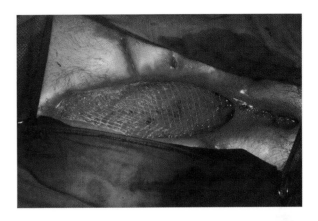

19. The intent of the operation has been

   (A) accomplish primary closure
   (B) establish primary intention healing
   (C) re-epithelialization
   (D) transfer soft tissue padding
   (E) establish second intention healing

20. The skin grafted has each of the features recommending its use **EXCEPT:**

   (A) covers more space with less graft
   (B) brings in new blood supply
   (C) contoured to defect
   (D) will not likely lift up from seroma
   (E) readily available

21. Long term features might include each of the following **EXCEPT:**

   (A)   Marjolin ulcer
   (B)   contracture
   (C)   darker pigmentation
   (D)   concave defect
   (E)   recurrent granulation

ANSWERS AND TUTORIAL ON ITEMS 19-21

The answers are: **19-C; 20-B; 21-A.**

   A split thickness skin graft is a ready source of skin for re-epithelialization which follows granulation and second intention healing. Rather than waiting for the prolonged contracture of this wound to the point where the advancing edges can re-epithelialize it over the granulation bed, the split thickness skin graft was taken from any cosmetically accessible site, and was meshed. This allows contouring and spreading over a wider defect than the donor site as well as allowing seroma to come through the graft without lifting it. The wound will both darken and contract, but will remain a concave defect, since no extra tissue padding or blood supply was brought in with the split thickness skin graft. It has no premalignant potential as would the Marjolin ulcer.

Items 22-24

This lesion has been making the patient aware of an odd taste for five months and in the last two months has interfered with speech.

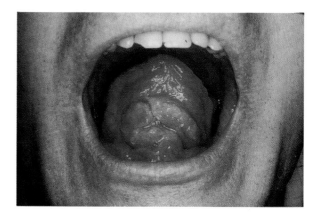

22. It is most probably

   (A)   congenital
   (B)   inflammatory
   (C)   benign
   (D)   malignant
   (E)   secretory

23. The histopathologic examination after biopsy would show

   (A)   adenocarcinoma
   (B)   squamous cell carcinoma
   (C)   leiomyosarcoma
   (D)   lipoma
   (E)   secretory cysts

24. Treatment will be limited to

(A) radiotherapy
(B) local excision
(C) incisional biopsy
(D) commando composite resection with radical neck dissection
(E) skin graft to anterior undersurface of the tongue

ANSWERS AND TUTORIAL ON ITEMS 22-24

The answers are: **22-D; 23-B; 24-D.**

There are some benign lesions that exist under the anterior surface of the tongue and adjacent structures such as ranula and epulis, and this is not one of them. This is an ulcerated form of squamous cell carcinoma proven by a small incisional biopsy in the planning for the several stage treatment that will involve a very extensive operation in order to get control of the margins and resurface the floor of the mouth following the neck dissection.

"Let me have a surgeon; I am cut to th' brains."

William Shakespeare (1564-1616)
King Lear IV, 6, 196

Items 25-27

This patient complained of symptoms that led to a barium swallow (A) and then to the finding (B) seen being repaired in the operating room.

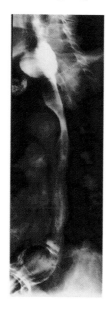

(A)

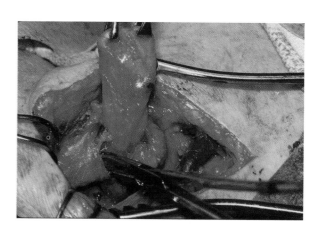

(B)

25. This finding is most probably

    (A) congenital
    (B) inflammatory
    (C) benign
    (D) malignant
    (E) infectious

26. An etiologic agent is

    (A) lye ingestion
    (B) ionizing radiation
    (C) tuberculosis
    (D) muscular propulsion
    (E) acid reflux

27. Adjunctive to excision will be treatment by

    (A) esophageal bougie dilatation
    (B) myotomy
    (C) corticosteroids
    (D) radiation
    (E) antibiotics

ANSWERS AND TUTORIAL ON ITEMS 25-27

The answers are: **25-C; 26-D; 27-B.**

The specific complaint this patient had when she presented pre-operatively was the regurgitation of food up to several hours after eating that was in no way digested. She said it had also caused her foul breath. The barium swallow shows a Zenker's diverticulum in the classic position. This is a pulsion diverticulum, occurring at the junction of the hypopharynx and esophageal muscles as the decussation allows a mucosal diverticulum to form between the muscular fibers. The diverticulum itself can be either excised, as it was here, or tacked in a position so that it is superior allowing dependant drainage.

Along with the operation to excise the diverticulum is an adjunctive procedure

10

to correct the underlying problem that gave rise to it, and that is by partial myotomy, relieving the constricting pressure that has given rise to the propulsion diverticulum originally.

Items 28-30

This is the surgical specimen removed from a woman with a 25 pound weight loss in four months, occult stool blood, and dysphagia with inability to belch or vomit.

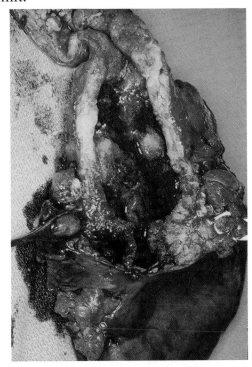

28.   From the gross appearance of the tumor, this is a cancer which is

(A)   Stage I
(B)   Stage II
(C)   Stage III
(D)   metastatic from a distant primary tumor
(E)   originating in smooth muscle

29.   The histology of this tumor is likely to be

(A)   lymphoma
(B)   adenocarcinoma
(C)   squamous cell carcinoma
(D)   leiomyosarcoma
(E)   amelanotic melanoma

30.   Its origin would appear to be from

(A)   distal third of esophagus
(B)   proximal stomach
(C)   lymphoid submucosa
(D)   muscular wall
(E)   submucosal metastases

ANSWERS AND TUTORIAL ON ITEMS 28-30

The answers are: **28-C; 29-B; 30-B.**

This is adenocarcinoma of the stomach originating in the gastroesophageal junction. The distal esophagus is involved with the adenocarcinoma which has "crawled up" proximally into the esophagus. The usual lining cells of the stomach are glandular, as opposed to the transition in the esophagus to squamous cells, so primary carcinoma arising on one side or the other would have characteristic cell type of origin with the boundary being at the hiatus. This boundary shifts when there is either glandular epithelium or squamous epithelium exposed in a primary milieu of the opposite type as happens with Barrett's esophagitis which is a columnar transition or also in re-epithelialization after inflammatory denuding of the esophagus in reflux esophagitis. In this case, however, it is all malignant epithelium that has spread over the margin, and that large tumor and the obstruction to which it gave rise are Stage III evidence of disease which is palliated by esophagogastrectomy.

Items 31-33

This upper GI barium study (A) is obtained in following-up a patient suspected of having unhealing ulcer. The patient underwent operation (B) revealing the disease seen in the specimen depicted.

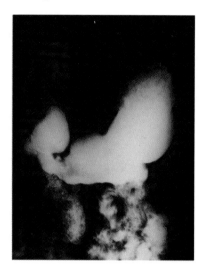

(A)

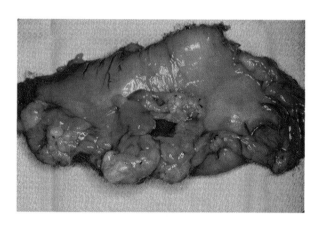

(B)

31.   The X-ray pattern reveals

(A)   previous Billroth-II gastrectomy
(B)   lesser curvature ulcer
(C)   *linnitis plastica*
(D)   gastroenteric fistula
(E)   gastric outlet obstruction

32.   The specimen photo is of the unopened distal (antral) stomach showing

(A)   malignant gastric ulcer
(B)   colon cancer metastatic to stomach
(C)   penetrating antral ulcer
(D)   extrinsic gastric obstruction
(E)   lymphoma in gastric wall

33.   To give this clinical appearance, the gastric ulcer must be

(A)   malignant
(B)   penetrating
(C)   atrophic
(D)   recurrent
(E)   originating outside mucosa

ANSWERS AND TUTORIAL ON ITEMS 31-33

The answers are: **31-D; 32-C; 33-B.**

This patient presented with her own spontaneous "dumping syndrome" after a protracted period of an unhealing ulcer. This complication developed which was a penetrating antral ulcer that communicated with the GI tract. That the ulcer penetrated did not mean that it was malignant, and she had successful resection of both the antrum and the fistula in the lower gut to which it was adherent and successful Billroth I gastroduodenostomy.

Items 34-36

This photo is taken during operation for uncontrolled upper gastrointestinal bleeding in a patient with sepsis, renal failure and pneumonia.

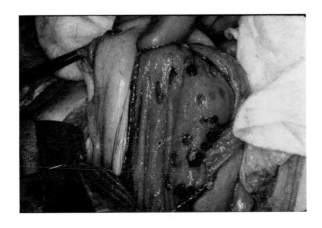

34.   This mucosal appearance is called

   (A)   Cushing ulcer
   (B)   stress ulcer
   (C)   Curling ulcer
   (D)   steroid ulcer
   (E)   aspirin-induced ulcer

35.   The location of such ulceration is typically

   (A)   antrum
   (B)   body and fundus
   (C)   duodenum
   (D)   lesser curvature
   (E)   pylorus

36.   Treatment would be by

   (A)   oversewing bleeding ulcers
   (B)   vagotomy
   (C) H_2-receptor antagonists
   (D)   compression balloon
   (E)   gastrectomy

ANSWERS AND TUTORIAL ON ITEMS 34-36

The answers are: **34-B; 35-B; 36-E.**

This patient developed uncontrollable GI bleeding in the ICU, complicated by failure in several organ systems. This condition is referred to as stress ulceration, and the only really effective way to treat it is to prevent it, since the patients have very high mortality associated with the underlying disease, and autodigestion of the stomach is just one more manifestation of multiple failing organ systems subsequent to sepsis and hypoperfusion.

The ulcers are typically multiple, undermined, and take the pattern of an erosive gastritis in the fundus and cardia of the body of the stomach — but they *skip* the *antrum*. Treatment is by the best operation that can possibly be done to control bleeding at one operative occasion, since there will not be an opportunity for a second procedure. This has meant gastrectomy in most of these patients. Since the mortality is high and the bleeding control difficult in these patients, attention has been directed toward prevention. The ICU patients who have had diligent attention to their gastric pH either by neutralization through instilled antacids or H_2-receptor antagonists have had a remarkably reduced incidence of this complication.

Items 37-39

A patient with unhealing gastric ulcer undergoes the Upper GI study shown here (A) and decision is made for operation. The unopened specimen is depicted (B).

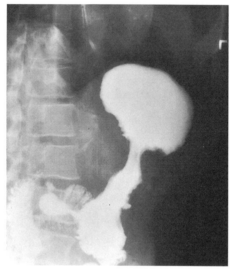

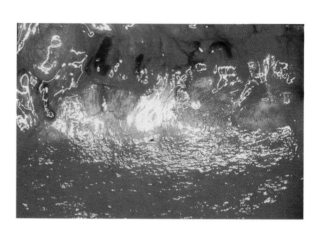

(A)   **(B)**

37.   Indication for operation was

    (A)   gastric total obstruction
    (B)   potential for curative resection
    (C)   debulking
    (D)   reduce portal hypertension
    (E)   denervate stomach

38.   X-ray and gross appearance suggest

    (A)   lesion limited to mucosa
    (B)   transmural involvement
    (C)   healed perforation
    (D)   lesion would have resolved with more time
    (E)   it is likely to be lymphoma

39.   Histopathology shows an adenocarcinoma and associated lymph nodes are negative. The patient's prognosis for 5 year survival is

    (A)   90%
    (B)   75%
    (C)   60%
    (D)   40%
    (E)   25%

ANSWERS AND TUTORIAL ON ITEMS 37-39

The answers are: **37-B; 38-B; 39-D.**

This patient has a malignant gastric ulcer. There are no X-ray signs of unresectability, and this operation was for curative intent. However, from the unopened specimen, you can see that the ulcer has penetrated to the serosa, and even though the lymph nodes are negative, this drops the survival at 5 years from 70% down to much less. When this is seen, it is important to recognize whether it is a healed scar that is present on the surface of the serosa or malignant penetration. In this case the latter was true. So the operable patient had the discovery of a resectable tumor and underwent a gastrectomy with curative intent, but has less than half a chance of being tumor free at 5 years even without lymph node involvement of this transmural gastric cancer.

Items 40-42

In the course of an operation for upper gastrointestinal bleeding, a 34 year-old woman has the discovery of the gastric lesions depicted.

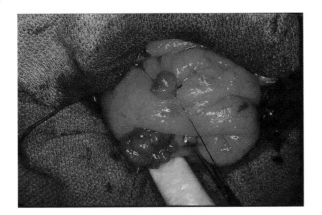

40.   The origin of these tumors is likely to be

(A)   mucosal
(B)   submucosal lymphatics
(C)   muscular wall
(D)   distant metastases
(E)   implants from an esophageal primary tumor

41.   Treatment of the lesions should be

(A)   total gastrectomy
(B)   simple excision
(C)   vagotomy
(D)   chemotherapy
(E) H_2-receptor antagonists

42.   The histopathologic report reveals

(A)   carcinoma *in situ*
(B)   benign gastric polyps
(C)   lymphoma
(D)   foreign body reaction
(E)   leiomyoma

ANSWERS AND TUTORIAL ON ITEMS 40-42

The answers are: **40-A; 41-B; 42-B.**

Most tumors of the stomach are malignant. This is one of the fortunate few mucosal lesions that turn out to be benign, and this woman had benign gastric polyps. The source of the GI bleeding was from duodenal ulcer, so there was no direct relationship in that the polyps were not bleeding. They otherwise might have been endoscopically removed as both biopsy and treatment. These mucosal lesions are worrisome, however, because they are rare among the greater number of gastric mucosal lesions that are malignant, and the appearance of such a lesion could not be dismissed without excision. However, simple excision is adequate therapy with a close follow-up for evidence of new lesions that may develop.

Items 43-45

This photograph shows the removed gall bladder sectioned to reveal its contents.

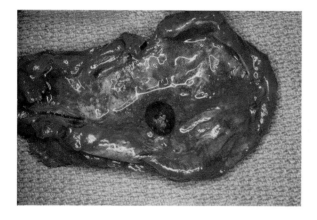

43.   This condition is

   (A)   emphysematous cholecystitis
   (B)   acute purulent cholecystitis
   (C)   chronic cholecystitis
   (D)   empyema of the gall bladder
   (E)   "milk of calcium" sludge formation

44.   This gall bladder likely was removed from a patient with

   (A)   diabetes
   (B)   melanoma
   (C)   hemolysis
   (D)   hypercholesterolemia
   (E)   Gilbert's syndrome

45.   If the gall bladder had not been removed, it would likely have

   (A)   perforated
   (B)   degenerated to carcinoma
   (C)   resolved completely
   (D)   become an intrahepatic abscess
   (E)   become chronic cholecystitis

ANSWERS AND TUTORIAL ON ITEMS 43-45

The answers are: **43-B; 44-C; 45-E.**

This specimen shows acute purulent cholecystitis. There is no great mural thickening of the gall bladder wall and any evidence of fibrosis is suggestive that inflammation has been going on for a long period of time. There is purulence in the mucosa. One large dark pigmented gallstone is also prominent. It is likely that the patient has a reason for making a pigmented gallstone and it would be likely that that would be hemolysis based in some underlying hematologic disorder. If acute cholecystitis is not treated, it will not necessarily go on to perforation, particularly if not gangrenous. Over time, repeated episodes of cholecystitis associated with the gallstone will cause the chronic cholecystitis changes referred to, including the very thickened and fibrotic gall bladder wall which will be even less effective in facilitating absorption of fluid and contrast concentration.

Items 46-48

Through an inflammatory subhepatic mass, a difficult dissection is carried out to identify anatomic structures when a collection of pus is encountered and collected as depicted here.

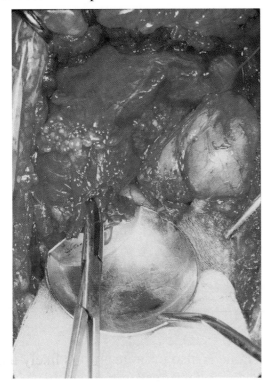

46.   The likely diagnosis is

    A)   adenocarcinoma of gall bladder
    (B)   pylephlebitis
    (C)   carcinoid
    (D)   empyema of the gall bladder
    (E)   gallstone ileus

47.   Patients with this condition often have associated

    (A)   second primary malignancies
    (B)   diabetes mellitus
    (C)   transplant
    (D)   hyperalimentation
    (E)   viral hepatitis

48.   If no further anatomic structures can be defined, it would be advisable to

    (A)   stop and close
    (B)   proceed with blind cholecystectomy
    (C)   perform cholecystostomy
    (D)   call for intraoperative endoscopic retrograde cholangiopancreatography
    (E)   open duodenum and proceed retrograde

ANSWERS AND TUTORIAL ON ITEMS 46-48

The answers are: **46-D; 47-B; 48-C.**

Operating in this subhepatic inflammatory mass is both tedious and dangerous. It is apparent that the patient has an empyema of the gall bladder, which has either perforated or is necrotic and walled off by surrounding omentum. This may be treated as an abscess and simple drainage of the abscess, conducting as much as possible of the purulent bile out of the gall bladder, might allow resolution of the densest component of this inflammatory reaction, particularly if the foreign body gall stones are also extracted. It is *not* a good idea to be dissecting into tissue in which no clear anatomic identification is possible. That would especially include coming up from the distal end of the biliary tree by working backward from the common duct entry at the ampulla. Duodenotomy is not indicated except for other indications, and in this instance, drainage of the empyema is the most effective first stage. If structures were easily identified and dissection could proceed safely, then cholecystectomy is a definitive treatment. But it should not be a definitive treatment at the cost of permanent biliary stenosis or worse complications in the patient in whom the surgeon proceeds blindly.

Items 49-51

This intra-operative view shows the gall bladder in a patient with painless jaundice.

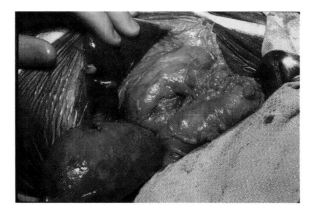

49. Clinical findings in such patients often include

(A) gallstones in gall bladder on ultrasound
(B) palpable nontender mass
(C) pus in the common duct
(D) impacted ampullary gallstone
(E) Klatzkin tumor

50. The primary biliary pathology in these cases is

(A) distal obstruction
(B) Corolli's disease
(C) reflux sclerosing cholangitis
(D) pigmented gallstones
(E) infection with enteric pathogens

51. Immediate cholecystectomy should *not* be carried out, because

(A) it is not primarily involved with the pathologic process
(B) it will fully recover form and function
(C) it makes subsequent exposure technically difficult
(D) retraction "handle" is lost to pull up the common duct
(E) it may be needed for biliary diversion

ANSWERS AND TUTORIAL ON ITEMS 49-51

The answers are: **49-B; 50-A; 51-E.**

A palpable nontender gall bladder in a patient with painless jaundice is Courvoisier's sign. The association is that gall bladder distension usually is on the basis of distal malignant obstruction rather than inflammation that is associated with stone obstruction. If there is sufficient stone formation to give distal biliary obstruction, that is an inflammatory condition that would probably have resulted in chronic cholecystitis with fibrotic contracture. A gall bladder not involved in inflammation or fibrosis is likely to be the innocent victim of a distal obstruction not of its own making. The most common cause of such obstruction is a malignancy in the head of the pancreas.

This clinical probability was well described by Courvoisier using a color print for one of the first times in a medical journal showing the deep jaundice of the patient. Since the gall bladder wall is noninflamed, though it is distended, the cystic duct may be open to the passage of bile. If the head of the pancreas is so well encased in tumor that decompression at that point cannot be achieved, the gall bladder may be needed as a conduit for diversion of the bile into the gut. Subsequently, the large and protruding palpable gall bladder should not be the first attack in the exploration, since it may be the biliary conduit necessary for palliation of the bile duct obstruction.

A patient with CT evidence of distal pancreatic mass who has normal amylase and bilirubin undergoes exploration with the findings indicated in this photograph.

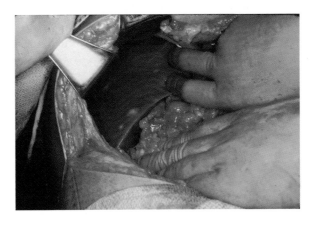

52.   Treatment should now consist of

(A)   pancreatic resection
(B)   gastrojejunostomy
(C)   cholecystojejunostomy
(D)   right hepatic lobe resection
(E)   biopsy of omental nodules

53.   Primary therapy for this patient would consist of

(A)   5-fluorouracil
(B)   analgesics
(C)   radiation
(D)   indwelling stents
(E)   debulking

54. Median survival could be estimated to approximate

(A) five years
(B) six months
(C) one year
(D) three years
(E) two years

ANSWERS AND TUTORIAL ON ITEMS 52-54

The answers are: **52-E; 53-B; 54-B.**

An honest initial appraisal for the current status of treatment for pancreatic carcinoma is that pancreatic cancer is primarily untreatable. That does not mean that it is not treated, but that surgery is very limited in its effectiveness except in highly select instances. In this patient, a distal pancreatic mass has been seen, and the patient is neither jaundiced nor has any evidence of obstruction to the gastric outlet or pancreatic inflow. For that reason, palliation is not possible without symptoms relieved by such procedures, and palliation in advance is not often a good idea, since it may create more problems than it may later solve. These potential problems may occur long after the patient's very limited life expectancy has passed. The patient here has both nodules in the omentum as well as hepatic metastases. It is not certain that these show up on CT, and in this case didn't. However, this is contraindication to resection, and without evidence of actual or eminent obstruction, palliation operations designed to relieve such obstruction would not be indicated.

The discussion with patient and family as appropriate would determine what their desires would be relative to treatment given the very limited prognosis and a median survival of around six months. If they wish to begin some form of chemotherapy with its attendant morbidity and its very limited probability of doing any tumor shrinkage or slowing of the rate of growth, that can be discussed with them along with the facts that this is not a very chemosensitive tumor, and in fact, that there is very little that one does for such a patient other than diagnosis, prognosis, and symptomatic relief to the degree possible.

"The medical student is likely to be one son (sic) of the family too weak to labor on the farm, too indolent to do any exercise, too stupid for the bar and too immoral for the pulpit."
Daniel Coit Gilman (1831-1908)

Items 55-57

A 38 year-old man becomes abruptly desperately ill with acute abdomen, elevated WBC, hypocalcemia and shock. He is resuscitated with crystalloid fluid and operation undertaken which shows exploration findings (A) and the specimen removed at that exploration depicted here (B). The resection is principally carried out with suction and lavage.

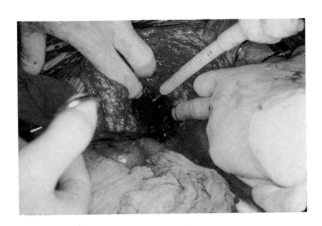

(A)

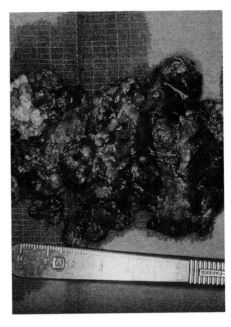

(B)

55.   The diagnosis is most probably

    (A)   necrotizing hemorrhage pancreatitis
    (B)   ruptured duodenal diverticulum
    (C)   aortic aneurysm rupture
    (D)   anterior perforating duodenal ulcer
    (E)   necrotic Hodgkin's lymphoma

56.   Postoperatively he will require rapid replacement of

    (A)   pancreatic enzymes
    (B)   insulin
    (C)   glucagon
    (D)   potassium
    (E)   calcium

57.   The likelihood is that this operation will

    (A)   cure the disease
    (B)   cause enteric fistulas
    (C)   lead to uncontrolled bleeding
    (D)   need repeating
    (E)   prevent septicemia

ANSWERS AND TUTORIAL ON ITEMS 55-57

The answers are: **55-A; 56-E; 57-D.**

Acute pancreatitis may take a fulminant form in which necrosis of retroperitoneal tissue and hemorrhage are prominent features. Occasionally,

21

destruction is so complete that pancreatic islet cell function is lost and the patient can become diabetic. However, insulin-secreting β-islet cells and glucagon-secreting α-cells are lost simultaneously. Thus, diabetes is a relatively easy problem to manage later, as it is with those who have had total surgical pancreatectomy. The most acute need that will be recognized postoperatively is the calcium depletion. He has saponified retroperitoneal fat and that is already reflected in hypocalcemia. For that reason, calcium infusion will be an urgent requirement in his postoperative support.

With the ongoing process not completely resolved by a single operation, it is likely this operation will have to be repeated. It is for this reason that some authors recommend the abdomen be left open and packing used so that no extensive re-operative approaches are needed each time the retroperitoneum is debrided of further devitalized tissue. For early aggressive operation and cleaning out as much devitalized tissue as can be achieved (often, as in this case, done principally with lavage and suction rather than sharp dissection from the chemical dissection that has already occurred) the mortality of early surgical management of pancreatitis is very high, since the mortality of this fulminant form of hemorrhagic pancreatitis is high no matter how it is treated.

A 24 year-old woman with fasting hypoglycemia undergoes arteriography (A) followed by operation with the findings depicted (B).

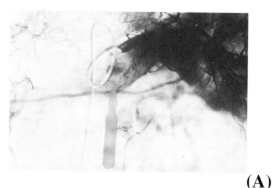

(A)

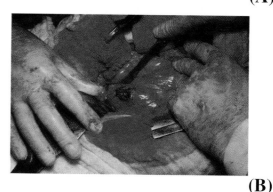

(B)

58.   The most likely tumor imaged by pancreatic arteriography is

  (A)   gastrinoma
  (B)   insulinoma
  (C)   VIPoma
  (D)   nesidioblastosis
  (E)   carcinoid

59.   The treatment should be

  (A)   total pancreatectomy
  (B)   excision of distal pancreas
  (C)   Whipple resection of head of pancreas
  (D)   subtotal wedge pancreatic resection
  (E)   enucleation

60. Following the procedure, her chance of cure is

(A) 10%
(B) 25%
(C) 50%
(D) 75%
(E) 95%

ANSWERS AND TUTORIAL ON ITEMS 58-60

The answers are: **58-B; 59-E; 60-E.**

This patient has insulinoma. Ninety percent of these are benign, solitary and resectable. It is for that reason that arteriography gives a very high yield as to the localization of the islet cell adenoma. Gastrinoma is not so easily localized, since in the majority of instances it is multiple, malignant and metastatic when first encountered. For that reason, there are many more failures of arteriography in gastrinoma and in the other tumors listed than there are in insulinoma (the most satisfactory diagnosis for which arteriographic pancreatic localization is employed).

Because of the nature of this tumor, simple enucleation is sufficient to yield a very high cure rate of this disease. This would not necessarily be the case for the other tumor types listed. If one lacked the ability to localize the tumor or if primary exploration did not reveal it on either operative sonography or careful palpation, one could attempt a blind subtotal pancreatic resection. Even then, the hypoglycemia symptoms can be managed medically, and the tumor symptoms can be controlled during its

slow growth. If it then grows up to arteriographic visualization stage, a limited resection is then possible for cure of the insulinoma.

Items 61-63

A 60 year-old man is referred for evaluation of a distended abdomen (depicted here) with fluid wave and an elevated alpha-fetoprotein. CT shows a large right liver mass.

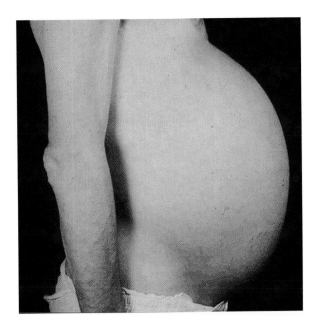

61. The patient's operability will be limited by what likely concomitant disease?

(A) secondary aldosteronism
(B) Laennec's cirrhosis
(C) pancreatitis
(D) congestive heart failure
(E) renal failure

23

62. One of the principle determinants of the reserve status that will define operability is

   (A) alpha-fetoprotein
   (B) serum albumin
   (C) Factor VIII
   (D) renal function
   (E) cardiac output

63. Resectability, if the patient is operable, can be facilitated in its determination by

   (A) ultrasonography
   (B) hepatic arteriogram
   (C) cavagram
   (D) chest X-ray
   (E) pulmonary function studies

ANSWERS AND TUTORIAL ON ITEMS 61-63

The answers are: **61-B; 62-B; 63-B.**

This patient has the classic clinical appearance of Laennec's cirrhosis. In this instance, the recurrent toxic injury to the hepatic cells has led to continuing scarring, regeneration within a firm and fibrous liver with islands of regenerating nodules. Because the hepatic insult has been metabolic and nutritional rather than focal, the damage is diffuse. For that reason, the estimation of the hepatic reserve will help determine whether the patient is operable. One such measurement that will be critically important is the serum albumin, since the liver is the principle manufacturer of serum albumin as well as prothrombins and other proteins vital for homeostasis and hemostasis. Of these factors, the one most useful in its measurement is the serum albumin.

If it is judged that the patient is operable, the next determination will have to be whether the hepatic tumor is resectable. This determination is often difficult because hepatoma originates in a liver that has underlying cirrhosis. The liver resection can be difficult. Arteriography is useful for determining the extent of spread of tumor and for determining how much hepatic tissue must be resected, and how much viable liver will remain after resection. If the liver resection required would be a trisegmentectomy on the basis of the vascular distribution, and the hepatic reserve is already considerably compromised, the nature of the underlying liver disease and the extent of the primary tumor may combine to make this patient inoperable and the tumor unresectable.

Items 64-66

During hysterectomy for menometrorrhagia, a firm mass in the left lateral lobe of the liver is noted in an asymptomatic patient, and surgical consultation is requested to see if the procedure should be modified or terminated. Because of the left lateral lobar position (A), a left lateral lobectomy is carried out for the sectioned specimen seen in (B)

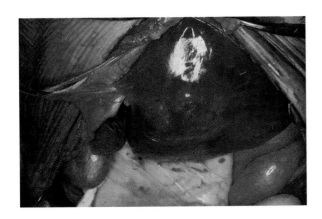

(A)

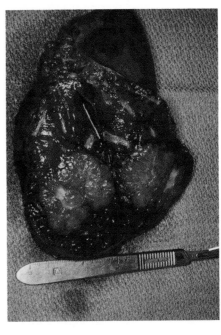

(B)

64. The mass is likely to be

    (A)   thrombosed cavernous hemangioma
    (B)   focal nodular hyperplasia
    (C)   infectious
    (D)   malignant primary
    (E)   metastasis

65. Four weeks following this resection, the patient's liver function will be

    (A)   normal
    (B)   90% of pre-operative level
    (C)   50% of pre-operative level
    (D)   alkaline phosphatase increased over normal
    (E)   LDH increased over normal

66. The liver lesion will probably

    (A)   recur
    (B)   occur again at a new site
    (C)   spread to lungs
    (D)   be cured
    (E)   be the source of carcinoid syndrome

ANSWERS AND TUTORIAL ON ITEMS 64-66

The answers are: **64-B; 65-A; 66-D.**

    This lesion is focal nodular hyperplasia, and its presentation in this patient is the most common way it comes to light. It has only a weak association with any prior history of birth control pill use, and very rarely does it cause bleeding intra-abdominally as a crisis. It is most often found incidentally, masquerading as a more worrisome intrahepatic tumor such as metastases.

This resection will no doubt resolve the problem, which is principally of differential diagnosis between this and those more worrisome lesions. Following left lateral lobectomy, the patient's liver function should return to normal quickly.

Items 67-69

An apartment burglar is shot by police in an exchange of gunfire, and the left upper quadrant injury is explored showing this left lateral lobe of liver wound.

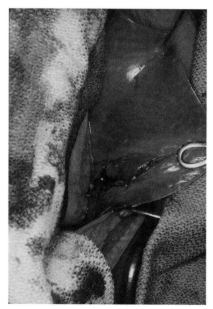

67.   Treatment should be by

   (A)   observing it
   (B)   draining it
   (C)   suturing it
   (D)   resecting it
   (E)   packing it

68.   The clinically significant later component of this injury might likely be

   (A)   loss of functioning liver
   (B)   infection
   (C)   leakage of bile
   (D)   portal vein thrombosis
   (E)   hemobilia

69.   If he has no evident sequelae at 4 weeks he requires

   (A)   follow-up arteriography
   (B)   follow-up liver scan
   (C)   CT
   (D)   ultrasound
   (E)   no specific follow-up

ANSWERS AND TUTORIAL ON ITEMS 67-69

The answers are: **67-D; 68-E; 69-E.**

The significant component of this penetrating injury is the perforation of the gut that lies behind the liver, in this case a through and through perforation of the stomach. This left lateral liver lobe injury may cause some peritoneal signs, but a more substantial component of liver is lost by a partial resection of this lobe. In suturing this lesion, as much liver would be defunctionalized and left *in situ* as would be removed in a relatively simple operation in removing this segment of the left lateral lobe. The significant component of that injury, therefore, is not so much the loss of liver or the risk of leakage or infection as the accumulation of any intrahepatic hematoma from some concomitant blunt injury from the deceleration of the missile. This intrahepatic liver hematoma can burst into the biliary tree and give the postoperative sequel of hemobilia. For that reason, the liver is searched for evidence of any blunt injury and hematoma following this penetrating wound. Follow-up of such patients is generally limited by the tolerance the patient has for making repeated medical visits, and often the patient is unavailable for follow-up by the same team of physicians if he is incarcerated in an institution. However, it is unlikely that he would require any specific follow-up if he were asymptomatic at 4 weeks following exploration.

Items 70-72

A Greek immigrant has developed a second primary colon cancer which is being investigated; the new operation he is undergoing (left colectomy), following the low anterior sigmoid resection 3 years earlier, begins with an exploration of the abdomen and firm cystic masses are found in 3 sites in the liver. A biopsy is carried out:

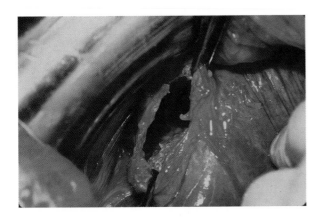

70. A complication of this unexpected encounter could be

   (A)   uncontrolled hemorrhage
   (B)   anaphylaxis
   (C)   contraindication of colon resection
   (D)   requires chemotherapy with 5-fluorouracil
   (E)   bile leakage

71. A longer term complication from this biopsy could be

   (A)   peritoneal carcinomatosis
   (B)   implant of multiple cysts
   (C)   septicemia
   (D)   jaundice
   (E)   cholecystitis

72. At the time of recognition, the area should be

   (A)   walled off with hypertonic topical-treatment-soaked pads
   (B)   excised with a margin of normal liver
   (C)   cauterized for control of hemostasis
   (D)   extended to inclusion of hepatic lobectomy
   (E)   resected *en bloc* with contiguous colon cancer

ANSWERS AND TUTORIAL ON ITEMS 70-72

The answers are: **70-B; 71-B; 72-A.**

This patient had careful examination of the liver on this occasion

27

of his second bowel resection, to ascertain whether metastases were present. When three nodules were found in the liver, it was thought that this was information for staging of the colon cancer, and the biopsy depicted was carried out. Although rare in the United States, the disease depicted is not rare world-wide, and the patient comes from an area of hydatid cyst endemia. Although the cysts were approached and opened without special precautions, an immediate recognition of this characteristic appearance led to walling off the contents of the abdomen to isolate the cysts, and hypertonic solutions were used to control the fluid that was contained in it. The lining was ablated in this one cyst, and the others were not opened. After careful hemostasis and control of this area with packing, again with gauze soaked in hypertonic solution with a final swabbing with formalin-soaked sponges inside the interior of the cyst, the procedure was then redirected to the colon resection which was carried out and the patient followed with appropriate antimicrobial therapy.

A possibility that can be avoided in this instance when recognition is made is that the spillage of the contents of the cyst into the peritoneum can give anaphylaxis. The long-term effect is that daughter cysts could be implanted in multiple locations throughout the peritoneal cavity spread by this unintended rupture. Hydatid cyst disease is due to *Echinococcus* and both the antigenic proteins from the protozoa and the implantation of viable organisms can give rise to anaphylaxis and disseminated hydatid disease.

"In surgery, eyes first and most; fingers next and little; tongue last and least."
Sir George Murray Humphrey (1820-1896)

28

Items 73-75

This 58 year-old had a palpable abdominal mass develop over several months before reporting to the clinic with a bizarre fever pattern. After testing, the liver mass depicted (A) was resected by right hepatectomy (B, C).

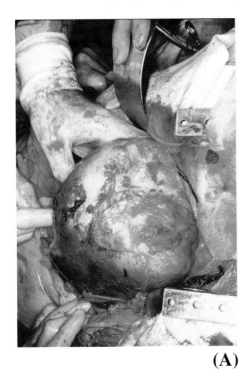

(A)

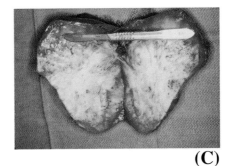

(B)

(C)

73. The fever is probably due to

   (A) septicemia
   (B) cholangitis
   (C) central nervous system metastases
   (D) para-oncologic mediators
   (E) pyogenic liver abscess

74. The tumor cell type is probably

   (A) hepatocellular carcinoma
   (B) metastatic colonic adenocarcinoma
   (C) epidermoid carcinoma
   (D) fibrosarcoma
   (E) gall bladder carcinoma

75. The hepatectomy would only slightly improve mean survival time if untreated of

   (A) 5 years
   (B) 3 years
   (C) 1 year
   (D) 9 months
   (E) 4 months

ANSWERS AND TUTORIAL ON ITEMS 73-75

The answers are: **73-D; 74-A; 75-E.**

This patient has a primary hepatocellular carcinoma. As many of them are, this was quite advanced when first detected. The detection was not by mass lesion effect, surprising as that might seem from its bulk, but from an unusual fever of unknown origin which following extensive testing could not be attributed to any known source. This pattern of bizarre fever is often associated with hepatoma, and is due to largely unknown mediators associated with the hepatoma. The extensive resection necessary for control of the primary tumor is appropriate as a curative treatment, but is rarely indicated for palliation, since the patient's survival with or without resection if it is not curative approximates 4 months.

Items 76-78

A 22 year-old woman had a sudden episode of shock brought on by abdominal pain with no antecedent trauma or warning signs. She had been in good health, with her only prior medication being oral progestational contraceptives. She underwent operation with the hepatic findings shown (A, B).

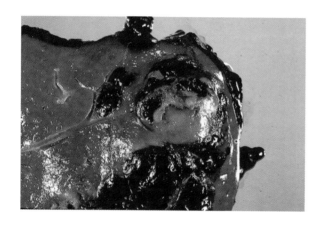

(A)

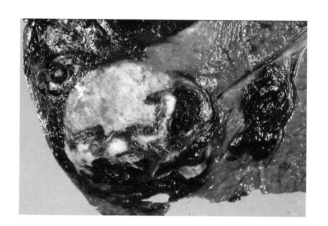

(B)

76. The tumor type is

(A) hepatocellular adenoma
(B) fibrolamellar carcinoma
(C) cavernous hemangioma
(D) focal nodular hyperplasia
(E) angiosarcoma

77. The presentation of this tumor is most often by

(A) spontaneous hemorrhage
(B) metastasis
(C) jaundice
(D) abdominal mass
(E) fever of unknown origin

78. The prognosis of the patient after liver resection of the tumor is

(A) actuarial
(B) limited by toxicity of follow-up chemotherapy
(C) dependent on radiosensitivity
(D) dependent on presence or absence of estrogen receptors
(E) less than 25% 5 year survival

ANSWERS AND TUTORIAL ON ITEMS 76-78

The answers are: **76-A; 77-A; 78-A.**

This young woman exhibits the classic "pill tumor". The presentation is also classic in that these patients frequently have no antecedent warning before an intra-abdominal hemorrhage brought on by the spontaneous rupture of these benign adenomas. Although they occur infrequently, they seem to occur in the setting of the use of oral contraceptive pills. They closely resemble focal nodular hyperplasia, but those latter tumors rarely rupture, are usually an incidental finding on exploration, and are only weakly associated with the use of oral contraceptives.

Resection in this instance was for control of bleeding. This having been successfully completed, the patient's survival is actuarial without adverse health impact either on the primary tumor or its treatment. The cell type of the "pill tumor" is that of hepatocellular adenoma.

"A physician who treats himself has a fool for a patient."

Sir William Osler (1849-1919)

Items 79-81

A 17 year-old is an unbelted backseat passenger in a collision in which she was found unconscious in the front seat with a scalp laceration, from her head having struck the dome light. She had left rib fractures visible on X-ray. Her hematocrit fell 8 points during observation over 90 minutes (which included the angiogram) (A). When she returned to consciousness complaining of pain in her left side and shoulder, she underwent operation with removal of the specimen (B).

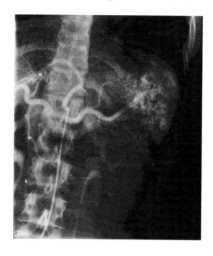

(A)

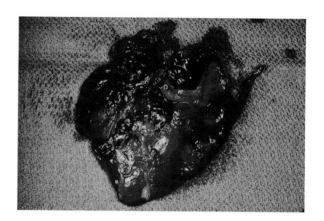

(B)

79.   The shoulder pain is probably from

    (A)   undiagnosed acromio-clavicular separation
    (B)   left clavicle fracture
    (C)   referred from left rib fractures
    (D)   left subphrenic irritation
    (E)   cutaneous cervical nerve stimulation referred from scalp laceration

80.   The hematocrit drop is probably due to

    (A)   dilution from crystalloid resuscitation
    (B)   scalp laceration hemorrhage
    (C)   antidiuretic hormone increase from closed head trauma
    (D)   intrathoracic blood loss from rib fractures
    (E)   hemoperitoneum

81.   Following operation she should receive

    (A)   γ-globulin
    (B)   pneumovax
    (C)   Tuftsin
    (D)   platelets
    (E)   fibrinogen

ANSWERS AND TUTORIAL ON ITEMS 79-81

The answers are: **79-D; 80-E; 81-B.**

Classic clinical features of a ruptured spleen include left neck and shoulder pain. This is from the referral of pain along the distribution of the collateral innervation of the phrenic nerve, which is from C-2, 3, and 4 levels of cervical spinal cord innervation. Blood under the left diaphragm can give this "Tice's sign", the classic for splenic rupture. In addition, any patient with left rib fractures has sustained translational energy enough to disrupt the spleen if the ribs have been broken. Furthermore, anyone other than a newborn child with a head injury and shock has to have the shock explained at some point of blood loss other than the head.

A young patient who has had splenectomy should have vaccination against infection from encapsulated grampositive organisms. Polyvalent vaccine against *Pneumococcus* is available as an agent that may help in decreasing the incidence of this lethal post-splenectomy syndrome. The patient would hardly need platelets, since one of the postoperative sequelae would be thrombocytosis. Although the spleen produces some humoral factors such as Tuftsin and is a source of some globulins, these should not be found deficient nor would they be available for administration in replacing them.

Items 82-84

A 37 year-old with known lymphoma has an increasing problem with bruising, gingival bleeding and a dropping hematocrit. He undergoes operation with the whole specimen (A) shown and cut section (B).

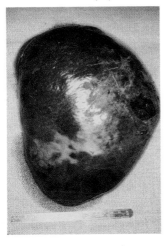

(A)

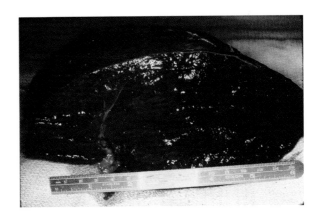

(B)

82. The indication for operation is

   (A) splenic infarct
   (B) massive splenomegaly
   (C) hypersplenism
   (D) anemia
   (E) pain

83. Platelets administered during operation should be given

   (A) following skin closure in the OR
   (B) one hour after recovery room arrival
   (C) before induction of anesthesia
   (D) at skin incision
   (E) after splenic artery is clamped

84. Left untreated, the biggest risk would be

   (A) splenic vein thrombosis
   (B) splenic infarct
   (C) rupture of the spleen
   (D) respiratory insufficiency
   (E) occult (e.g., intracranial) hemorrhage

ANSWERS AND TUTORIAL ON ITEMS 82-84

The answers are: 82-C; 83-E; 84-E.

This patient has histiocytic lymphoma, and his recent clinical complications are those of hypersplenism. Platelets are very useful as adjunct to operation for hypersplenism, but are most useful when they are given and can remain in the circulation — which they can't be as long as the splenic artery conducts them to splenic filtration out of circulation. Because the single most important feature of hypersplenism in this patient is platelet insufficient in numbers or inadequate in function to prevent spontaneous hemorrhage with minimal or unrecognized trauma, the indication for operation is to reduce this likelihood, since the ease of bruising in the skin surface shows what might be possible in anatomic places where it would do more damage, such as the eye or the central nervous system.

"The profession of medicine is distinguished from all others by its <u>singular beneficence.</u>"
Sir William Osler (1849-1919)

Items 85-87

A 26 year-old woman complains of early satiety and increasing girth. Sonography reveals a startling finding (A), which is followed in 2 weeks by CT (B) after her complaints include abdominal pain. At operation, a mass is found (C), which is sectioned (D).

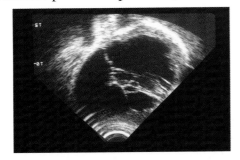

(A)

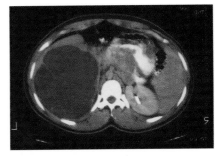

(B)

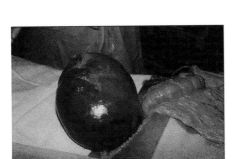

(C)

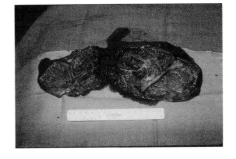

(D)

85. The likely origin of this lesion is

(A) hematogenous sepsis
(B) *Echinococcus granulosus*
(C) congenital
(D) hypersplenism
(E) lymphoma

86. The most likely risk from this finding if untreated would be

(A) thrombocytopenia
(B) rupture
(C) splenic vein thrombosis
(D) amyloidosis
(E) pancreatitis

87. This condition under ordinary circumstances is usually

(A) self limited
(B) pre-malignant
(C) an emergency
(D) associated with portal hypertension
(E) presenting as sepsis

ANSWERS AND TUTORIAL ON ITEMS 85-87

The answers are: **85-C; 86-B; 87-A.**

This patient has a splenic cyst of amazing dimensions. Not only is it easy to see why her complaints of early satiety have been prominent, it is also easy to see that the most likely event involved in the occurrence of any trauma directed to the abdomen is a rupture of this very large cyst. Most such cysts are self limited, and do not achieve these dimensions. The conditions listed are not related to splenic cysts, which most usually behave in a very benign fashion without causing complication other than a startling finding as on this patient's X-ray and sonography.

Items 88-90

A 27 year-old man has acute abdominal pain with two recognized prior episodes of occult GI bleeding without a source recognized at that time through upper and lower endoscopy. At exploration, findings are as exhibited.

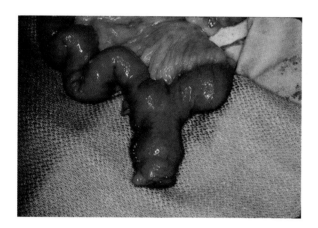

88.   The patient has an ulcer in the

   (A)   duodenum
   (B)   proximal ileum
   (C)   diverticulum
   (D)   distal ileum
   (E)   gastric antrum

89.   GI bleeding episode came from prior associated

   (A)   ulcerative colitis
   (B)   ileal ulcer
   (C)   duodenal ulcer
   (D)   hemorrhoids
   (E)   colon tumor

90.   Treatment is by

   (A)   vagotomy
   (B)   H$_2$-receptor antagonists
   (C)   resection
   (D)   oversewing the ulcer
   (E)   endoscopic laser

ANSWERS AND TUTORIAL ON ITEMS 88-90

The answers are: **88-D; 89-B; 90-C.**

This patient has a Meckel's diverticulum. The prior episodes are often referred to as "bleeding Meckel's diverticulum," but the bleeding is not from the Meckel's diverticulum. The ectopic gastric mucosa sometimes found in Meckel's diverticulum can give low pH peptic juices with acid injury in the ileum. Bleeding ulcers are typically adjacent to the Meckel's diverticulum and, therefore, are often downstream in the distal ileum. Treatment is simply resection of the Meckel's diverticulum and its "ectopic" gastric mucosa with the adjacent ulcer.

Items 91-93

A 50 year-old man with a WBC of 45,000 cells/mm³ after a 10 year course of untreated chronic lymphocytic leukemia complains of a tender abdominal mass. At elective operation depicted in (A), a specimen is removed (B).

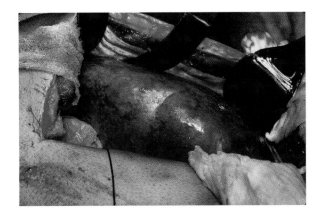

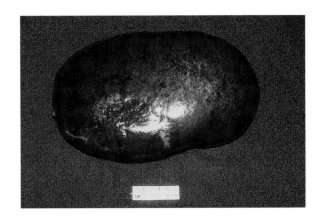

(A)

(B)

91. The most significant hazard of such an operation is:

    (A) uncontrolled hemorrhage
    (B) splenosis
    (C) removing most of blood-forming cells
    (D) postoperative meningococcemia
    (E) intravascular thrombosis

92. A patient undergoing this operation should receive each of the following **EXCEPT:**

    (A) heparin anticoagulation
    (B) pneumovax
    (C) prophylactic antibiotics
    (D) packed cell transfusion
    (E) aspirin

93. Each of the following sequelae after splenectomy is considered a preventable complication **EXCEPT:**

    (A) left lower lobe atelectasis
    (B) subphrenic abscess
    (C) thrombocytosis
    (D) re-operation for bleeding
    (E) pneumococcal septicemia

ANSWERS AND TUTORIAL ON ITEMS 91-93

The answers are: **91-C; 92-A; 93-C.**

 A patient who has myeloproliferative disorder can frequently "pack" bone marrow, replacing all blood-forming potential within the bone marrow by extramedullary sites. In this case, myeloid metaplasia means that the principle source of the patient's blood-forming cells is the spleen. At this level of splenic size increase, however, the very size of the spleen becomes a problem for the patient, and the risk potential for serious visceral disruption is increased, particularly in a patient who has decreased quantity or quality of platelets and an anemia to start with.

Splenectomy, especially for hematologic disorders, is followed by an inordinately high rate of bleeding causing re-operation. For that reason, heparin anticoagulation should not be given in association with this operation. It is true that thrombocytosis typically occurs following splenectomy, but not so immediately and not with such consequences of thrombosis or viscous blood flow as to outweigh the risks associated with excess bleeding from heparinization.

Thrombocytosis is an expected consequence of splenectomy, and is not, therefore, considered a complication. For only much higher levels of platelets circulating in patients who were normal before the splenectomy (such as trauma victims) is any treatment directed to the thrombocytosis, such as aspirin or other antiplatelet agents, being given when the platelet count is near 1 million cells/mm^3. For a patient with a hematologic abnormality, these platelets are not likely to be as prone to cause thrombosis as normal platelets might. Immediately after the splenectomy, the concern should be higher for control of bleeding than it would be for the prevention of clotting, which rules out heparin anticoagulation.

"Take as a career something that in its difficulty requires resolve, in its complexity brains, and in its accomplishment gives lasting satisfaction."

Alan Gregg (1890-1957)

Items 94-96

A 54 year-old man presented intermittent symptoms of bowel obstruction. Ultrasound suggested a solid mass distinct from the pancreas, and barium swallow (A) suggested a defect at the third portion of duodenum. At exploration (B) a mass was resected (C) with a cut section (D) revealing intrinsic tumor.

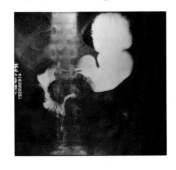

(A)

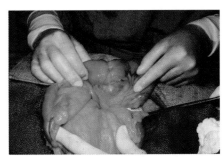

(B)

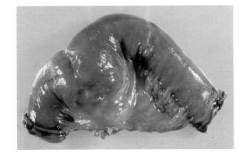

(C)

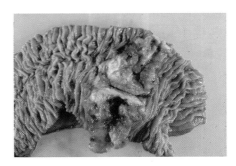

(D)

94. The most likely source of a tumor in the small bowel is

    (A)   lymphoma
    (B)   melanoma
    (C)   metastatic
    (D)   epidermoid
    (E)   primary

95. The lesion depicted here appears to be mucosal in origin, which would suggest the tumor is

    (A)   lymphoma
    (B)   melanoma
    (C)   metastatic
    (D)   epidermoid
    (E)   primary

96. Such a tumor's principle feature in presentation would be

    (A)   occult blood loss
    (B)   jaundice
    (C)   pancreatitis
    (D)   bowel obstruction
    (E)   portal hypertension

ANSWERS AND TUTORIAL ON ITEMS 94-96

The answers are: **94-C; 95-E; 96-D.**

    Most small bowel tumors are metastatic from some other site. This is a highly unusual primary adenocarcinoma of the small bowel. As seen in the barium image, it does appear to be an intrinsic bowel primary tumor with obstruction to flow. This is confirmed on the operating room exposure and examination of the specimen. Some primary bowel tumors can be from the muscularis externa, but this one is of primary mucosal origin, and primary bowel adenocarcinoma remains on the list of causes of primary bowel obstruction, but should not rank very high on such a list, since it is a rare lesion.

Items 97-99

A 64 year-old patient with *polycythemia rubra vera* enters the ER with abdominal pain, an elevated WBC and LDH, and a doughy mass on abdominal exam. At operation, the findings depicted are seen.

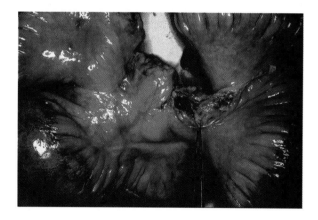

97.   The origin of this problem is

    (A)   vegetations on defective heart valves
    (B)   mural cardiac thrombosis
    (C)   celiac syndrome
    (D)   mesenteric venous
    (E)   mesenteric arterial

98.   The patient's treatment at this point is principally

    (A)   bowel resection
    (B)   systemic anticoagulation
    (C)   caval umbrella filter
    (D)   thrombectomy
    (E)   cardiac valve replacement

99.   Untreated, the problem would proceed to all of the following **EXCEPT:**

    (A)   perforation
    (B)   pulmonary thromboembolism
    (C)   bowel necrosis
    (D)   sepsis
    (E)   portal vein thrombosis

ANSWERS AND TUTORIAL ON ITEMS 97-99

The answers are: **97-D; 98-A; 99-B.**

This patient has hyperviscosity, and the thrombogenic factors that attend this condition give rise to venous thrombosis on the mesenteric venous side. When a "mesenteric vascular accident" is referred to in analogy to "stroke", arterial phenomena are frequently interpreted as being meant by this remark, but gut arterial phenomena are rare. Venous, not arterial, problems predominate. But when a venous problem is mentioned, remember that this is mesenteric venous which does not flow into the vena cava, so thromboembolism into the cava and pulmonary arterial embolus is not a consequence. For that reason, caval umbrella filtration or other techniques designed to prevent thromboembolic phenomena are not helpful. The treatment of this condition is by bowel resection, since thrombectomy and re-establishing blood flow in thrombectomized veins is futile.

Items 100-102

A 37 year-old man exhibited signs of intermittent small bowel obstruction. Following one of these episodes which was more severe than previous ones had been, he is taken to the OR for exploration which is depicted.

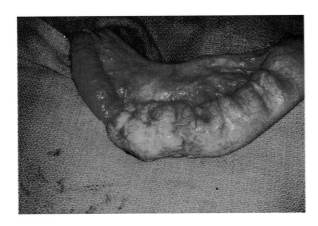

100. The likely source of this problem is in the

    (A)   mesenteric vein
    (B)   mucosa
    (C)   submucosa
    (D)   muscular wall
    (E)   mesenteric artery

101. The bowel's appearance is

    (A)   nonviable
    (B)   venous congestion
    (C)   edematous
    (D)   necrotic
    (E)   infarction

102. Adjunctive treatment will be with

    (A)   corticosteroids
    (B)   sulfadiazine
    (C)   radiation
    (D)   chemotherapy
    (E)   hyperosmotic infusion

ANSWERS AND TUTORIAL ON ITEMS 100-102

The answers are: **100-C; 101-C; 102-D.**

    This patient has a primary small bowel lymphoma. As you can see from the clear demarcation of the bowel, the submucosa lymphatics are "packed" with lymphoma cells at the site of the lymphoma, which is anatomically quite limited at the site of this disease. The bowel is neither congested with venous blood nor infarcted from a lack of arterial blood supply. Instead, it is thickened and edematous from lymphoid hyperplasia and edematous from lymphatic transudation. The treatment of this disease will likely be by resection of this area of bowel, and then primary chemotherapy according to combination drug treatment plan for this lymphoma.

Items 103-105

A 71 year-old woman was being evaluated for transient ischemic attacks. She had a heart murmur and carotid atherosclerosis, with no ulcerated plaques seen on arteriography. As that finding was being investigated, acute abdominal pain brought her to operation (A) where these depicted findings (B) were discovered.

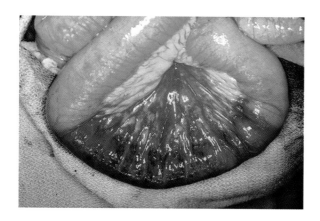

(A)

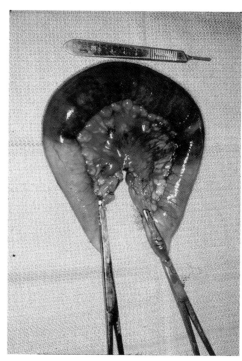

(B)

103. The likely origin of this problem is

    (A)   mesenteric venous
    (B)   cardiac
    (C)   intestinal lymphatics
    (D)   peritoneal adhesions
    (E)   abdominal aorta

104. Adjunctive therapy recommended to follow this operation should be

    (A)   carotid endarterectomy
    (B)   heparin anticoagulation
    (C)   caval umbrella filtration
    (D)   superior mesenteric endarterectomy
    (E)   abdominal aneurysmectomy

105. Recovery of gut function is likely because

    (A)   the disease is definitively treated by resection
    (B)   recurrence is unlikely
    (C)   the gut is not the primary site of pathology
    (D)   good collateral circulation is likely
    (E)   patients in whom this illness occurs are otherwise healthy

ANSWERS AND TUTORIAL ON ITEMS 103-105

The answers are: **103-B; 104-B; 105-C.**

This patient has experienced an arterial thromboembolus, the exception, rather than the rule, in mesenteric vascular events. In this instance it is cardiac in origin, and had been reflected in other arterial perfusion beds by the transient ischemic attacks for which she was being evaluated when this episode occurred. Adjunctive therapy in this instance would include heparin anticoagulation and further evaluation of the cardiac defect that has probably given rise to the embolic phenomena. A contraindication to heparinization would be any evidence of recent infarction in the central nervous system. Since the gut is not the primary site of pathology, it is likely that the gut will recover function following resection of the component that had been embolized.

Items 106-108

A 60 year-old patient with distended abdomen and a pattern of late bowel obstruction undergoes delayed laparotomy with the findings displayed.

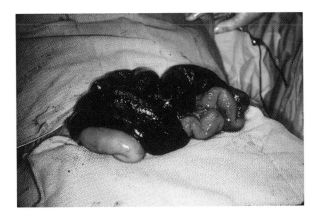

106. The bowel condition shown here shows

(A) proximal normal gut
(B) distal normal gut
(C) proximal and distal unobstructed gut
(D) midgut infarction
(E) total bowel infarction

107. Treatment should include

(A) wrapping warm packs around gut
(B) aorta-mesenteric arterial graft
(C) colostomy
(D) Doppler mesenteric demarcation
(E) resection of entire bowel

108. This operative finding is compatible with all of the following **EXCEPT:**

(A) mesenteric venous thrombosis
(B) mesenteric arterial occlusion
(C) low-flow ischemic bowel
(D) normal postoperative recovery
(E) high grade bowel obstruction

ANSWERS AND TUTORIAL ON ITEMS 106-108

The answers are: **106-D; 107-D; 108-D.**

The picture represented here is a small bowel infarction. Almost all the gut seen is nonviable, with possible distal

43

margins that appear to be borderline viable, but certainly not normal. Increasing the aerobic demand of the bowel by wrapping it in warm pads would be a way of tipping over ischemic bowel into infarction. A better way to determine whatever bowel still has some degree of blood flow would be with Doppler demarcation.

There is no colon visible in the specimen exposed, and colostomy would not be appropriate unless there is some evidence of devitalization of the colon involved. Resection of the entire bowel would not be a good idea. This would remove some areas of bowel that could potentially recover, and there is no effective way of supporting, long- term, anyone who has no bowel absorptive surface. For that reason, patients are often treated with multiple-stage procedures resecting only that gut which is clearly non- viable, and giving the benefit of doubt to any other areas, coming back at a second look to see if they are declared viable or definitely not so. With this degree of dead bowel, whatever its cause, the patient has very little likelihood of a normal postoperative recovery, and frequently the gut is just in advance of the rest of the body organs in this downhill spiral.

Items 109-111

A patient undergoing operation for cholecystitis is found to have this appearance of the distal ileum.

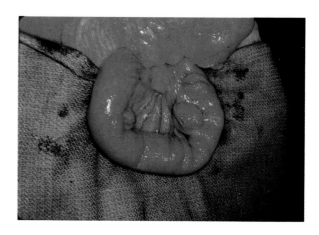

109. This pattern is consistent with each of the following **EXCEPT:**

   (A)   congenital origin
   (B)   atherosclerosis
   (C)   multiple Meckel's diverticula
   (D)   ileal diverticulosis
   (E)   asymptomatic patient

110. Treatment of this condition may be limited to

   (A)   resection of all involved bowel
   (B)   antibiotics by vein
   (C)   oral antibiotics
   (D)   no treatment
   (E)   local excision

111. If the patient should become symptomatic, problems that could develop include each of the following **EXCEPT:**

(A) perforation
(B) bacterial overgrowth
(C) malignant degeneration
(D) diverticulitis
(E) fistula formation

ANSWERS AND TUTORIAL ON ITEMS 109-111

The answers are: **109-C; 110-D; 111-C.**

The clear distinction between bowel diverticula and Meckel's diverticulum is that the Meckel's diverticulum is on the antimesenteric border, whereas ileal diverticula are clearly on the mesenteric side. This is true for diverticulosis of most types, including that which is congenital. Of that which is acquired, atherosclerosis represents the large component in etiology.

It is also likely that the patient would be asymptomatic unless there are second order complications of the ileal diverticulosis. For that reason treatment of the condition itself might be no treatment at all. If some symptoms did develop, however, one of the sources would not be malignant degeneration, and that would not be a reason for suggesting that an asymptomatic patient undergo resection of the involved bowel.

"The glory of medicine is that it is constantly moving forward, that there is always more to learn."

William J. Mayo (1861-1939)

A 23 year-old man had symptoms of partial bowel obstruction, and on physical examination a mobile firm abdominal mass was palpable. At operation the appearance of the mass is seen in (A) and after resection the intact mass (B) and cut section (C) are examined.

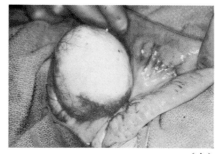

(A)

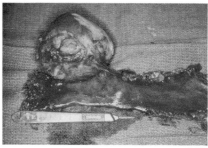

(B)

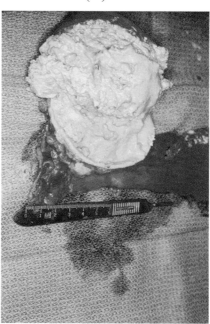

(C)

112. The origin of this mass is likely to be

 (A) traumatic
 (B) congenital
 (C) infectious
 (D) malignant
 (E) vascular

113. The lining of the mass is most probably

 (A) mucosa
 (B) epidermoid
 (C) inflammatory
 (D) infected
 (E) smooth muscle cell

114. Upon the resection and re-anastomosis done following the mass's removal, you would expect

 (A) suture line recurrence
 (B) metastases
 (C) new primary lesions
 (D) a cure
 (E) associated neoplasms

ANSWERS AND TUTORIAL ON ITEMS 112-114

The answers are: **112-B; 113-A; 114-D.**

This young man has a mesenteric cyst. The cyst was rather late in presentation with minimal symptoms of bowel obstruction, but one of the reasons that late presentation is more likely than it would be if the bowel wall gave rise to this lesion is that growth of the mass in the mesentery is unlikely to interrupt the flow of the contents of the bowel until it impinges directly upon the bowel or causes other structures to adhere to it. The origin of most mesenteric cysts is congenital. The lining is that of the structures adjacent to it, and the secretary mucosa has accumulated the debris of secretions from the lining cells. There are some parasitic or other communicable forms of mesenteric cystic disease, but for the congenital variety, new primary lesions would not be expected and the patient should experience a cure.

Items 115-117

A 51 year-old woman had a colon polyp removed by sigmoidoscopy. The frond-like pattern seen on this section (A) caused concern and a resection of the sigmoid colon was performed with a second polyp seen in micrographic pattern (B).

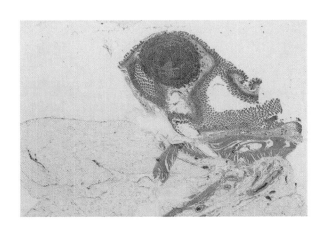

(A)

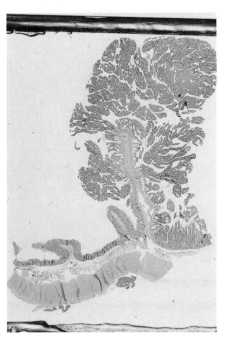

(B)

115. This appearance is compatible with a diagnosis of

    (A)   adenomatous polyp
    (B)   villous adenoma
    (C)   colonic pseudopolyp
    (D)   familial polyposis
    (E)   juvenile polyposis

116. The problem for which resection was indicated is

    (A)   inadequate margin
    (B)   inflammatory potential
    (C)   carcinoid
    (D)   adenocarcinoma in specimen
    (E)   necrotic specimen

117. Following this resection, one would expect her prognosis for 5 year survival to be

(A) 95%
(B) 80%
(C) 60%
(D) 40%
(E) 25%

ANSWERS AND TUTORIAL ON ITEMS 115-117

The answers are: **115-B; 116-D; 117-A.**

These life size cut sections of colonic polyps are those of villous adenomata. In the stalk, but not in the base, adenocarcinoma limited to the mucosa and not involving the margins is the indication for the resection of this villous adenoma. No further therapy would be necessary and a very good prognosis would be highly likely for a patient with a disease limited to this minimal origin in a resected villous adenoma.

"An expert is a man who tells you a simple thing in a confused way in such a fashion as to make you think the confusion is your own fault."

William B. Castle (1897-1990)

Items 118-120

A 60 year-old woman had acute peritoneal signs with fever and left upper quadrant tenderness over a palpable mass. The barium enema (A) suggested a splenic flexure obstruction, and she underwent operation (B), revealing a pericolic abscess surrounded by omentum (C) adherent to the stomach. On section (D), a tumor is shown.

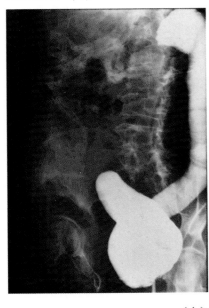

(A)

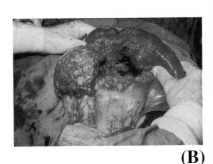

(B)

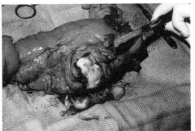

(C)

(D)

118. If left untreated this tumor would most likely have produced

    (A)   gastro-colic fistula
    (B)   colo-colic bypass
    (C)   diverticulitis
    (D)   pseudocyst
    (E)   pulmonary metastases

119. Resection of this tumor with a margin of stomach's greater curvature showed 2 positive nodes. This patient's prognosis is chiefly a function of

    (A)   primary tumor size
    (B)   positive lymph nodes
    (C)   perforation into the peritoneum
    (D)   adherence to the stomach
    (E)   Duke's class level of invasion

120. Colon resection in this case achieved all of the following **EXCEPT:**

    (A)   relief of colon obstruction
    (B)   high probability of cure
    (C)   decreased potential for bleeding
    (D)   debulking of large necrotic tumor
    (E)   removing septic focus in abdomen

ANSWERS AND TUTORIAL ON ITEMS 118-120

The answers are: **118-A; 119-C; 120-B.**

    This finding is of a large penetrating colonic adenocarcinoma that is perforated into the abdomen with a pericolic abscess. The omentum has walled off this intra-abdominal sepsis, and the purulence as well as the outgrowth of the adenocarcinoma have attached the colon to the stomach. Resection of the tumor is actually accomplished with a margin of stomach. This would have led to a gastrocolic fistula and would have been demonstrated from either a positive barium enema or an upper GI study which would have shown communication of the upper and lower gastrointestinal tract.

The perforation into the peritoneum is a sign of advanced disease, and it is a worse indicator than Duke's classification as to the probability of peritoneal and more distant spread. Operation, therefore, has a very good and useful purpose in relieving obstruction, decreasing probability of tumor bleeding, repairing the probable gastro-colic fistula and removing the septic focus around the perforated colon. High probability of cure would have to be reserved for patients with those lesions with localized disease and not that which has had both transmural and lymphatic regional spread and also spread into areas where typical metastases would not occur, such as the perforated colon cancer exposed to the peritoneum.

Items 121-123

After workup for occult blood in the stool, a 54 year-old woman has right hemicolectomy with the specimen shown. This specimen shows an ulcerative adenocarcinoma with extension through the muscularis mucosae and negative nodes.

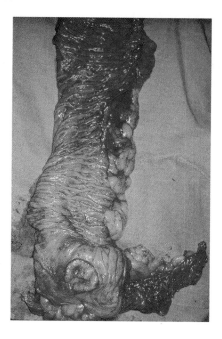

121. This would represent Duke's Stage

(A) A
(B) B_1
(C) B_2
(D) C_1
(E) D

122. This early detection and treatment for a cecal colon carcinoma would have a 5 year survival prognosis of

(A) 98%
(B) 85%
(C) 60%
(D) 30%
(E) 5%

123. Following this treatment, she should undergo serial screening with each of the following **EXCEPT:**

(A) CEA determinations
(B) stool guaiac
(C) liver CT scan
(D) colonoscopy
(E) digital rectal exam

ANSWERS AND TUTORIAL ON ITEMS 121-123

The answers are: **121-C; 122-B; 123-C.**

A colon adenocarcinoma that extends through the muscularis mucosae as the extent of this local invasion without nodes that are positive represents Duke's Stage B_2. Survival free of disease should be 85% for such a lesion given the treatment of right hemicolectomy. Serial determinations of CEA and a search for a new primary or recurrent tumor using stool guaiac, rectal examination, and colonoscopy would be appropriate, but the liver CT scan would only be done for reason of a positive screen on one of these serial follow-up tests, and would be done for cause of suspicion of such findings and not as a primary follow-up screening method.

"One of the essential qualities of the clinician is interest in humanity, for the secret of the care of the patient is in caring for the patient."

Francis Weld Peabody (1881-1927)

<u>**Items 124-126**</u>

A 60 year-old man has acute abdominal crampy pain and obstipation. A barium enema finding suggests complete obstruction at the sigmoid colon. At operation a finding (A) is revealed, for which a low anterior resection is carried out, (B) revealing a tumor in cut section.

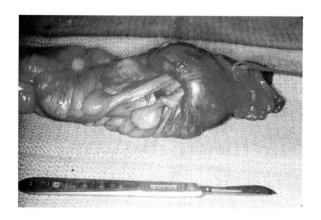

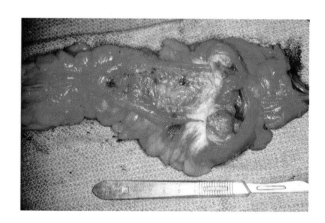

(A) **(B)**

124.   This bowel obstruction is due to

   (A)   peritoneal adhesions
   (B)   internal hernia
   (C)   total tumor occlusion
   (D)   intussusception
   (E)   ischemic colitis

125.   The probable next sign of this process would have been

   (A)   perforation
   (B)   bloody mucoid stool
   (C)   infarction
   (D)   spontaneous reduction
   (E)   hepatic metastases

126.   The likely involvement of the primary bowel tumor component in this process was

   (A)   polypoid
   (B)   annular
   (C)   mesenteric lymph nodes
   (D)   intramural
   (E)   extraserosal

ANSWERS AND TUTORIAL ON ITEMS 124-126

The answers are: **124-D; 125-B; 126-A.**

The findings in this case are those of a classic adult intussusception with a polypoid adenocarcinoma acting as a lead point. Besides the obvious signs of a worsening bowel obstruction, a characteristic clinical finding is the passage of bloody mucoid stool. Annular configuration of sigmoid colon adenocarcinoma may be more characteristic, but this form of "napkin ring" bowel constriction is less likely to set up the acute bowel obstruction as presented in this patient, and intussusception in the adult is more characteristically due to a polypoid adenocarcinoma lead point.

Items 127-129

A 48 year-old woman has had diarrhea, muscle weakness, and one episode of lower GI bleeding. A large polypoid mass is found on barium enema examination leading to a sleeve resection of the colon with the polypoid lesion depicted after repeated sigmoidoscopic biopsy was benign.

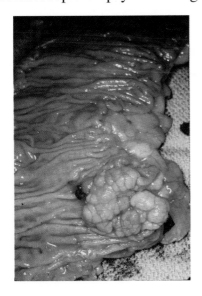

127. The history and appearance of such a lesion are most compatible with

    (A)   polypoid adenoma
    (B)   lymphoma
    (C)   villous adenoma
    (D)   carcinoid
    (E)   leiomyoma

128. Sleeve resection of the colon bearing the polyp was selected as an appropriate operation for each of the following reasons **EXCEPT:**

    (A)   lymph node dissection *en bloc* is unnecessary
    (B)   standard anatomic colon operations are harder to do
    (C)   the lesion is limited to the mucosa
    (D)   there is no need for wide margins
    (E)   the lesions are not usually multiple

129. The principle reason for removing this lesion is

    (A)   premalignant potential
    (B)   secretory diarrhea
    (C)   tendency to intussusception
    (D)   can cause extensive hemorrhage
    (E)   recurrence

ANSWERS AND TUTORIAL ON ITEMS 127-129

The answers are: **127-C; 128-B; 129-A.**

This patient exhibits a large villous adenoma with a characteristic clinical history leading to its discovery by both barium enema and sigmoidoscopic examination. Repeated biopsies showed no malignant degeneration, but endoscopic removal was not possible because of its size and pedicle. Because this is a benign lesion, the colon bearing this lesion was resected by a sleeve resection rather than a standard anatomic colon procedure which is designed to encompass the venous and lymphatic drainage of the lesion, unnecessary in this case because there would be little likelihood of metastatic potential from a benign lesion. No wide margins are needed and the lesions are not typically multiple, so this was a conservative colon resection for a large lesion that was not only symptomatic, but also has a high degree of malignant potential, and consequently operation is indicated. The operation for any benign colon polyp is different from that for a malignant tumor of the colon when that is confidently predicted pre-operatively as it was in this instance; otherwise, a standard colon operation as for adenocarcinoma would be appropriate if the nature of the lesion were indeterminate.

An 80 year-old man had subtotal resection of extensive right colonic adenocarcinoma with a large caliber drain placed in the right retroperitoneal space 10 months before. For the last few weeks the drain site has been enlarging and fecal contents have been leaking through it.

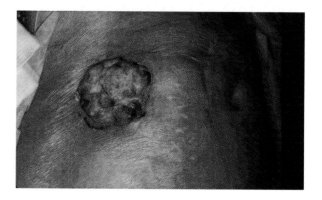

130.   This most likely represents

   (A)   a retroperitoneal abscess
   (B)   retained foreign body
   (C)   malignant fistula track
   (D)   post-pancreatitis drainage
   (E)   bowel necrosis

131.   Without distal evidence of obstruction what is likely to happen if this a fistula?

   (A)   it will close spontaneously
   (B)   it will extrude foreign body before closing
   (C)   it will respond to extensive incision and drainage
   (D)   radiation will cause it to close
   (E)   it will continue

132. The exception to spontaneous closure of colonic fistulae represented in this instance is

(A) distal obstruction
(B) malignant epithelium
(C) foreign body granulation
(D) radiation fibrosis
(E) inflammatory bowel disease

ANSWERS AND TUTORIAL ON ITEMS 130-132

The answers are: **130-C; 131-E; 132-B.**

This man has a malignant fistula from incomplete resection of extensive right colon cancer. The adenocarcinoma has advanced out the drain track, and this has maintained an open colon fistula from the suture line which was positive for malignant tumor. The "law of the fistula" states that most gastrointestinal fistulae should close unless there is distal obstruction. That may be present in this case as well, since we know that there is residual intra-abdominal disease; however, he was passing stool normally at the time his fistula remained open. The exceptions to the rule that the fistulae should close in the absence of distal obstruction include foreign body, some primary inflammatory process such as inflammatory bowel disease, radiation, and infection. Another reason that a fistula should remain open is that it is lined with mucosa, and in this instance malignant mucosa. This means that a well lubricated shunt is a possible diversion without cicatrization and the increased resistance to flow that would favor normal GI tract route and the Ohm's Law bypass of the fistula. The malignant epithelium will keep the fistula tract open, and the fistula can be expected to continue.

"A physician is obligated to consider more than a diseased organ, more even than the whole man — he must view the man in his world."

Harvey Cushing (1869-1939)

Items 133-135

After 4 attempts at endoscopic removal in stages, a large sessile polyp was still present in the sigmoid colon, and concern was expressed about perforation with a fifth attempt at endoscopic removal. Open polypectomy was carried out. This was the only colon lesion visible on barium enema in this 46 year-old woman.

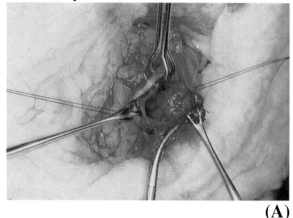

(A)

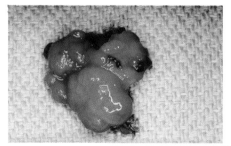

(B)

133. The best reason for aggressively pursuing the complete excision of this polyp is that

(A) the large size suggests malignancy
(B) it might obstruct
(C) it might perforate the bowel wall
(D) it might cause severe bleeding
(E) it might obscure other adjacent lesions

134. Should malignancy be present in such a polyp, the pathologist should examine most closely is the

(A) lymphatics
(B) mesenteric veins
(C) stalk of the polyp
(D) frond-like tip
(E) crypts of the mucosa

135. The polypectomy would be adequate therapy if carcinoma were found to be present in the

(A) stalk of the polyp
(B) resection margin
(C) mucosa at the tip
(D) submucosa at the base
(E) muscularis externa in the adjacent wall

ANSWERS AND TUTORIAL ON ITEMS 133-135

The answers are: **133-A; 134-C; 135-C.**

This polypectomy has removed the large colon polyp, and the concern about such a polyp is that the larger ones are often associated with malignancy. There is a long- standing controversy whether adenocarcinoma of the colon arises *de novo*, or from antecedent benign polyps, but there is an association of carcinoma and colonic polyps. The indication, therefore, for this colon polyp removal is to thoroughly examine it, and to check the areas that would be most likely to have malignant degeneration and those that might be of greatest clinical concern, potentially requiring further therapy than the polypectomy. For that reason, the most intense scrutiny should be of the stalk of the polyp, since any malignancy in the frond-like superficial surface of the tip of the polyp might still be adequately treated by the polypectomy; whereas, invasion of the stalk would cause the recommendation that a colon resection encompassing adjacent muscular wall and lymphatics be carried out in follow-up, should malignancy be discovered in this large polyp.

Items 136-138

The sigmoid colon was removed from a patient who had sigmoidoscopic diagnosis of colon cancer. The cut section of the specimen is shown.

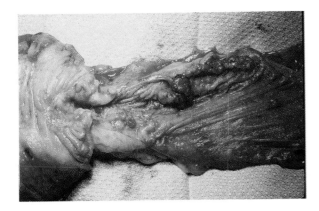

136. The mucosa of the specimen shows

    (A)   multiple polyps
    (B)   multiple malignancies
    (C)   metastatic lesions
    (D)   neuromas of myenteric plexus
    (E)   pseudomembranous colitis

137. The association of polyps and colon cancer is

    (A)   cause and effect
    (B)   chance association
    (C)   genetically co-determined in families
    (D)   a response to the same toxic stimuli
    (E)   unknown

138. This appearance of the specimen may suggest all of the following **EXCEPT:**

    (A)   follow-up endoscopy should be done annually
    (B)   stool testing for occult blood should be semi-annual
    (C)   the patient is a sporadic individual case of familial polyposis
    (D)   CEA follow-up is appropriate
    (E)   annual physical exam should include digital rectal exam

ANSWERS AND TUTORIAL ON ITEMS 136-138

The answers are: **136-A; 137-C; 138-C.**

The resected colon specimen from this individual shows both polyps and colon cancer. The association of polyps and colon cancer is known to be genetically co-determined in families; however, there is controversy about the association in sporadic cases not involved in such families. The patient should be followed with each available technique to detect new primary cancers or recurrence of the one resected. The specimen does not show the classic familial polyposis syndrome, and it is unlikely that a patient would be a sporadic individual case of familial polyposis.

Items 139-141

A woman with acute abdominal pain, a right abdominal mass and X-ray evidence of obstruction is operated upon with the findings seen in the intact specimen (A) and its cut section (B).

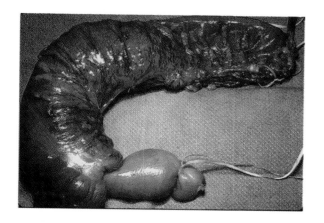

(A)

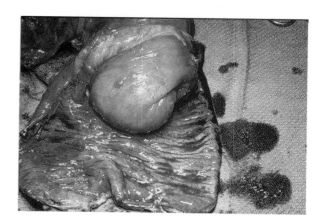

(B)

139.   This represents a clinical condition of

    (A)   cecal volvulus
    (B)   cecal intussusception
    (C)   mesenteric venous occlusive disease
    (D)   colonic pseudo-obstruction
    (E)   paralytic ileus

140.   The feature to be looked for in adults who acquire this condition is

    (A)   faulty fusion fascia
    (B)   inflammatory bowel disease
    (C)   a lead point
    (D)   mesenteric vascular antecedent obstruction
    (E)   radiation enteritis

141.   The likely source of initial pathology in this case is

    (A)   adenocarcinoma
    (B)   lipoma
    (C)   polyp
    (D)   Crohn's disease
    (E)   ischemic colitis

ANSWERS AND TUTORIAL ON ITEMS 139-141

The answers are: **139-B; 140-C; 141-A.**

This woman presents with complete bowel obstruction from cecal intussusception. The bowel is shown telescoped upon itself, and almost always in adults this results from a "lead point" in the bowel. In an older adult the most likely source of such a lead point would be a primary cancer of the gut, and in this case it was a cecal carcinoma that lead the intussusception.

Items 142-144

A 25 year-old man had a 10 year history of a known bowel problem and presented with obstipation. The X-ray (A) shows his problem and (B) a specimen of resected colon is also shown.

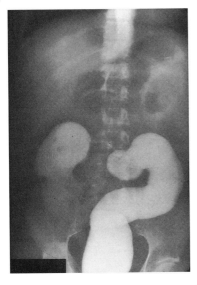

(A)

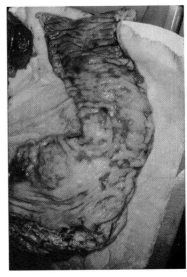

(B)

142.   The barium enema shows multiple findings consistent with

(A)   Crohn's disease
(B)   ulcerative colitis
(C)   familial polyposis
(D)   pseudomembranous colitis
(E)   radiation fibrosis

143.   The resected specimen confirms this X-ray appearance of

(A)   multiple polyposis
(B)   carcinoma
(C)   radiation fibrosis
(D)   pseudopolyps
(E)   diverticulosis

144.   The X-ray and specimen reveal a pattern most consistent with

(A)   "apple core" constricting carcinoma
(B)   "lead pipe" contracted colon
(C)   pericolic abscess
(D)   fistula
(E)   benign stricture

ANSWERS AND TUTORIAL ON ITEMS 142-144

The answers are: **142-B; 143-D; 144-E.**

This patient had ulcerative colitis, a problem that was known and under treatment for a decade. Although the disease seemed stable, there was increasing obstipation with the barium enema revealing a stricture in the midtransverse colon and what appeared to be filling defects just distal to the area of the stricture. There is a concern for malignant degeneration of the colon in patients with longstanding ulcerative colitis, but that incidence of malignancy generally increases following 10 years of treatment for ulcerative colitis, and some of the other features of the disease are seen in the X-ray and specimen.

The area of stricture is not so much the heaped up mucosal margin of an "apple core" lesion as a long benign stricture of the midtransverse colon which it turned out to be, and the filling defects that were thought to represent polyps are seen to be pseudopolyps on the cut section of colon. These are areas of colonic mucosa with ulceration around them making them appear to be polypoid, despite the relative normalcy of these islands of mucosa. This patient underwent resection of the colon for complications of his ulcerative colitis, including the benign stricture that was causing bowel obstruction and the continuing ulceration. No malignant degeneration had as yet occurred.

"The patient may well be safer with a physician who is naturally wise than with one who is artificially learned."

Sir Theodore Fox (1899-1984)

Items 145-147

A 58 year-old man had chronic renal failure and a distended abdomen when he developed acute abdominal pain. The abdominal X-ray (A) showed a finding later confirmed at operation (B) with a specimen resected (C).

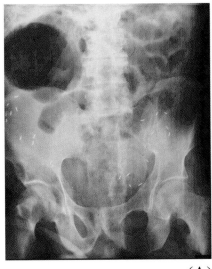

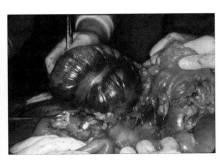

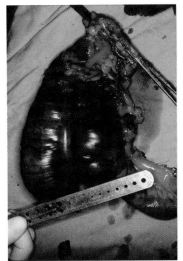

(A)   **(B)**   **(C)**

145. This condition is known as

    (A)   uremic colitis
    (B)   paralytic ileus
    (C)   mesenteric arterial embolus
    (D)   hereditary telangiectasia
    (E)   cecal volvulus

146. The bowel in this condition requires

    (A)   revascularization
    (B)   pacemaker stimulation
    (C)   prostigmine
    (D)   resection
    (E)   anticoagulants

147. If diagnosed very early, management might be possible by

    (A)   rectal tube
    (B)   sigmoidoscopy
    (C)   colonoscopy
    (D)   abdominal massage
    (E)   anticoagulation

ANSWERS AND TUTORIAL ON ITEMS 145-147

The answers are: **145-E; 146-D; 147-C.**

The X-ray and operating room findings of cecal volvulus show that it is a very dilated distension of the cecum with a twist in its redundant mesentery. In this case, the volvulus has proceeded to strangulation and infarction of the gut, and no amount of warming, stimulation, revascularization, or any other therapy will bring back necrosis to function, so the infarcted bowel is resected. Had this condition been diagnosed early, manipulation of the cecum before massive dilatation might have been possible, although not safe, if massive distention had occurred. Perforation of a very dilated cecum is possible by endoscopic tube manipulation. Rectal tubes or sigmoidoscope examination would not be of benefit to decompress a twisted cecum for which colonoscopy would be the only appropriate endoscopic route.

Items 148-150

An 18 year-old presented with painful rectal piles that recently had become troublesome with bleeding, soiling clothes by spotting, and with painful sphincter spasm. The appearance of the peri-anal findings is shown.

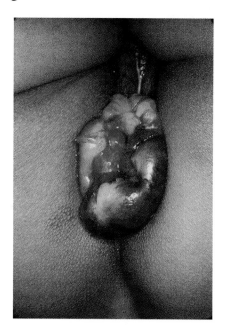

148. The condition seen is described as

(A) fistula *in ano*
(B) thrombosed hemorrhoids
(C) fissure *in ano*
(D) squamous cell carcinoma of anus
(E) perineal melanoma

149. The most painful component of this condition is known as

(A) Bowen's dysplasia
(B) proctitis
(C) tenesmus
(D) prolapse
(E) crypt abscess

150. This condition may be exacerbated by each of the following **EXCEPT:**

(A) pregnancy
(B) portal thrombosis
(C) trauma
(D) Sitz baths
(E) straining at stool

ANSWERS AND TUTORIAL ON ITEMS 148-150

The answers are: **148-B; 149-C; 150-D.**

This young woman had a very painful experience with thrombosed hemorrhoids. Thrombosis can occasionally lead to infarction of the overlying mucosa in the case of internal hemorrhoids or skin in the case of external hemorrhoids, and spontaneous passage of a blood clot through surface necrosis. This is usually accompanied by some bleeding. Although there are nerve endings in the skin which can be associated with painful stimuli before necrosis in which case the nerve endings in the necrotic segment are no longer functioning as afferent nerve endings, but there is no somatic innervation of the internal hemorrhoids. When prolapsed, however, and when the inflammation has set in, involuntary spasm of the voluntary skeletal muscle gives the very painful sphincter contraction known as tenesmus. This condition can be brought about by local factors that cause inflammation such as proctitis or trauma; or, can be brought on by acute increase in hemorrhoidal venous pressure such as with increased intra-abdominal pressure (pregnancy, straining at stool) or portal venous thrombosis. Sitz baths should make the condition better rather than exacerbate it by relaxing the sphincter spasm and stimulating blood flow to help relieve the congestion in the area in which hemorrhoidal venous thrombosis is not complete.

Items151-153

A college student enters the health center with acute onset of right lower quadrant pain with an elevated WBC count. Point tenderness of the right lower quadrant includes a fullness that seemed to be a tender mass. He recalls having two episodes that were similar but not as severe within the past four months.

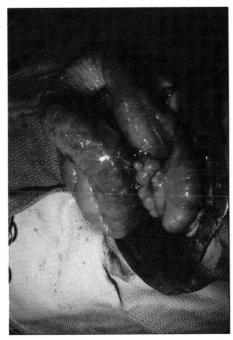

151.   The pre-operative diagnosis is

    (A)   acute appendicitis
    (B)   appendiceal abscess
    (C)   cecal volvulus
    (D)   regional enteritis
    (E)   amebic colitis

152.   Treatment should be

    (A)   appendectomy
    (B)   resection of all involved gut
    (C)   antibiotics
    (D)   ileostomy
    (E)   cecostomy

153.   In long term follow-up, he should undergo

    (A)   elective bowel resection
    (B)   semi-annual colonoscopy
    (C)   bowel-conserving management of complications
    (D)   corticosteroid treatment
    (E)   long-term parenteral antibiotics

ANSWERS AND TUTORIAL ON ITEMS 151-153

The answers are: **151-D; 152-A; 153-C.**

This student entered the health service with what would be a typical story for appendicitis except it had been repeated several times over four months. This might possibly be true for appendicitis with rupture and an appendiceal abscess, but the physical findings were also notable. A tender mass in the right lower quadrant suggests that there might an involvement of bowel in some primary process rather than in a peritoneal reaction to a primary inflammatory source in the appendix. This is compatible with Crohn's disease, since the terminal ileum is a site frequently involved with regional enteritis.

In a counterintuitive response, the treatment of regional enteritis is by appendectomy. The regional enteritis is not treated by operation; the complications of enteritis are. Should he have recurrent episodes of abdominal pain, a situation that is expected as the rule rather than the exception, one would not want to overlook appendicitis in someone with a previously confirmed diagnosis of regional enteritis; and, therefore, the appendix is removed. In the presence of a great deal of inflammatory bowel disease, this is sometimes worrisome for the possibility of fistula formation, a complication that is higher in frequency with regional enteritis. However, the disaster of having appendicitis progress to rupture in a patient who might otherwise have temporizing on any acute abdominal pain is worth this additional risk of appendectomy.

The patient should not undergo bowel resection, since the treatment of regional enteritis is medical and not surgical. The treatment of some complications of enteritis is surgical, and none of those obtained with respect to this patient at this time. However, it is likely that he may develop these in the future, particularly if medical therapy is unsuccessful in controlling the disease. For that reason, one would wish to be very conservative about managing the bowel, lest he have repeated resections and the sacrifice of more viable bowel and absorptive surface. In operating on a patient with regional enteritis, particularly following the original diagnosis, one is always thinking of the *next* operation. Particularly in someone who is young, one does not wish to compromise or sacrifice much bowel, because the patient may have a cumulative risk of bowel loss from later complications of the disease.

In the instance of this patient, after the operative confirmation of regional enteritis and an incidental appendectomy (which showed only peri-appendicitis) he went on to successful medical management of the enteritis with only one relapse through therapy with sulfadiazine and diet control. The relapse was additionally treated medically with a short-term corticosteroid treatment, and no surgically correctable complications of the recurrent enteritis occurred. Consequently, he retained all of the functional bowel minus the appendix.

"At the very moment when, at sunset, we were making our way through a herd of hippopotamuses, there flashed upon my mind, unforeseen and unsought, the phrase 'Reverence for Life'. The iron door had yielded; the path in the thicket had become visible."
Albert Schweitzer (1875-1965)

Items 154-156

A 17 year-old comes to the emergency room with abdominal pain of seven hours duration. Abdominal examination shows right lower quadrant tenderness. WBC is minimally elevated, but abdominal X-ray suggests a finding. At laparotomy, an inflamed appendix (A) was removed, with (B) specimen opened.

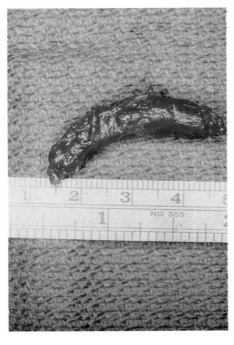

(A)

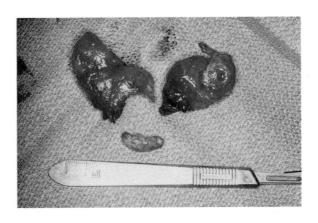

(B)

154. The X-ray finding helpful in diagnosis of appendicitis in this instance is

    (A)   sentinel loop
    (B)   free air in the abdomen
    (C)   stepladder bowel gas pattern
    (D)   gas-filled level in peri-appendiceal space
    (E)   appendicolith

155. This finding is associated with

    (A)   carcinoid
    (B)   intestinal worms
    (C)   perforation
    (D)   higher incidence of appendicitis
    (E)   appendiceal carcinoma

156. On the basis of the X-ray finding without abdominal pain, recommendation would be for

    (A)   urgent appendectomy
    (B)   incidental appendectomy
    (C)   lithotripsy
    (D)   colonoscopy
    (E)   right hemicolectomy

ANSWERS AND TUTORIAL ON ITEMS 154-156

The answers are: **154-E; 155-D; 156-B.**

This patient has appendicitis, without gangrenous infarction or perforation as later stage complications. A small loop of bowel that is paralytic and lies adjacent to an inflamed appendix is called a sentinel loop. It is not always present, and when visible is not an indication for operation. However, occasionally an appendicolith is visible on flat abdominal X-ray, and does assist in the diagnosis of appendicitis, since it is associated with a much higher incidence of appendicitis when present. Free air in the abdomen or a gas-fluid level in a peri-appendiceal space would not be expected nor would the stepladder pattern of bowel obstruction. The appendix is not perforated nor is there any peri-appendiceal abscess.

The appendicolith itself is a foreign body inside the appendix and because of its higher association with appendicitis at a rate greater than that of the population at large, the X-ray finding of an appendicolith even in a patient without abdominal pain would lead to a recommendation for incidental appendectomy at some elective procedure that is otherwise being undertaken that may have been the reason for the abdominal film that made the incidental discovery. At present there is no available lithotripsy for appendicoliths nor would it be likely that colonoscopy could reach to the level of the appendiceal lumen. Right hemicolectomy is a treatment for diseases quite beyond that of an appendicolith-associated appendicitis.

Items 157-159

A 55 year-old woman presents to the emergency room with right lower quadrant pain, a moderate elevation in white blood count, and a positive stool guaiac. The only aberration from classic clinical history for appendicitis was duration of just over 24 hours and the feeling of right lower quadrant fullness. Findings at laparotomy are shown.

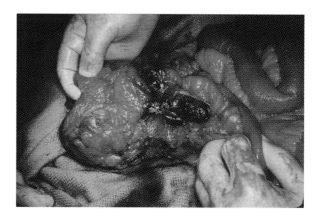

157.   The appendix in this patient exhibits

(A)   perforation
(B)   carcinoid
(C)   retrocecal position
(D)   normalcy
(E)   gangrene

158.   The associated lesion might include all the following **EXCEPT:**

(A)   carcinoid
(B)   cecal carcinoma
(C)   appendicolith
(D)   appendiceal Crohn's disease
(E)   intestinal parasites

159. Treatment for this condition is

   (A) right hemicolectomy
   (B) appendectomy
   (C) radiotherapy
   (D) chemotherapy
   (E) somatostatin analogs

ANSWERS AND TUTORIAL ON ITEMS 157-159

The answers are: **157-E; 158-D; 159-A.**

This patient presented with the findings of appendicitis. The causes for appendicitis include inflammation from obstruction (whether that be of mucosal swelling with lymphoid submucosal expansion, intestinal parasites, and appendicolith), a tumor of carcinoid or lymphoma origin, or even adenocarcinoma of the cecum, which this happens to represent. The appendix exhibits gangrene from the occlusion of its blood supply as well as the obstruction of its lumen from this tumor. The treatment for this condition is right hemicolectomy, designed for the therapy of the cecal carcinoma more than for the gangrenous appendix, but the appendix represents the emergency component of this operation which might be otherwise carried out in a patient following a colon preparation and more definitive diagnosis with staging.

"In surgery all operations are recorded as successful if the patient can be got out of the hospital or nursing home alive, though the subsequent history of the case may be such as would make an honest surgeon vow never to recommend or perform the operation again."
George Bernard Shaw (1856-1950)

Items 160-162

A 40 year-old woman with diabetes mellitus experienced a severe soft tissue infection in the perineum and buttock during an extended period when her blood sugar was uncontrolled. After radical debridement of the necrotizing fasciitis, she had the wound shown in (A) at four weeks and (B) in eight weeks.

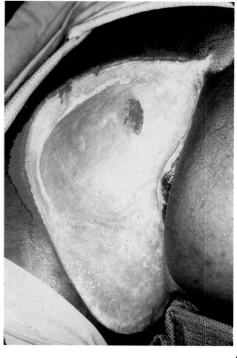

(A)

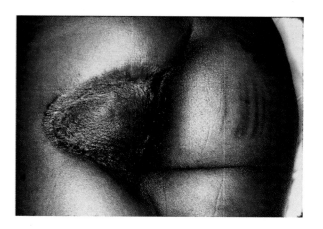

(B)

160. The healing process shown at four weeks is called

(A) epithelialization
(B) contraction
(C) granulation
(D) primary intention
(E) tertiary intention

161. The end result depicted at eight weeks results from

(A) full thickness skin graft
(B) composite myocutaneous flap
(C) primary intention
(D) split thickness skin graft
(E) secondary intention

162. The wound will be expected to further

(A) fill in new subcutaneous tissue
(B) contract centripetally
(C) change color to match surrounding skin
(D) slough the rejected graft
(E) bruise easily

ANSWERS AND TUTORIAL ON ITEMS 160-162

The answers are: **160-C; 161-D; 162-B.**

68

This patient has the healing stage of an open wound after the debridement of the necrotizing fasciitis, the very serious but not unknown complication of diabetes out of control with the mixed synergistic flora found in the area of the perineum and buttocks. The first picture is that of granulation tissue without epithelialization. Some degree of contraction may have begun, but not nearly so much as will be evident at four weeks. The skin was not closed by primary intention, and there is no evidence of immediate intentional closure on the photograph exhibited.

The result seen eight weeks later is that of re-epithelialization using a split thickness skin graft. A split thickness skin graft allows further contraction, and is not used to fill the subsurface defect for which composite subcutaneous tissue such as muscle would be more appropriate. For that reason it will continuously have the depression seen in the second photograph as the wound continues to contract centripetally. The wound will not change color to match the surrounding skin nor will it reject the autograft of the split thickness skin graft.

Epithelialization and further contraction was the intention in performing the skin graft. Later reconstruction would have to remove that epithelium and transfer in tissue to fill the defect if that were desired. In this patient's case, the wound seen in eight weeks was at the end stage of this process, since her diabetes had represented a serious threat to her. It was that complication of necrotizing fasciitis which had her diabetes out of control, and this is not an area of primary cosmetic concern. There is still abundant soft tissue between the split thickness skin graft and the bony prominences, so that new tissue transfer into this defect and reconstruction was not desired by the patient.

"Complete freedom from disease ... is almost incompatible with the process of living."
René J. Dubos (1901-1986)

Items 163-165

A 78 year-old woman had nausea and vomiting in her nursing home when examined and found to have an incarcerated femoral hernia. At operation the hernia was reduced only after laparotomy, and the bowel is shown in (A) and (B).

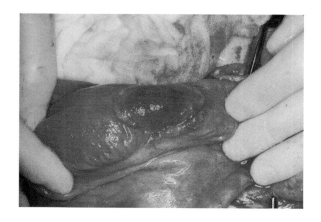

(A)

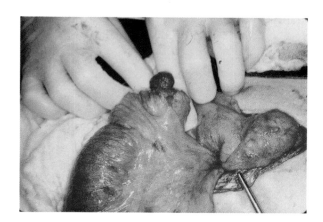

(B)

163. The most likely complication to follow next if the incarceration were untreated would have been

  (A) hemorrhage
  (B) complete bowel obstruction
  (C) blind loop syndrome
  (D) strangulation
  (E) perforation

164. This complication is highest in which type of hernia?

  (A) femoral
  (B) indirect inguinal
  (C) direct inguinal
  (D) sliding hiatal
  (E) umbilical

165. This partial bowel wall type of hernia is called

  (A) Spigelian
  (B) Richter's
  (C) McVay's
  (D) Schuldeiss lumbar
  (E) Bassini

ANSWERS AND TUTORIAL ON ITEMS 163-165

The answers are: **163-E; 164-A; 165-B.**

  This type of hernia is the Richter's hernia. This shows the result of incarceration of a portion of the bowel

70

wall without the full bowel circumference entrapment. With this incarceration, the strangulation is only a partial component of the bowel circumference. Perforation is the most likely next step. Indeed, that perforation might make the incarceration reducible when the incarcerated component of the bowel becomes necrotic and falls away, resulting in soilage of the peritoneum. The femoral hernia has the highest rate of Richter's hernia, as was true in this patient's case. The Spigelian hernia enters the abdominal wall at the *linea semilunaris* and exits lower down the rectus sheath, and is rarer than the Richter's hernia. The other names listed are names of techniques for repair of hernia and not of hernia types.

Items 166-168

A 30 year-old man with a long-standing bulge in his groin is seen for evaluation and repair. It is non-tender, but non-reducible. The patient claims to be asymptomatic.

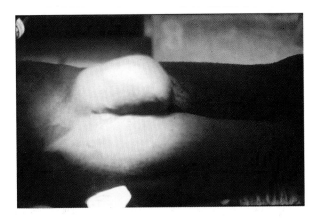

166. The most likely diagnosis is

    (A)   lipoma of groin
    (B)   incarcerated inguinal hernia
    (C)   sliding inguinal hernia
    (D)   lymphoma
    (E)   abscess

167. The correct approach to this mass should be

    (A)   incision and drainage
    (B)   needle biopsy
    (C)   laparotomy
    (D)   open excisional biopsy
    (E)   laparoscopy

168. The next most likely event if treatment is not carried out immediately would be

    (A)   hemorrhage
    (B)   perforation
    (C)   complete bowel obstruction
    (D)   spontaneous drainage
    (E)   it would persist as it appears now

ANSWERS AND TUTORIAL ON ITEMS 166-168

The answers are: **166-C; 167-C; 168-E.**

    The patient presenting with such a mass might exhibit irreducibility if it were a lipoma or lymphoma (both of which are likely to be non-tender). Incarceration and abscess would also be irreducible but tender. Since the patient is asymptomatic, and the mass has been present for a long time, it is likely that this represents a sliding inguinal hernia. The correct approach for such a mass should be repair by laparotomy. That would enable the return of the viscera back into the peritoneal cavity along with the sliding component of the hernia which likely contains the blood supply from the retroperitoneum.

If patients' sliding hernias are not repaired, it is very likely that they would persist as in this patient since sliding hernia is not typically strangulating. Hemorrhage, perforation and bowel obstruction are unlikely complications unless some further process should occur that might compromise blood supply, which is less likely in sliding hernia than it would be in incarcerated hernia without part of the sac being constituted by the bowel wall.

Items 169-171

An 82 year-old woman is brought from a nursing home with abrupt onset of nausea and vomiting. The irreducible groin mass here is discovered on physical examination. It had not been noted at the time of nursing home admission eight months earlier.

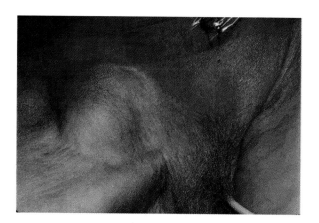

169. True statements about this kind of groin mass include

 (A) it is more common in women than in men
 (B) it is most often incarcerated
 (C) it does not require surgical repair
 (D) it most often has a sliding component
 (E) it is usually malignant

170. Treatment of this condition should be

 (A) a truss
 (B) an urgent operation
 (C) laparoscopy
 (D) colonoscopy
 (E) vascular resection and prosthesis

171. The complication most likely to happen next if untreated would be

 (A) hemorrhage
 (B) perforation
 (C) complete bowel obstruction
 (D) malignant degeneration
 (E) thrombosis

ANSWERS AND TUTORIAL ON ITEMS 169-171

The answers are: **169-A; 170-B; 171-C.**

This patient has a femoral hernia, and it is true that they are more common in women than in men, even though indirect inguinal hernia is more common than femoral hernia in women because of higher frequency overall. Femoral hernias may incarcerate, and do so more frequently than indirect inguinal hernias. Not all femoral hernias present as incarceration. However, incarceration does require urgent surgical repair and not management with some other means such as a truss. Bowel obstruction, progressing to complete obstruction is likely if the full bowel circumference is involved in the hernia rather than the partial thickness found in a Richter's hernia.

Items 172-174

This 32 year-old woman has a clinical finding pictured here. It is soft and reducible.

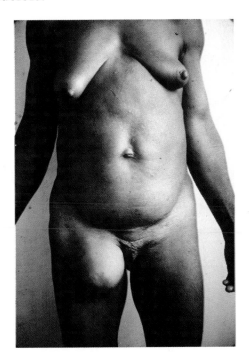

172. This defect is most likely a

    (A)   direct inguinal hernia
    (B)   indirect inguinal hernia
    (C)   Spigelian hernia
    (D)   femoral hernia
    (E)   Richter's hernia

173. This condition should be treated by

    (A)   urgent operation
    (B)   a truss
    (C)   elective operation
    (D)   incision and drainage
    (E)   a relaxing incision

174. This condition is most likely due to

    (A)   a lead point
    (B)   a collagen defect
    (C)   increased intra-abdominal pressure
    (D)   a congenital abnormality
    (E)   trauma

ANSWERS AND TUTORIAL ON ITEMS 172-174

The answers are: **172-D; 174-C; 174-C.**

    This African patient has a classic large reducible femoral hernia. Because of the higher frequency of incarceration in femoral hernias, elective operation would be advised. This hernia is probably acquired from increased intra-abdominal pressure, likely associated with pregnancy in this instance, and is unlikely to be associated with trauma or a collagen defect or some form of "lead point".

Items 175-177

A 60 year-old woman had a painless mass appear at the right angle of the jaw. The appearance of the mass (A) is confirmed by operative exploration (B).

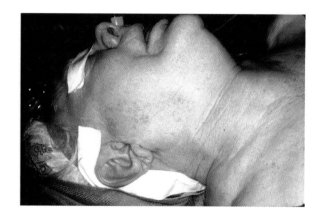

(A)

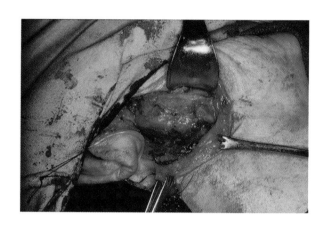

(B)

175.   The finding is

    (A)   vascular in origin
    (B)   neural derivative
    (C)   superficial glandular
    (D)   deep glandular
    (E)   lymphatic

176.   The probable histology of the mass is

    (A)   benign neoplasm
    (B)   inflammatory
    (C)   malignant neoplasm
    (D)   hematologic
    (E)   nerve sheath

177.   Treatment should be by

    (A)   radiotherapy
    (B)   superficial gland resection
    (C)   chemotherapy
    (D)   radical composite resection
    (E)   biopsy only

ANSWERS AND TUTORIAL ON ITEMS 175-177

The answers are: **175-C; 176-A; 177-B.**

This patient has the clinical appearance of a superficial parotid tumor, confirmed at operative exploration. The most likely histology of the mass is that of a benign neoplasm. Because of the benign nature of the neoplasm, although it might tend toward local recurrence if not completely excised, superficial gland resection is the treatment carried out. There is no need for radical surgical resection and sacrifice of the facial nerve nor adjunctive chemo- or radiotherapy, but the mass should also not be ignored or biopsied only. Complete excision by superficial parotidectomy is followed by a highly successful control rate.

Items 178-180

A 42 year-old man has recurrent headaches and nausea following resection of a brain tumor 2 years before. Arteriography (A) showed a finding confirmed at operation (B) with the removal of a lesion (C)

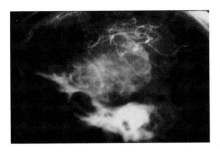 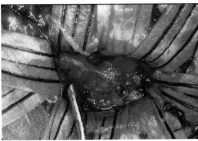 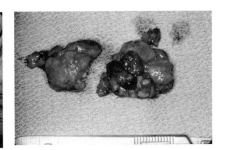

(A)	**(B)**	**(C)**

178. The nature of this mass is

    (A)   inflammatory
    (B)   metastatic
    (C)   dural in origin
    (D)   vascular in origin
    (E)   neuronal in origin

179. Prognosis for 5 year survival of incomplete resection of such a lesion is

    (A)   less than 5%
    (B)   10%
    (C)   25%
    (D)   50%
    (E)   greater than 75%

180. If recurrence appears, it would most likely be by

    (A)   hematogenous spread
    (B)   lymphatic metastases
    (C)   pulmonary nodules
    (D)   hepatic metastases
    (E)   local spread

ANSWERS AND TUTORIAL ON ITEMS 178-180

The answers are: **178-C; 179-E; 180-E.**

This patient has a 2 year course from the prior operation that he had for a brain tumor. Some brain tumors are much more rapidly growing than that, and this would likely rule out some of the most malignant of the brain tumors. That local resection is attempted again is also suggestive of the nature of this lesion which originates in the dura mater. This patient has a recurrent meningioma. Even incomplete resection of this lesion would likely give a prognosis of greater than 75% at five years. The recurrence of such a lesion is usually local rather than metastatic in some fashion, rarely if ever leaving the skull through hematogenous or lymphatic routes. Local recurrence should be treated by repeat operation as in this instance.

Items 181-183

A 48 year-old man had fallen and struck his head 6 months earlier, and presented 3 months after injury with forgetfulness, astereognosis, and lateralizing signs. Operation revealed a collection of fluid described as "old engine oil".

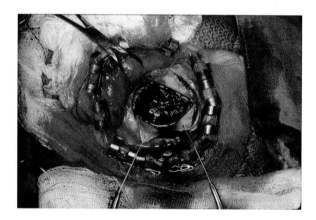

181. The source of this fluid would be

(A) bridging veins
(B) middle cerebral artery
(C) arterial aneurysm
(D) middle meningeal artery
(E) meningeal tumor

182. The location of this fluid collection is

(A) inner table of the skull
(B) subdural
(C) epidural
(D) intracerebral
(E) arteriovenous malformation

183. Prognosis following operation should be

(A) nearly complete recovery
(B) 10% 5 year survival
(C) stable neurologic deficit without progression
(D) 50% 5 year survival
(E) probable recurrence within 2 years

ANSWERS AND TUTORIAL ON ITEMS 181-183

The answers are: **181-A; 182-B; 183-A.**

This patient has the classical clinical presentation of a subdural hematoma. The time course and the nature of the injury relate to the tear in the bridging veins that give rise to this collection of blood and the operative appearance of "old engine oil" confirm this as subdural hematoma. Following drainage of this collection, recovery should be nearly complete if there were no prior neurologic difficulties that gave rise to the fall in the first place.

76

Items 184-186

A 34 year-old man developed incontinence, foot drop and weakness in the legs. X-rays (A and B) were done and operation (C and D) carried out with resection of a mass (E).

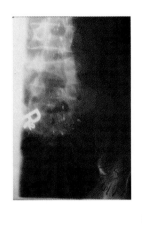

(A)

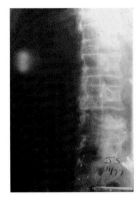

(B)

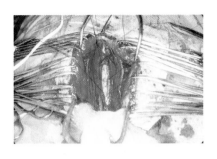

(C)

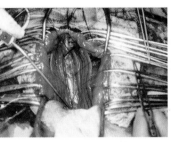

(D)

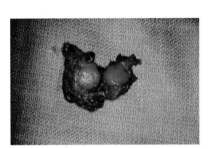

(E)

184. This mass is located in the

    (A)   cauda equina
    (B)   epidural space
    (C)   paraspinal neural arch
    (D)   skeletal spine
    (E)   blood vessels

185. Treatment of this condition is by

    (A)   surgical excision
    (B)   radiotherapy
    (C)   further search for the primary site
    (D)   local infusion therapy
    (E)   systemic chemotherapy

186. Functional postoperative status expected would be

    (A)   fixed neurologic deficit
    (B)   progressive deterioration from level at time of operation
    (C)   arrest of degeneration, but no recovery of lost function
    (D)   immediate restoration to full function
    (E)   gradual recovery to nearly full function

ANSWERS AND TUTORIAL ON ITEMS 184-186

The answers are: **184-A; 185-A; 186-E.**

This patient has an intraspinal tumor originating after the spinal cord and in the region of the cauda equina. This means that it is near the region of peripheral nerve trunks rather than the central nervous system and the regenerative capacity of peripheral nerves is better than that very limited recovery potential within the central nervous system. Surgical excision is the treatment of this mass, and with decompression, the deficits that the patient had experienced that brought him to diagnosis and treatment are likely to gradually recover to nearly full function.

Items 187-189

A 28 year-old woman had loss of position sense, sensation and motor skills in her upper extremities gradually increasing over months. CT showed a mass in the cervical spine with the attenuation coefficients of lipid. Operation revealed a cervical cord (A and B) with a mass (C), removed intact (D).

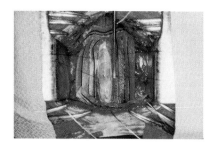

(A)

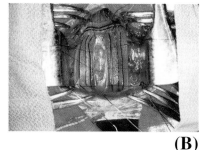

(B)

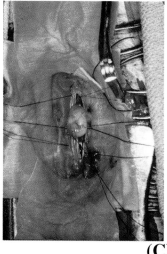

(C)

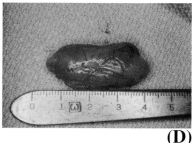

(D)

187. The clinical features and appearance are most compatible with

(A) lymphoma
(B) ependymoma
(C) lipoma
(D) glioma
(E) hematoma

188. Location of the tumor is

(A) paraspinal
(B) epidural
(C) subdural
(D) intramedullary
(E) intrasyringeal

189. Recovery potential postoperatively is expected to be

    (A)   fixed neurologic deficit
    (B)   progressive deterioration from level at time of operation
    (C)   arrest of degeneration, but no recovery of lost function
    (D)   immediate restoration of full function
    (E)   gradual recovery to nearly full function

ANSWERS AND TUTORIAL ON ITEMS 187-189

The answers are: **187-C; 188-C; 189-E.**

This young woman has an acquired intraspinal block from a soft encapsulated, benign tumor. However, the position of this benign tumor was in the confined space of the cervical spine and had given rise to neurologic deficits. The appearance and consistency of this tumor are those of lipoma, and because of its subdural position as seen in the operative exploration, even with its soft consistency, it had caused compressive symptoms. The excision of this mass and the decompression of the spine within the canal without the space-occupying presence of this lipoma can be expected to allow gradual recovery to nearly full function.

"Doctors are men who prescribe medicines of which they know little to cure diseases of which they know less in human beings of which they know nothing."
Voltaire (1694-1778)

Items 190-192

A 20 year-old man is brought to the emergency room after having been shot at a range of six feet in the left lower extremity. The wound appears as shown (A and B) and (C, D, E, and F) debridement is carried out in the operating room.

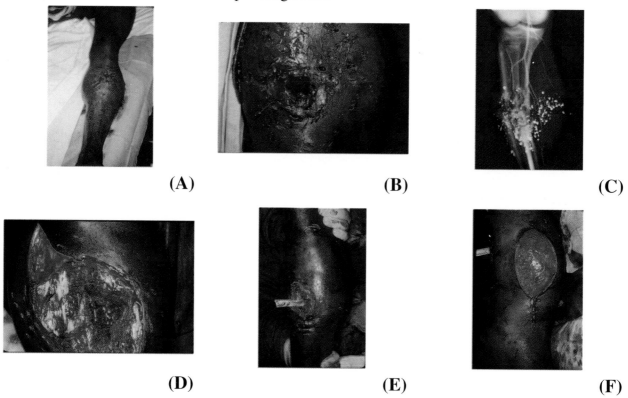

(A) (B) (C)

(D) (E) (F)

190. The kind of weapon used as evident in this gunshot wound was

(A) low velocity handgun
(B) high velocity handgun
(C) high powered rifle
(D) shotgun
(E) hollow-point bullet

191. The highest priority in evaluation of the injury is determination of

(A) fracture of tibia
(B) fracture of fibula
(C) involvement of knee joint
(D) function of soleus muscle
(E) neurovascular integrity

192. Following debridement, each of the following operating room procedures is appropriate **EXCEPT:**

(A) primary closure
(B) external fixator bone stabilization
(C) saline irrigation
(D) systemic antibiotics
(E) packing wound with dressing material

ANSWERS AND TUTORIAL ON ITEMS 190-192

The answers are: **190-D; 191-E; 192-A.**

This patient has a short range shotgun wound, evident from the multiple points of entry. The large mass of the shot charge even with the low velocity of the shotgun missiles spread out over the wider space gives very great tissue destruction, with nearly 100% of the energy of the shot after it has left the muzzle absorbed in causing tissue injury. This injury is likely to be translated into fractures, and extensive soft tissue destruction. The highest priority will be determination of neurovascular integrity. Of the treatments that follow debridement of this wound, the inappropriate option is primary closure, which would be ill-advised even if it were possible.

Items 193-195

A burglary suspect was surprised by police upon exiting from a locked building, setting off an alarm. When he pulled out a weapon, he was shot in the abdomen at a range of 20 feet. The ileum is shown here at laparotomy.

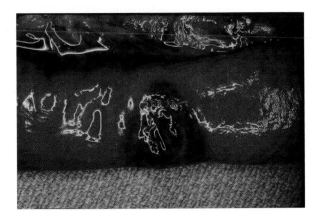

193. The weapon that caused this gunshot injury was

(A) low velocity handgun bullet
(B) high velocity handgun bullet
(C) shotgun
(D) high powered rifle
(E) hollow point bullet

194. The injury sustained can be described as

(A) blunt only
(B) penetrating only
(C) blunt and penetrating
(D) septic
(E) non-contaminated

195. Treatment should be by

(A) simple closure of the hole
(B) resection of the bowel segment
(C) ileostomy
(D) debridement and drainage
(E) ileocolostomy

ANSWERS AND TUTORIAL ON ITEMS 193-195

The answers are: **193-A; 194-C; 195-B.**

This patient is injured by a police round. The objective of the handguns that police are issued is to instantly immobilize a personal threat to their own safety, and this is accomplished with a handgun with such power to immobilize the assailant, but not to assassinate him at some long range while he attempts to make an escape. This .38 calibre gunshot wound is found to have penetrated the abdomen and also to have perforated the bowel. But as can be clearly seen around the penetrating injury there is a rim of devitalized tissue, which had suffered from the shock of the passing missile. Its elastic limit has been exceeded and this area of the wound channel has been devitalized. This penetrating injury, therefore, had a blunt component, and other viscera not in the direct missile track (e.g., the spleen, nearby arteries that may have had intimal flaps raised in their disruption and other evidence of blunt and penetrating injury) must be examined for evidence of disruption. In the instance of this injury site, if a higher velocity weapon had been used, one might consider checking the chest viscera for blunt injury from the translation of higher velocity wound channels in the abdomen. The important feature here is to recognize that a penetrating injury of the viscera in the wound track may constitute a blunt injury to tissues outside the channel. For that reason, simple closure of perforation is inappropriate as treatment of what is obviously a penetrating wound without a recognition of the blunt component. The devitalized area of bowel around the perforation would have to be excised, and the probable method for doing so would be simple resection of this bowel segment.

A 40 year-old worker for the gas company was investigating a complaint of a gas leak when an electrical short in a high voltage circuit nearby caused a spark ignition and explosion in the confined space where he was working. You see him in the ER on admission.

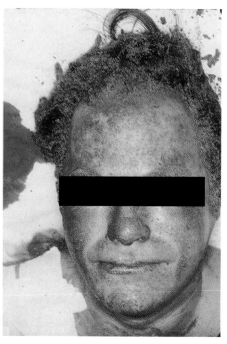

196.   The chief concern at this point would be

   (A)   cosmetic result
   (B)   donor sites for grafting
   (C)   antibiotics for sepsis
   (D)   inhalation burn
   (E)   tetanus prophylaxis

197.   The extent of the burn that is visible is probably

   (A)   9%
   (B)   18%
   (C)   1%
   (D)   36%
   (E)   54%

198. The depth and thickness of the burn visible is probably

(A) 50% full thickness 50% partial thickness
(B) 75% full thickness 25% partial thickness
(C) 100% partial thickness
(D) 100% full thickness
(E) it cannot be determined at this time

ANSWERS AND TUTORIAL ON ITEMS 196-198

The answers are: **196-D; 197-A; 198-E.**

This patient has suffered an explosion with a flash burn visible on the head. The frontal exposure that is seen here gives a 9% estimate as to the surface that is burned by the "rule of nines". However, the skin burn is indeterminate as far as the depth of the burn injury at this time, and the chief concern is not the skin burn or its subsequent cosmetic result or varying techniques of its management. The life-threatening injury in a flash burn with explosion is inhalation burn. The hot gases that resulted from the explosion would have been inhaled in the confined space. As a consequence, inhalation burn would be the single most urgent priority in this patient's management.

"If an operation is difficult, you are not performing it correctly."
Sign over O.R. door, Robert E. Gross
(Boston Children's Hospital Medical Center)

Items 199-201

A woman working in a laundry has her hand caught in a mangle. At the time of the emergency room visit (A) the injury is depicted, and is seen again at two weeks (B) when she returns for follow-up treatment.

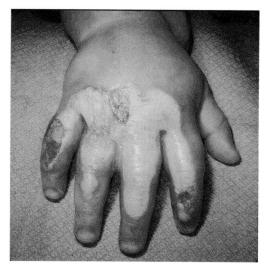

(A)

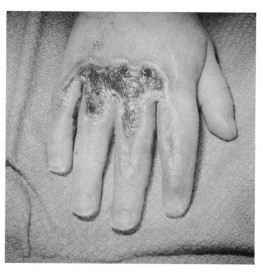

(B)

199. The first concern in the initial presentation would be

 (A) tetanus prophylaxis status
 (B) antibiotics for sepsis
 (C) evaluation of crush component of injury
 (D) immediate debridement of dead tissue
 (E) resurfacing with skin graft

200. As evident at 2 weeks, the proportion of the burn at original presentation was

 (A) 50% full thickness 50% partial thickness
 (B) 100% full thickness
 (C) 100% partial thickness
 (D) indeterminate even at 2 weeks
 (E) 90% full thickness 10% partial thickness

201. The most important endpoint in management of this injury will be

 (A) color match of graft with surrounding skin
 (B) coverage of extensor tendons
 (C) healed alignment of fractures
 (D) functional capability of the hand
 (E) minimized cosmetic soft tissue scarring

ANSWERS AND TUTORIAL ON ITEMS 199-201

The answers are: **199-C; 200-A; 201-D.**

This patient had the unfortunate combination of both thermal burn and mechanical injury to the hand, and injury in both bone and soft tissue components. On the initial evaluation, the burn injury is rather immediately apparent, although its extent in terms of depth is "declared" over time in observation. What is not immediately apparent but must be checked for at the time of presentation is the extent of the crush component of the injury. For that reason, X-ray of the hand should be obtained as well as a check on neurovascular components of each finger.

Over time, it is apparent that half of the burn wound was full thickness and half partial thickness, since the wound has shrunken about 50% of its original magnitude, which has happened faster than contraction could have taken place if the whole burn was originally full thickness tissue destruction of the skin of this hand.

The most important long-term objective in the management of hand injury generally is the functional capability of the hand. Whatever the hand looks like, so long as it functions well with limited disability, sacrifices in form and appearance would be made to maximize function. No cosmetically motivated treatment is acceptable that gives good appearance at a sacrifice of function in hand injury.

Items 202-204

A young woman enters the emergency room with complaint of fever and a painful puncture in her finger with tenderness radiating up her arm to a tender nodule in her axilla since gardening last week.

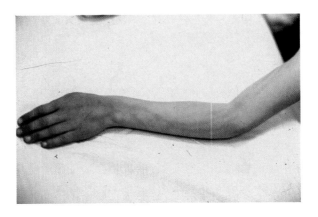

202.   The photograph shows

(A)   lymphedema of the arm
(B)   suppurative thrombophlebitis
(C)   lymphangitis
(D)   Volkmann's ischemic contracture
(E)   Raynaud's phenomenon

203.   This phenomenon in this setting is often associated with

(A)   tetanus
(B)   *Staphylococcus*
(C)   basophilic virus
(D)   mycobacteria
(E)   sporotrichosis

204. Treatment would be by

   (A) incising and drainage, finger only
   (B) wide filleting of fascial compartments of forearm
   (C) hyperbaric oxygen
   (D) specific antibiotic
   (E) no treatment needed

ANSWERS AND TUTORIAL ON ITEMS 202-204

The answers are: **202-C; 203-E; 204-D.**

This patient exhibits the streaking of lymphangitis ascending up the arm. During inflammation is about the only time we are aware of these lymphatic channels through such graphic display when inflamed.

The injury described is quite typically that of an outdoor kind of puncture wound, such as a rose thorn penetration in a finger. All such punctures from outdoor environments should bring to mind tetanus as an organism to be covered, but multiple other organisms reside in such soils as well, especially spore-forming organisms. This injury as described is classic for sporotrichosis, and treatment would be by antibiotics specific for this microbe. Other agents such as the basophilic virus of catscratch fever or atypical mycobacteria present in the soil would require differing antimicrobial coverage.

Items 205-207

A 35 year-old woman is involved as right front seat passenger in a head-on automobile collision. She is seen in the emergency room with a tender abdomen with the appearance shown here.

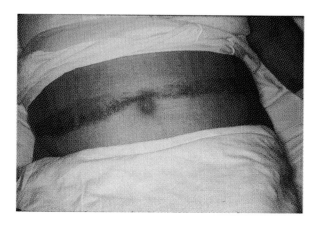

205. A likely injury she may have sustained would be

   (A) perforated colon
   (B) ruptured spleen
   (C) mesenteric vascular avulsion
   (D) fractured pelvis
   (E) pneumothorax

206. She obviously had a considerable deceleration force spread out over surface and time in what constitutes

   (A) penetrating trauma
   (B) torsion injury
   (C) blunt trauma
   (D) hypertension
   (E) vertical deceleration

207. Each of the following clinical indicators of intra-abdominal injury is useful **EXCEPT:**

(A) abdominal tenderness
(B) paracentesis
(C) CT scan
(D) peritoneal lavage
(E) arteriography

ANSWERS AND TUTORIAL ON ITEMS 205-207

The answers are: **205-B; 206-C; 207-A.**

This patient was obviously wearing her seat belt! The bruise around the abdomen from the mark of the seat belt shows that she sustained a considerable deceleration force, and at least as evident from the soft tissue of the abdomen superficially, this constituted a significant blunt trauma. In blunt trauma to the abdomen, some of the more sensitive tissues and organs may be disrupted, and a ruptured spleen would be the most likely visceral injury sustained from this vehicular blunt trauma. The other injuries listed are possible, but probably the spleen would rupture before any of the others attain a threshold clinical injury significance.

With respect to evaluation of such an abdominal injury, each of the invasive or radiographic studies may be helpful. However, one cannot follow abdominal tenderness in a patient who already has evidence of a significant abdominal wall injury. It is unlikely that her abdomen would be nontender even without any translation of this force into the viscera beneath this very large surface bruise from the secondary impact with a seat belt.

"At the beginning, disease is easy to cure but difficult to diagnose; but as time passes, not having been recognized or treated at the onset, it becomes easy to diagnose but difficult to cure."

Machiavelli, The Prince 1519

Items 208-210

A 63 year-old woman had screening mammography after a normal physical examination and a suspicious left breast finding was suggested. She underwent needle localization (A) with mammogram (B) and excisional biopsy with specimen mammogram (C) confirming the excision.

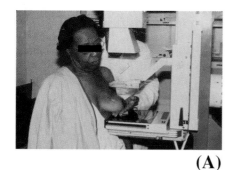

(A)

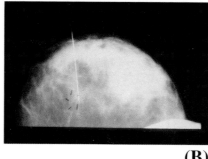

(C)

(B)

208. Needle localization is helpful for breast biopsy principally for the reason that

 (A) less breast tissue needs to be excised
 (B) it can be carried out under local anesthesia
 (C) the histologic diagnosis is made easier
 (D) the mammographically detected lesion is clinically nonpalpable
 (E) benign from malignant breast masses are easily distinguished using mammography

209. The best feature of screening mammography is that

 (A) fewer biopsies are required
 (B) it can be repeated twice annually in high risk patients
 (C) it decreases the death rate from breast cancer
 (D) it is highly cost-effective
 (E) it makes earlier diagnosis of smaller lesions possible

88

210. Screening mammography is indicated in which patient?

(A)　a 28 year-old woman identified as "high risk"

(B)　a 55 year-old woman with a 4 cm right breast mass

(C)　a 52 year-old woman with a positive family history

(D)　a 40 year-old woman who has never had a "baseline" mammogram

(E)　annually in a 30 year-old whose mother died of the disease

ANSWERS AND TUTORIAL ON ITEMS 208-210

The answers are: **208-D; 209-E; 210-C.**

The procedure illustrated is that of needle localization and specimen mammography of mammographically detected breast calcifications in a patient screened by mammography, meaning that they are asymptomatic patients identified as at risk for having the disease. Needle localization is helpful in finding lesions identified by mammography that are not clinically palpable. If anything, this increases the number of biopsies required, and quite a large number of these biopsies will be for benign disease that would otherwise not be appreciated by being palpated by either the patient or the physician.

Mammography should not be repeated at very frequent intervals, particularly in younger age groups, and it is not remarkably cost-effective. Mammography and other diagnostic and treatment methods that have been intensified as the incidence of breast cancer increases in the population have not changed the death rate from breast cancer. Screening mammography is indicated in patients who are at high risk and at such an age that the benefit will exceed any risks and cost factored in to case finding. For example, patients less than 50 are rarely appropriate in age for screening mammography, even for "baseline" findings.

Patients who have identified breast masses do not need mammography of the dominant breast mass, because the dominant breast mass will have to be removed whether or not mammographically identified as nonsuspicious. The only indication for mammography in such an instance is to avoid overlooking any other area of the breast during biopsy where nonpalpable lesions exist. The finding of a palpable breast mass is not the indication for mammography generally, and especially not for mammography designated as "screening". The utility of specimen mammography is to be sure that the mammographically suggested lesion has been successfully excised, since it would not be palpable for that confirmation.

Items 211-213

After 6 years of failing kidneys, a patient enters end-stage renal disease and is started on dialysis. He undergoes nephrectomy (A) for hypertension. Six months later, a renal allograft is implanted (B) which functions 6 years. Following recurrent treatment for episodes of rejection, the rejected allograft is explored (C) and removed (D).

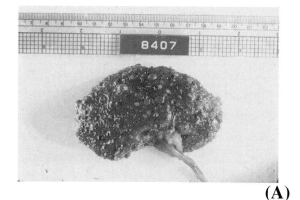

(A)

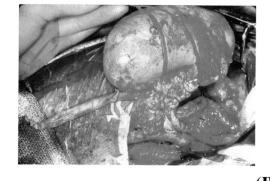

(B)

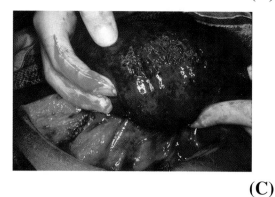

(C)

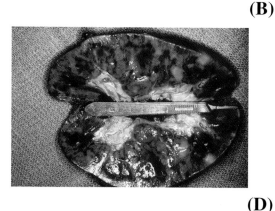

(D)

211. The patient's native kidney (A) and graft (D) are of different size for each of the following reasons **EXCEPT:**

   (A) the patient's kidney is a contracted scar
   (B) the graft has undergone hypertrophy
   (C) there was a size discrepancy between donor and recipient kidney
   (D) the graft is swollen because of rejection inflammation
   (E) the grafted kidney has acute bacterial nephritis

212. Indications for removing either the native or transplanted kidney when it is nonfunctional include each of the following **EXCEPT:**

   (A) mild, easily drug-managed hypertension
   (B) focus of sepsis
   (C) polycystic or enlarged mass
   (D) access to vessels for repeat transplant
   (E) focus of primary malignancy

213. In the event of glomerulonephritis as a cause for the primary renal failure, as in this case, an immune response in addition to rejection that may be acquired later by the allograft is

(A) Goodpasture's syndrome
(B) recurrent glomerulonephritis
(C) hyperacute rejection
(D) graft versus host reaction
(E) polyarteritis nodosa

ANSWERS AND TUTORIAL ON ITEMS 211-213

The answers are: **211-E; 212-A; 213-B.**

The grafted kidney takes over the function of both native kidneys once they are functionally destroyed. In this patient's instance, the end-stage renal disease has left contracted small native kidneys which were removed as the source of uncontrolled hypertension. The same indications for removal of a rejected allograft hold as for the native kidneys, and that would not include easily drug-managed hypertension, but would be indication for nephrectomy if there were a source of sepsis, or a focus of malignancy, or the implanted kidney was obscuring the vessels needed for a repeat transplant.

If the patient's native kidneys have suffered glomerulonephritis, one of the possible fates of the transplant kidney after it has been in position for a prolonged period of time is a recurrence of glomerulonephritis in the graft. For that reason, immunosuppressive therapy that has been used for transplant graft acceptance has been employed in primary treatment of glomerulonephritis to see if there might be benefit to a reduced

immune response to the patient's own kidneys that seem to be identified as "non-self" in the acquiring of this disease.

Items 214-216

An 18 year-old woman is admitted to the ER with hypertensive encephalopathy, at first thought to be related to hallucinogens. On physical examination, an abdominal bruit is heard and an angiogram (A) obtained, before operation, which is depicted in (B).

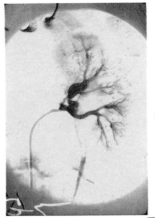

(A)

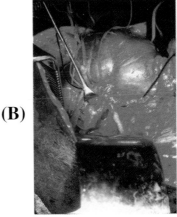

(B)

214. The likely source of the problem is

(A) atherosclerotic stenosis
(B) renal artery aneurysm
(C) fibromuscular hyperplasia
(D) retroperitoneal fibrosis
(E) renal artery embolus

215. The lesion in the renal artery is apparently chronic because of the appearance of

    (A)   collateral blood flow
    (B)   post-stenotic dilatation
    (C)   diminished size of kidney
    (D)   cortical thinning
    (E)   long irregular segment of tight stenosis

216. The lesion is most likely to result in

    (A)   low renin hypertension
    (B)   salt-losing syndrome
    (C)   resistance to angiotensin converting enzyme inhibitor therapy
    (D)   secondary aldosteronism
    (E)   recurrence after bypass graft

ANSWERS AND TUTORIAL ON ITEMS 214-216

The answers are: **214-C; 215-B; 216-D.**

This young patient has very little likelihood of developing atherosclerosis unless she were part of a kindred with unusual lipid disorder. This is the pattern most likely seen in fibromuscular hyperplasia. In this form of renal arterial stenotic hypertension, post-stenotic dilatation is evident as seen on the angiogram. Renal vascular hypertension is a syndrome of secondary aldosteronism, and is driven by high renin levels. Management of high renin hypertension can be done with drug therapy, and in this instance, renal bypass by aorto- renal graft bypass procedure gave a highly satisfactory result in both blood pressure reduction to normal as well as salvage of renal function on the affected side.

"Real knowledge is to know the extent of one's ignorance."

Confucius (Analects II, 7)

Items 217-219

A 55 year-old man had intermittent petechial skin lesions of his feet (A) and "splinter" hemorrhages under toe-nails. He had a palpable pulsating abdominal mass studied angiographically (B).

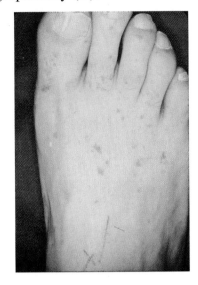

(A)

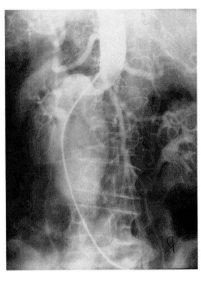

(B)

217. The lesions depicted in (A) are caused by

(A) thrombocytopenia
(B) bacteremia
(C) telangiectasia
(D) collagen vascular disease
(E) atheroemboli

218. The X-ray (B) depicts a

(A) Leriche syndrome
(B) abdominal aortic aneurysm
(C) aortic dissection
(D) renal arterial occlusion
(E) mesenteric vascular occlusion

219. This clinical presentation is known as

(A) adult vasculogenic impotence
(B) trash foot
(C) abdominal angina
(D) "marching" aortic dissection
(E) adult coarctation of aorta

ANSWERS AND TUTORIAL ON ITEMS 217-219

The answers are: **217-E; 218-B; 219-B.**

This patient has the classic clinical presentation of "trash foot". This is the distal end artery impact of atheroemboli thrown from a large abdominal aortic aneurysm seen in the angiogram. The very large size of the abdominal aneurysm is certainly an indication for its resection and replacement, but that is made even more urgent by the risk to limb of the "trashing" with the atheroemboli which are impacting in the end vessels of the lower extremities.

93

Items 220-222

A 52 year-old man had painless hematuria and a palpable flank mass on examination. Sonogram (A) showed a mass with arteriogram (B) and cavagram (C) following this study and preceding the OR exploration (D).

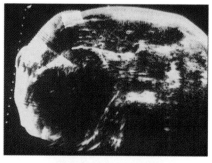

(A)

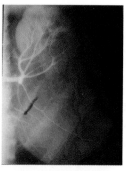

(B)

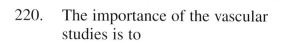

(C)

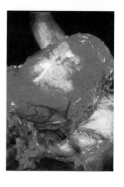

(D)

220. The importance of the vascular studies is to

  (A) plan subtotal nephrectomy
  (B) delineate Gerota's fascia for tumor bloc
  (C) reveal hepatic metastases
  (D) demonstrate intravenous extension
  (E) place venous occlusion-coil

221. The tumor in this case is most likely

  (A) renal cyst
  (B) Wilms' tumor
  (C) hypernephroma
  (D) metastatic
  (E) epidermoid

222. Early components of the operation will include each of the following steps **EXCEPT:**

  (A) low ligation of the ureter
  (B) arterial ligation
  (C) biopsy of the tumor mass
  (D) control of intravenous extension
  (E) *en bloc* dissection

ANSWERS AND TUTORIAL ON ITEMS 220-222

The answers are: **220-D; 221-C; 222-C.**

This patient has a large hypernephroma. The important

components of this hypernephroma are seen on the cavagram with an intravenous extension. Should the kidney be removed and this tumor thrombus within the cava be persistent, not only could the tumor disseminate through this hematogenous means, but also the thrombus and tumor embolus itself can be a problem as can any pulmonary embolus. During the dissection of this tumor, early arterial ligation will help control bleeding and early control of the venous extension of the tumor will limit the spread of this tumor which will be dissected *en bloc*.

What will not take place is biopsy of this tumor mass. The biopsy would violate the "bloc", and the pattern of X-ray leaves little doubt as to the nature of this mass. The biopsy would not change treatment as far as the radical *en bloc* nephrectomy is concerned, and the definitive diagnosis will be obtained by histology of the resected specimen.

Items 223-225

A 20 year-old man has a painless testicular mass demonstrated in an army induction physical, and undergoes operation with the specimen depicted delivered from the operative field.

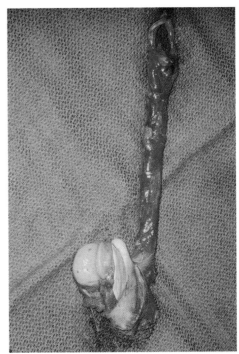

223. The appropriate incision for this exploration is in the

   (A)   scrotum
   (B)   groin
   (C)   flank
   (D)   abdomen
   (E)   thoraco-abdominal region

224. The nature of the mass is most likely

   (A)   hydrocele
   (B)   spermatocele
   (C)   seminoma
   (D)   teratoma
   (E)   metastatic

225. Follow-up therapy would likely include

(A) radiotherapy
(B) estrogen
(C) mithromycin
(D) contralateral orchiectomy
(E) 5-Fluorouracil

ANSWERS AND TUTORIAL ON ITEMS 223-225

The answers are: **223-B; 224-C; 225-A.**

The appropriate incision for scrotal mass is exploration via a groin incision, and not in the scrotum. The reason for this is that the early control of venous effluent and lymphatic extension should be obtained before the mobilization of the mass itself. As seen here, the dissection from the groin achieves control of the spermatic cord and then the section of the testicular mass reveals a primary testicular tumor, which is in all likelihood a seminoma. This is not only the characteristic appearance of the seminoma but it is the most frequent primary testicular malignancy. Seminoma is radiosensitive, so follow-up therapy would likely include radiotherapy.

A 19 year-old woman is seen in the emergency room with right lower quadrant pain, a drop in hematocrit and a positive Gravindex test with last menstrual period 50 days earlier. In sonography of the abdomen, a mass is seen interpreted as an ovarian cyst. At operation the specimen depicted is removed.

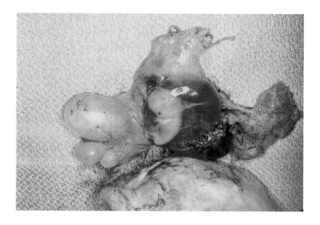

226. The nature of the ovarian mass is

(A) corpus luteum cyst
(B) teratoma
(C) adenocarcinoma
(D) Stein-Levanthal ovary
(E) endometrioma

227. The risk of highest immediate significance to the patient is

(A) torsion of the cyst
(B) hemorrhage
(C) metastatic spread
(D) endometriosis
(E) infertility

228. In the future, the most probable life-threatening risk the patient faces would be

(A) tubal abscess
(B) torsion ovarian cyst
(C) carcinoma of ovary
(D) uterine carcinoma
(E) ectopic pregnancy

ANSWERS AND TUTORIAL ON ITEMS 226-228

The answers are: **226-A; 227-B; 228-E.**

This patient presents with a finding that should never be ignored in the emergency room and must always be thought of in any reproductive-age female. She has a ruptured ectopic pregnancy. The nature of the ovarian mass is that of corpus luteum cyst, which comes along with the pregnancy. The very vascular nature of a tubal (the most common kind of ectopic) pregnancy with a placental implantation in surrounding tissues makes hemorrhage a very high likelihood and in a volume of bleeding sufficient to cause shock in the patient. With the excision of this tube and adjacent structures, "cross-over" from the opposite ovary to the remaining tube may lead to a higher incidence of ectopic pregnancy in the future following operation for this primary instance of it.

"Between a good doctor and a bad doctor, there's a world of difference, but between a good doctor and no doctor, there is little difference."

Otto Loew

Items 229-231

A 30 year-old woman had a sensation of fullness of the abdomen "like my last pregnancy". A palpable abdominal mass was present. At operation she had the large mass (A) removed and (B) sectioned.

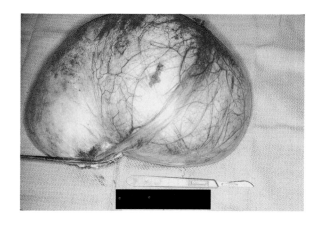

(A)

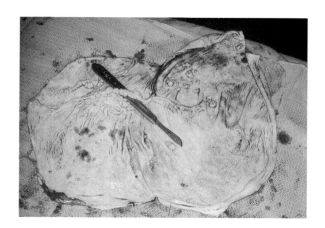

(B)

229.   The mass most likely represents

    (A)   cystadenocarcinoma
    (B)   simple ovarian cyst
    (C)   corpus luteum cyst
    (D)   cystic teratoma
    (E)   hydatid cyst

230.   The most important indication for removal of this mass is to

    (A)   prevent malignant degeneration
    (B)   decrease likelihood of metastases
    (C)   relieve symptoms of mass effect
    (D)   prevent rupture and spill of fluid into peritoneum
    (E)   prevent torsion

231.   In follow-up, the patient should be checked for

    (A)   elevated human chorionic gonadotrophin
    (B)   malignant ascites
    (C)   ectopic pregnancy
    (D)   contralateral ovarian cyst development
    (E)   daughter cysts throughout peritoneum

ANSWERS AND TUTORIAL ON ITEMS 229-231

The answers are: **229-B; 230-C; 231-D.**

This patient has a very large but simple ovarian cyst. Its very presence gives rise to considerable mass symptoms, and that would be indication for its removal. Following excision of this cyst, contralateral ovarian cyst development must be watched for. However, this is neither infectious nor malignant, and the measures designed for monitoring of patients with either of these conditions are not appropriate for this patient.

Items 232-234

A 20 year-old woman is seen in the emergency room with acute abdominal pain. She is 8 days from her last menstrual period, and has a negative Gravindex. She has a right tender adnexal mass and X-ray shows the outline of a mass with opaque objects on the film within the mass. At operation the mass depicted is removed.

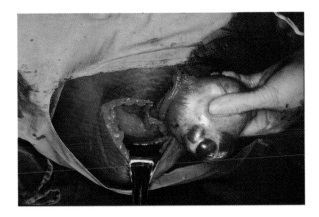

232. The most likely diagnosis is

    (A)   lithopedion
    (B)   ruptured ectopic pregnancy
    (C)   torsion ovarian teratoma
    (D)   infarcted endometrioma
    (E)   uterine fibroid

233. The opaque objects on X-ray film may likely represent

    (A)   teeth
    (B)   fetal bones
    (C)   calcified fibroid
    (D)   intrauterine contraceptive device
    (E)   organizing hematoma

234. The nature of the mass is

    (A)   malignant tumor
    (B)   infectious cyst
    (C)   inflammatory collection
    (D)   luteinal phase
    (E)   benign neoplasm

ANSWERS AND TUTORIAL ON ITEMS 232-234

The answers are: **232-C; 233-A; 234-E.**

    This young woman has the classic presentation of ovarian teratoma. The ovarian teratoma is twisted because of its weight and range of positions in the abdomen, giving rise to a torsion of the ovarian teratoma which would be indication for operation. As unlikely as it might seem originally, the opaque objects on the X-ray film would most likely represent teeth! That is because teeth, hair, and other epidermoid structures are fairly common in teratomas, and the teeth are the most radiopaque components and when present can be diagnostic of ovarian teratoma. Although these may have components within each of three germ layers and one or more of these may be malignant, the most common presentation in this age group and under these circumstances is that of a benign neoplasm.

Items 235-237

A 40 year-old woman had a pelvic mass first described as uterine fibroids. With abdominal distension and ascites, this was re-evaluated and operation undertaken with the total abdominal hysterectomy and bilateral salpingo-oophorectomy specimen shown here.

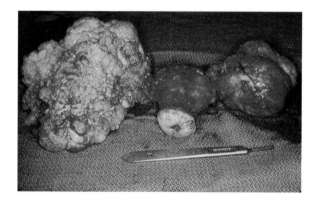

235. The specimen shown most likely represents

    (A)   bilateral ovarian cysts
    (B)   Stage III ovarian carcinoma
    (C)   endometriosis
    (D)   tubo-ovarian abscess
    (E)   ectopic pregnancy

236. Additional components of the operation would include

    (A)   omentectomy
    (B)   splenectomy
    (C)   liver biopsy
    (D)   colostomy
    (E)   hepatic artery cannulation

237. The follow-up pattern predicted for the patient is

    (A)   very low likelihood of response to chemotherapy
    (B)   high response to chemotherapy and 90% 5 year survival
    (C)   30% response to chemotherapy and 60% 5 year survival
    (D)   high initial response to chemotherapy but early recurrence
    (E)   60% response to radiotherapy and 60% 5 year survival

ANSWERS AND TUTORIAL ON ITEMS 235-237

The answers are: **235-B; 236-A; 237-D.**

This patient has bilateral ovarian adenocarcinoma presenting in Stage III. In addition to the total abdominal hysterectomy and removal of both ovaries and tubes, omentectomy is an additional component of the operation, since ovarian carcinoma is really a disease of the peritoneum. Debulking as much tumor as can be found in addition to that which is located within the gynecologic organs would be helpful in order to get the best effect of chemotherapy. Chemotherapy is likely to produce a favorable response rate initially, and despite this very high initial response rate to chemotherapy, early recurrence is likely, with a limited prognosis following the chemotherapy which will be used as an adjunct to this operation.

Items 238-240

A gravida 3, para 2 woman enters labor with normal delivery of a 8 pound Apgar 9 infant. The afterbirth is spontaneously passed, although after a delay, and it is shown here.

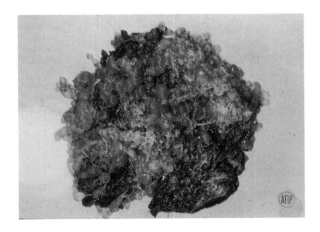

238. The findings indicate

(A) normal placenta
(B) retained segment of placenta
(C) hydatidiform mole
(D) invasive choriocarcinoma
(E) chorioamnionitis

239. The patient should have which study in follow-up

(A) CT of liver
(B) pelvic sonography
(C) endometrial biopsy
(D) human chorionic gonadotrophin (hCG) measurement
(E) D and C (dilatation and curettage)

240. The patient should be advised to

(A) undergo immediate total abdominal hysterectomy
(B) avoid pregnancy
(C) undergo monthly checkups with pap smears
(D) undergo tubal ligation
(E) begin chemotherapy

ANSWERS AND TUTORIAL ON ITEMS 238-240

The answers are: **238-C; 239-D; 240-B.**

The specimen shown here is that of the patient's placenta and it represents a hydatidiform mole. To determine whether this represents an invasive mole, one of the earlier stages of the malignant placental tumors that include choriocarcinoma and other trophoblastic neoplasms, human chorionic gonadotrophin (hCG) assay after pregnancy is helpful. The patient should be advised to avoid pregnancy, since pregnancy itself will give an hCG elevation, and that would lose the utility of this hCG marker as a proxy for recurrent tumor. Under the circumstances of recurrence, the patient would be advised to undergo hysterectomy as the possibility that this mole might have been invasive would be sustained by evidence of its recurrence.

Items 241-243

A 40 year-old woman asked evaluation for and removal of a large lump on her left thigh (A). It was soft and mobile without pulsation or fixation. It "shelled out" (B) and is shown intact (C) after removal.

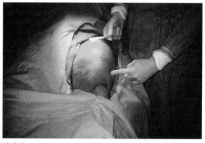

(A)

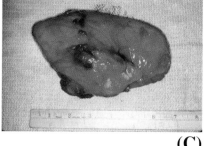

(C)

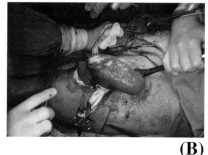

(B)

241.   The likely diagnosis is

    (A)   fibroma
    (B)   liposarcoma
    (C)   abscess
    (D)   lipoma
    (E)   neurilemmoma

242.   Follow-up treatment to be recommended is

    (A)   chest X-ray
    (B)   liver scan
    (C)   antibiotic
    (D)   chemotherapy
    (E)   routine examination

243.   Such lesions are often

    (A)   multiple
    (B)   malignant
    (C)   metastatic
    (D)   necrotic
    (E)   painful

ANSWERS AND TUTORIAL ON ITEMS 241-243

The answers are: **241-D; 242-E; 243-A.**

This patient has a large lipoma of her thigh. This soft, supple mass still has a capsule around it, and is capable of "shelling out". Most such lesions occur rather commonly in the population at large and many are multiple in any given patient. Routine examination and follow-up is all that is necessary, without specific invasive monitoring in order to determine recurrence.

Items 244-246

A 72 year-old woman had osteoarthritis with left knee more severely involved than the right. After prolonged consideration while maintained on steroid therapy, she underwent operation on her left knee depicted.

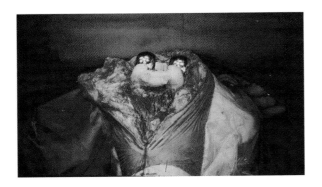

244. Each of the following adjuncts to operation is indicated **EXCEPT:**

    (A)   antibiotic prophylaxis
    (B)   corticosteroid replacement
    (C)   thromboembolism prophylaxis
    (D)   prolonged bed rest
    (E)   physical therapy

245. A likely subsequent operation will be to

    (A)   remove the hardware from left knee
    (B)   drain infected hematoma
    (C)   release contracture of left hip
    (D)   place vena cava filter
    (E)   replace right knee

246. The most serious debilitating surgical complication for which extraordinary preventive measures are directed is

    (A)   deep venous thrombosis
    (B)   atelectasis
    (C)   joint infection
    (D)   three unit blood loss
    (E)   decubital ulcers

ANSWERS AND TUTORIAL ON ITEMS 244-246

The answers are: **244-D; 245-E; 246-C.**

This patient is undergoing a total knee prosthetic replacement. Because of her prolonged steroid therapy she will surely require steroid treatment as coverage for her operation. Antibiotic prophylaxis and thromboembolism prevention are certainly components of her therapy, but prolonged bedrest is not. The reason is that most patients who have this operation are going to be severely debilitated by a prolonged period of bedrest and must be mobilized early. This is also part of the physical therapy of the prosthetic knee replacement. It is likely that she will undergo subsequent replacement of the opposite knee, which will become even more burdensome to her when the newly rehabilitated function of the operated knee is apparent. It is highly unlikely that she will develop a joint infection, for which extraordinary means are expended to prevent this very serious debilitating surgical complication.

Items 247-249

A 25 year-old had a 9 year history of recurrent infections in both axillae, which her younger sister has also had for four years starting at the same age. She has had multiple incision and drainage treatments and returns to the outpatient clinic with the condition seen here.

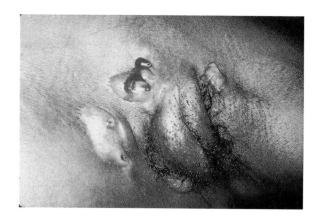

247. This condition is most likely representative of

   (A) IV drug abuse
   (B) mastitis of axillary tail of Spence
   (C) resistant *Pseudomonas* infection
   (D) necrotizing fasciitis
   (E) *hidradenitis suppurativa*

248. This condition is related to the

   (A) lymph nodes
   (B) eccrine sweat glands
   (C) apocrine sweat glands
   (D) deodorant hypersensitivity dermatitis
   (E) fixed drug eruption

249. It is best treated at this stage by

   (A) antibiotics
   (B) incision and drainage
   (C) radiotherapy
   (D) excision of all infected skin areas
   (E) topical antiseptics

ANSWERS AND TUTORIAL ON ITEMS 247-249

The answers are: **247-E; 248-C; 249-D.**

This patient has *hidradenitis suppurativa*, a problem that develops in some patients following menarche and at the time of apocrine sweat gland development in which this syndrome is based. It often occurs in families and other problems apparent in this instance, may involve other areas of the body than the axilla, particularly the groin and perineum. The abscesses are frequent and recurrent, and incision and drainage is appropriate as therapy for any given abscess. However, over time, the recurrence is so debilitating that it is worthwhile for some patients to have all of the affected skin with apocrine sweat gland contents removed and rotation flap grafts or other form of resurfacing to replace the affected skin areas.

Items 250-252

One of the emergency room "regulars" is seen for a very distended and puffy hand and fever. His upper arm and forearm are seen in this photograph at the time of examination.

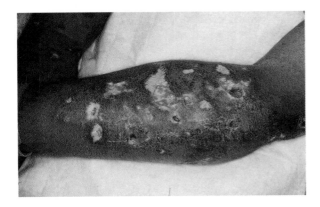

250. The underlying diagnosis is

    (A)   chronic granulomatous disease
    (B)   heroin addiction
    (C)   mycosis fungoides
    (D)   histoplasmosis
    (E)   epidermoid carcinoma

251. One of the systemic complications of this condition is

    (A)   tricuspid valvulitis
    (B)   glomerulonephritis
    (C)   urosepsis
    (D)   hepatic metastasis
    (E)   aplastic anemia

252. Each of the following is an actual complication of the condition portrayed **EXCEPT:**

    (A)   osteomyelitis
    (B)   digital gangrene
    (C)   Volkmann's ischemic contracture
    (D)   clostridial septicemia
    (E)   carcinogenesis

ANSWERS AND TUTORIAL ON ITEMS 250-252

The answers are: **250-B; 251-A; 252-E.**

This patient is a "skin popper" injecting heroin and the excipient with which it is mixed under the subcutaneous tissue. This is often done in search for a vein, which veins are often obliterated early in the course of the addiction. For that reason, the patient then may seek out arterial injection sites, both for vascular access and also for the special sensation known as a "hand trip" or "flash" which may be partly due to the drug, but in a large part is due to catecholamine release and excipient embolization. Some of the excipients with which the heroin powder is mixed include quinine and talc. The former aids oxidation-reduction potential favoring anaerobic organisms and clostridial septicemia is a possibility. Because of the arterial embolization and ischemia, Volkmann's ischemic contracture is possible, as well as bone infections, osteomyelitis, and soft tissue destruction. Of all the complications reported, that include right heart valvulitis and migratory pulmonary emboli, carcinogenesis of the infected area is not likely amid all the other sequelae of drug abuse.

Items 253-255

A 60 year-old patient had a "coin lesion" in the right apex on chest X-ray. PPD skin test was positive, and bronchial washings were negative. Following antimicrobial therapy, right upper lobectomy was carried out and the cut specimen is shown in this photograph.

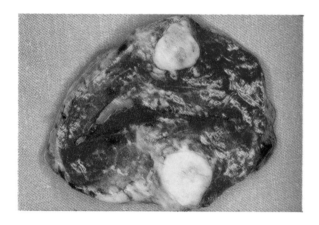

253.   The specimen shows what is likely a

(A)   hamartoma of the lung
(B)   tuberculous granuloma
(C)   adenocarcinoma
(D)   "scar carcinoma" of the lung
(E)   epidermoid carcinoma

254.   Operation was carried out to

(A)   keep this lesion from spreading
(B)   rule out malignancy
(C)   prevent later carcinogenesis
(D)   facilitate antimicrobial therapy
(E)   prevent cavitation

255.   The differential diagnosis of solitary coin lesions includes each of the following **EXCEPT:**

(A)   carcinoma of the lung
(B)   metastatic adenocarcinoma
(C)   fungal infection
(D)   sarcoid
(E)   hamartoma

ANSWERS AND TUTORIAL ON ITEMS 253-255

The answers are: **253-B; 254-B; 255-D.**

This patient has a tuberculous granuloma, located in its usual position in the lung. The operation was to rule out malignancy in a coin lesion. Since the diagnosis of a coin lesion has a differential that includes carcinoma of the lung in that which will most likely be treated by operation, the differential also considered is that of the other options listed with the exception of sarcoid. Sarcoid does not give a coin lesion but is largely a butterfly pattern along the hilum of lymphatic involvement.

Items 256-258

A 60 year-old woman with exertional dyspnea and shortness of breath at rest has dusky fingernails as seen in (A). A chest X-ray reveals bilateral findings with a large central mass in the right lung. The patient was not operated on, but treated with short-term chemotherapy, with death in a few weeks from the pulmonary disease depicted in (B).

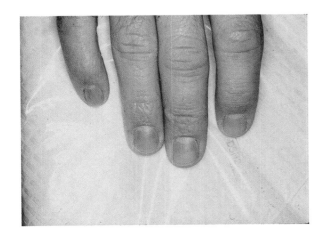

(A)

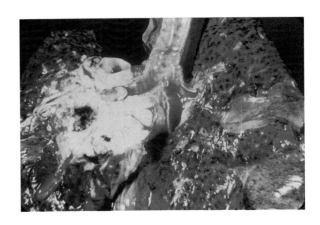

(B)

256. The primary reason the patient was *not* operated on was

    (A) unresectability
    (B) inoperability
    (C) probable cell type
    (D) involvement of mainstem bronchus
    (E) mediastinal nodes positive

257. The most likely type of tumor is

    (A) bronchogenic carcinoma
    (B) adenocarcinoma
    (C) small cell carcinoma
    (D) metastatic
    (E) chondrosarcoma

258. From 1987 and each year thereafter, the most frequent cause of cancer deaths in US women has been

    (A) breast cancer
    (B) colon cancer
    (C) ovarian cancer
    (D) lung cancer
    (E) cervical cancer

ANSWERS AND TUTORIAL ON ITEMS 256-258

The answers are: **256-B; 257-A; 258-D.**

    This woman has shortness of breath at rest as well as exertional dyspnea with the cyanotic nail beds portrayed. The chest X- ray showed a large central mass in the right lung at the time that it was a resectable lesion, but the patient was not operated upon but begun on short-term chemotherapy. The reason the patient was not operated on was not unresectability of the tumor but inoperability of the patient. As seen in the pattern of margins clustered around the bronchus, the most highly probable form of cancer is bronchogenic carcinoma. It is a mark of some unfortunate progress in equality that since 1987 and every year thereafter lung cancer has been the most common cause of cancer deaths in US women, passing breast cancer in each of the last eight years.

Items 259-261

A patient with end-stage renal failure supported by dialysis developed increasing congestive heart failure and chest pain. The patient died before thoracotomy could be carried out, and the heart is shown after the pericardium is opened.

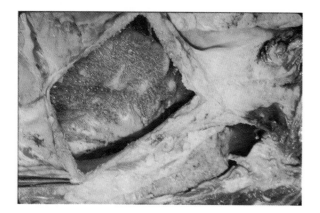

259.   The diagnosis most likely is

(A)   miliary tuberculosis
(B)   candidemia
(C)   viral pericarditis
(D)   fibrinous pericarditis
(E)   mesothelioma

260.   Treatment for this condition would be

(A)   pericardiocentesis
(B)   intracavitary steroid injection
(C)   pericardial window
(D)   pericardiectomy
(E)   amphotericin B

261.   The congestive failure is due to

(A)   low output
(B)   high pulmonary vascular resistance
(C)   myocardiopathy
(D)   valvular stenosis
(E)   low filling pressure

ANSWERS AND TUTORIAL ON ITEMS 259-261

The answers are: **259-D; 260-D; 261-A.**

This patient has uremic fibrinous pericarditis. Because of the encasement of the pericardium, only a very low filling on venous return is possible and the patient experiences low output congestive failure. Treatment for this would not be instillation of anything into the pericardium, so much as relief of the "coeurasse" encasing the heart. The myocardium is adequate to function if it had a filling volume of blood it could eject, but fibrinous pericarditis is a restriction of the cardiac output based in this limitation on venous filling. Early in the disease, a pericardial "window" allows drainage of this uremic pericarditis; however, late in the development in which fibrinous pericarditis occurs and the pericardial sac stiffens to become an encasement, this restrictive pericarditis on the basis of its fibrinous nature is best treated by pericardiectomy.

Items 262-264

A young woman with atypical signs of obstruction and one episode of upper GI bleeding is studied for possible ulcer, and is found to have the X-ray appearance seen on the 2 radiographs; she undergoes operation with the findings shown *in situ* and in comparison with the pre-operative X-ray.

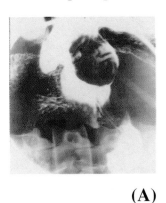

(A)

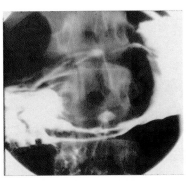

(B)

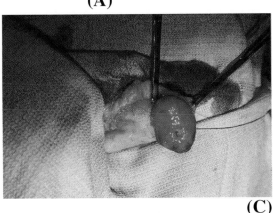

(C)

(D)

262. The origin of the tumor is likely to be

    (A)   mucosal
    (B)   submucosal lymphatics
    (C)   foreign body
    (D)   muscular wall
    (E)   distant metastasis

263. The histopathology of the tumor indicates

    (A)   gastric adenocarcinoma
    (B)   squamous cell carcinoma
    (C)   leiomyoma
    (D)   lymphoma
    (E)   inflammatory

264. The prognosis following operation is

   (A)   90% 5 year survival
   (B)   actuarial
   (C)   10% 5 year survival
   (D)   50% 5 year survival
   (E)   guarded, dependent or multiple primaries evolving

ANSWERS AND TUTORIAL ON ITEMS 262-264

The answers are: **262-D; 263-C; 264-B.**

Given this young patient's age, she is a less likely candidate for the adenocarcinoma more common in older age groups. Nonetheless, she has evidence of solid, partially obstructing tumor fixed to the bowel wall. This leads to the possibility that this might be an intramural neoplasm. Lower in the GI tract, carcinoid and lymphoma might be on the list of possibilities, but at this higher level leiomyoma — a smooth muscle tumor — is a leading candidate in the differential diagnosis.

This woman turned out to have leiomyoma — a fortunate lesion that is benign and presenting only because of the intermittent but increasing pattern of obstruction. With resection of this lesion, her prognosis is unrestricted by this bowel wall disease and her survival is actuarial.

"My definition of an educated man is the fellow who knows the right thing to do at the time it has to be done... you can be sincere and still be stupid."

Charles Kettering (Sloan-Kettering)

Items 265-267

The barium swallow depicted here for this 32 year-old was ordered for reasons of three months dysphagia with sensation of food "sticking" in throat.

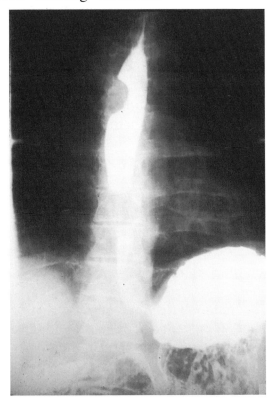

265.   The condition is most likely

    (A)   congenital
    (B)   inflammatory
    (C)   benign
    (D)   malignant
    (E)   foreign body

266.   The treatment is limited to

    (A)   radiation
    (B)   total esophagectomy
    (C)   colon interposition
    (D)   excision
    (E)   dilatation with bougie

267.   The probable complication if untreated might be

    (A)   rupture of the esophagus
    (B)   exsanguinating hemorrhage
    (C)   obstruction
    (D)   malignant degeneration
    (E)   metastases

ANSWERS AND TUTORIAL ON ITEMS 265-267

The answers are: **265-C; 266-D; 267-C.**

This relatively young patient entered with what looked like a ball-bearing under the mucosa when studied in fluoroscopy during barium swallow. The smooth and round contour makes it likely that this is not a malignant tumor, and, in fact, it had never occasioned bleeding or any other problem than the "sticking" sensation. The patient's age was not appropriate for the highest risk group for esophageal carcinoma, and there had been no prior corrosive or other ingestion suggesting an inflammatory reaction. This is one of the benign (unfortunately rare for this anatomic location, but fortunately common in younger age groups) conditions that are fixable, and the treatment here is by local excision. It is a leiomyoma. If this had progressed, one of the possibilities might have been hemorrhage, but more likely would have been obstruction which would have probably been antecedent to hemorrhage. These are unlikely to be degenerating into leiomyosarcoma, which are thought to arise primarily as malignant tumors rather than to undergo degeneration from a benign tumor.

Items 268-270

This barium swallow was ordered to evaluate the condition of a patient with symptoms of hiatal hernia.

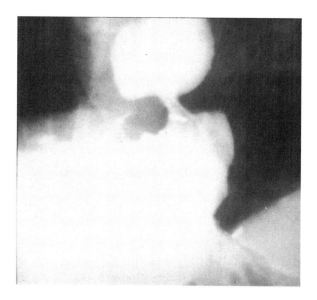

268. The lesion demonstrated is probably

    (A)   congenital
    (B)   inflammatory
    (C)   malignant
    (D)   not serious
    (E)   responsive to radiation

269. Treatment of this condition employs each of the following **EXCEPT:**

    (A)   H$_2$-receptor antagonists
    (B)   operation
    (C)   endoscopy
    (D)   radiation
    (E)   bouginage

270. The therapy will have to include a plan to

    (A)   replace the esophagus
    (B)   pull the stomach up into the chest
    (C)   control systemic spread of disease
    (D)   prevent acid reflux
    (E)   achieve wide margins around the disease

ANSWERS AND TUTORIAL ON ITEMS 268-270

The answers are: **268-B; 269-D; 270-D.**

This patient has esophageal stricture from acid reflux peptic esophagitis. The stenosis is the indication for operation, but simultaneously, some method to prevent acid reflux should take place to minimize recurrence. In this instance, that can be surgical if there will be a surgical treatment for the stenosis, but medical therapy is often employed as adjunct to or in place of operation for the hyperacidity. That includes each of the options listed with the exception of radiation, which would not be appropriate for a benign condition and would cause further fibrotic stenosis.

Items 271-273

This barium swallow radiograph was obtained in a 62 year-old patient who was being evaluated for malignancy after a screening chest X-ray showed left pleural effusion.

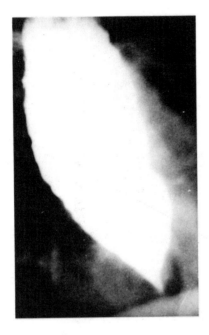

271. The condition depicted here is most compatible with

   (A) esophageal carcinoma
   (B) esophageal varices
   (C) Barrett's esophagus
   (D) normal esophagogram
   (E) achalasia

272. Treatment of this condition includes

   (A) chemotherapy
   (B) myotomy
   (C) antacids
   (D) corticosteroids
   (E) esophagectomy

273. This condition acquired in adults may likely be associated with

   (A) carcinoma
   (B) acid reflux
   (C) portal hypertension
   (D) ingestion of caustics
   (E) candidiasis

ANSWERS AND TUTORIAL ON ITEMS 271-273

The answers are: **271-E; 272-B; 273-A.**

This barium swallow shows the characteristic "beak" appearance of achalasia. Failure of relaxation of the esophagus has caused proximal dilatation. This is seen in congenital cases in which the myenteric plexus may be absent, or it may be acquired in adults who have a specific form of tropical disease (Chagas' disease — trypanosomiasis). Another cause of the acquired syndrome in adults is associated carcinoma, and the patient who had this achalasia was being investigated for a left pleural effusion that was found to be malignant, based in a bronchogenic squamous cell carcinoma.

Items 274-276

A mobile filling defect is discovered on upper GI and is depicted in this radiograph of an institutionalized psychiatric patient.

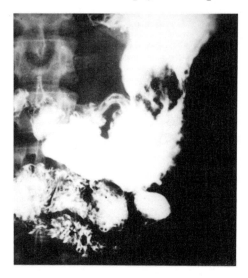

274.   This lesion is often composed of

    (A)   lymphoid tissue
    (B)   myxomatous connective tissue
    (C)   smooth muscle
    (D)   goblet cells
    (E)   hair

275.   Associated conditions may include

    (A)   lymphoma
    (B)   pica
    (C)   cardiac defects
    (D)   hereditary syndrome
    (E)   hyperacidity

276.   Treatment is by

    (A)   gastrectomy
    (B)   vagotomy
    (C)   lavage
    (D)   endoscopic removal
    (E)   antacids

ANSWERS AND TUTORIAL ON ITEMS 274-276

The answers are: **274-E; 275-B; 276-D.**

That the object discovered in the stomach is mobile without apparent fixation to the mucosa suggests that it could be a foreign body, and in a way it is. It is composed of undigestible bits of matter in the stomach called a bezoar and in this instance it is composed predominately of hair, so it is a trichobezoar. This may be seen in patients with a habit of compulsively chewing on their hair or with other habits of ingesting things that are not digestible (pica) in which case the nature of the bezoar takes on the characteristics of whatever is ingested. Gastrotomy used to be necessary with the excision of these bezoars if they became "ball valve" obstruction; now they are broken up and delivered endoscopically.

"Diseases desperate grown by desperate appliance are reliev'd, or not at all."
William Shakespeare (1564-1616)
Hamlet IV, iii, 9

Items 277-279

A barium enema is obtained on a patient with known gastric adenocarcinoma. The result is shown here.

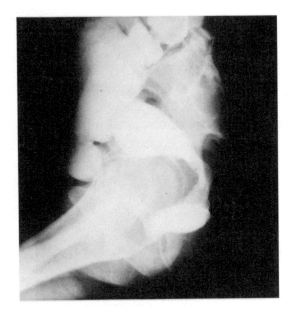

277. The likely cause of the lesion depicted is

   (A)   primary adenocarcinoma of the rectum
   (B)   colonic pseudo-obstruction
   (C)   metastasis from distant primary tumor
   (D)   denervation of myenteric plexus
   (E)   mucositis complication of chemotherapy

278. If biopsy diagnosis of carcinoma were obtained of the lesion shown, it would be

   (A)   Duke's C
   (B)   new primary
   (C)   Stage II
   (D)   Stage IV
   (E)   radiotherapy indication

279. Treatment that should be performed now is

   (A)   diverting colostomy
   (B)   abdominoperineal resection
   (C)   combination chemotherapy
   (D)   symptomatic
   (E)   gastrectomy

ANSWERS AND TUTORIAL ON ITEMS 277-279

The answers are: **277-C; 278-D; 279-D**.

This X-ray depicts the "Krukenberg tumor" or "rectal shelf". In this instance, the disease identified was that of gastric adenocarcinoma that had fallen to the inferior part of the peritoneal cavity and implanted there growing extramurally to compress the rectal lumen. By definition, this is Stage IV disease, since the primary adenocarcinoma has escaped not only through all layers of the stomach wall, but into distant metastatic sites. It is for that reason that treatment should be symptomatic, since there is no effective therapy for disease either in its primary or secondary location.

Items 280-282

On a chest X-ray, a radiologist spots densities confirmed on the subsequent radiographs depicted here

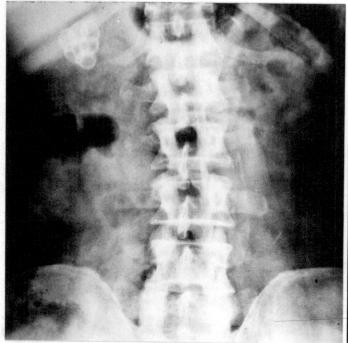

280. The location of these densities is likely to be in

    (A)   renal pelvis
    (B)   ureter
    (C)   gall bladder
    (D)   common bile duct
    (E)   rib

281. The diagnosis is likely to be

    (A)   urate stones
    (B)   calcium oxalate stones
    (C)   chondroma
    (D)   pigmented stones
    (E)   calcium cholesterol stones

282. Plain radiographic appearance of these defects happens

    (A)   over 90% of the time
    (B)   50%
    (C)   under 10%
    (D)   only if surrounded by gas
    (E)   if infected

ANSWERS AND TUTORIAL ON ITEMS 280-282

The answers are: **280-C; 281-E; 282-C**.

This is a fortunate incidental pickup in an asymptomatic patient of a "mulberry cluster" of stones with a rim of calcium that allowed their visualization on X-ray. They are in the gall bladder and not the

116

urinary collecting system. Most gall stones cannot be visualized without displacing contrast material, so this radiographic evidence was quite fortunate. The very presence, however, of asymptomatic gallstones does not mean they have to be removed, but is a valuable piece of information for the patient to carry along with the stones in the event that symptoms develop at a later time.

Items 283-285

A patient with jaundice and occasional elevated amylase undergoes endoscopic retrograde cholangiopancreaticography (ERCP) when amylase has returned to normal and the X-ray depicted here is taken.

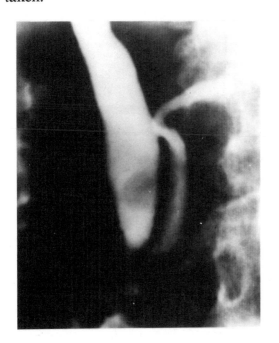

283. The anatomic appearance depicted supports the mechanism of clinical problems associated with

    (A) reflux cholangitis
    (B) Odditis
    (C) common channel theory
    (D) ball valve obstruction
    (E) cholangiocarcinoma

284. The patient's jaundice is probably due to

    (A) hepatitis
    (B) cholecystitis
    (C) hemolysis
    (D) choledocholithiasis
    (E) peri-ampullary carcinoma

285. Treatment should include

    (A) pancreatic biopsy
    (B) biliary diversion
    (C) choledocholithotomy
    (D) pancreaticoduodenectomy (Whipple procedure)
    (E) pancreaticojejunostomy (Puestow procedure)

ANSWERS AND TUTORIAL ON ITEMS 283-285

The answers are: **283-C; 284-D; 285-C**.

This X-ray taken at the time of ERCP shows contrast injection which fortuitously gives visualization of the pancreatic duct as well as the common bile duct. The free reflux from one system to the other might support the common channel theory and explain why inflammation at the ampulla might give rise to conjoined problems or that one might be etiologic of the inflammation in the other system.

The other finding of this ERCP is the cause for the patient's jaundice. We know the patient has had elevations of the bilirubin and periodic elevations of the amylase, and in the common duct opacification we notice a common duct stone. This should be treated by removing that stone from the common duct, if possible, by grasping it from the ERCP endoscopic procedure, and if not, a choledocholithotomy will be necessary. It is sometimes thought that if the stone cannot be grasped and delivered, dilating by sphincterotomy or some form of sphincteroplasty will allow the spontaneous passage of this stone. That depends on the size of the stone and the condition of the patient, and it might be worth the try in the event that a closed endoscopic procedure is not successful in removing the stone.

Items 286-288

This cholangiogram is obtained intra-operatively following cholecystectomy.

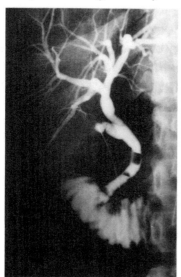

118

286. It shows

   (A)   total common duct obstruction
   (B)   massively dilated intrahepatic biliary tree
   (C)   absence of cystic duct
   (D)   contrast defects in common duct
   (E)   no evidence of hepatic duct dilatation

287. The most likely reason for the findings is

   (A)   air bubble
   (B)   blood clot
   (C)   improper mixing of contrast
   (D)   inflammatory polyp
   (E)   retained stones

288. Operation will now involve

   (A)   T-tube
   (B)   liver splitting hepatico-jejunostomy
   (C)   duodenotomy
   (D)   pancreatic biopsy
   (E)   sphincterotomy

ANSWERS AND TUTORIAL ON ITEMS 286-288

The answers are: **286-D; 287-E; 288-A.**

This X-ray shows the reason that intraoperative cholangiography is done. Through the cannulated cystic duct that is visualized, contrast flows freely from an apparently normal upper biliary tree into the duodenum. But along the way, there are several irregular filling defects.

Because of the irregularity, they cannot be air bubbles, and because of their multiple positions in an unmanipulated common bile duct, it is unlikely that they are inflammatory or a blood clot. The single most likely reason is that gallstones have passed from the gallbladder into the common bile duct and have not passed the ampulla. This cholangiogram, therefore, is indication for a common bile duct exploration, which will entail T-tube diversion at closure.

Items 289-291

This film is taken from an upper GI series done in follow-up postoperatively on an asymptomatic patient who had had jaundice when first seen 8 months before.

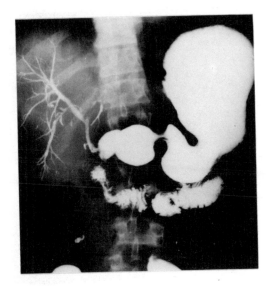

289.   The X-ray shows

(A)   alkaline reflux gastritis
(B)   postoperative defect following hepatic resection
(C)   blind loop syndrome
(D)   choledochoduodenostomy
(E)   calcific pancreatitis

290.   This situation is most likely going to lead to

(A)   severe ascending cholangitis
(B)   gas forming organisms in biliary tree
(C)   recurrent obstructive jaundice
(D)   gastric outlet obstruction
(E)   continued anicteric recovery of function

291.   If this finding did not follow operation, it might be indicative of

(A)   gallstone ileus
(B)   cholangiocarcinoma
(C)   necrotizing pancreatitis
(D)   persistent cholecystitis
(E)   salmonellosis

ANSWERS AND TUTORIAL ON ITEMS 289-291

The answers are: **289-D; 290-E; 291-A**.

This startling film shows free reflux of barium into an apparently normal biliary tree. Since this is postoperatively, we recognize this as the normal consequence of choledocoduodenostomy. If this had happened spontaneously, it might mean that a fistula had developed between the common duct and duodenum or some destruction of the sphincter of Oddi had occurred to allow for free reflux of barium. Since there is reflux freely into, and low pressure drainage out of, the common bile duct, ascending cholangitis should not be a major problem. Therefore, the likely continuing course is that of anicteric recovery of function. Gallstone ileus

119

requires a connection between the biliary tree and the gut bypassing the ampulla, and this might be compatible with that story had it happened spontaneously; however, most of those communications are from the gallbladder to the GI tract rather than from the common duct. If there had been retained stones resident in the common duct and it was dilated, such a fistula could give rise to gallstone ileus.

Items 292-294

A patient with persistently elevated amylase has the upper GI X-ray findings depicted (A), and in follow-up has the sonogram shown (B).

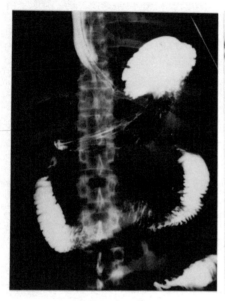
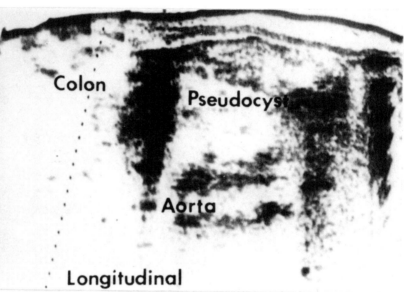

292. The barium study demonstrates all of the following findings **EXCEPT**:

    (A)   widened C-loop
    (B)   edema of surrounding bowel
    (C)   displacement of retro-peritoneal structures
    (D)   calcific pancreatitis
    (E)   passage of barium through jejunum

293. Sonography indicates all of the following **EXCEPT**:

    (A)   prominent abdominal mass
    (B)   cystic fluid collection
    (C)   thick capsule walling off fluid collection
    (D)   displacement of colon
    (E)   proximity to retroperitoneal great vessels

294. Such findings indicate

(A) immediate operation
(B) incision and drainage
(C) temporizing if patient is stable
(D) multiple antibiotic administration
(E) early recovery

ANSWERS AND TUTORIAL ON ITEMS 292-294

The answers are: **292-D; 293-C; 294-C**.

This patient has significant destructive pancreatitis. It is evident that he is in the early stages of pseudocyst formation. There is a collection of inflammatory fluid but without much evidence of a pseudocyst lining that contains this fluid. The inflammatory extension of this process is evident throughout the retroperitoneum on the very much displaced upper GI barium contrast. No evidence of calcification is noted in the bed of the pancreas, so it is likely that this is an acute, possibly even fulminant process, and not a chronic persisting one.

Since there is no thick pseudo-capsule to hold sutures for enteric internal drainage, temporizing on this patient might permit the development of such a structure. If that does not develop, and the patient has an operation that is too early for internal diversion, external drainage and the creation of a pancreatic fistula will take place. If the patient remains stable and the inflammatory process can progress to a mature pseudocyst, this will be a much better outcome for definitive one stage repair by internal diversion without all the attendant complications of fluid and electrolyte imbalance and autodigestion of skin surface as well as failure of containment of the inflammatory process from interruption of an immature pseudocyst during its formation.

Items 295-297

This cholangiogram is done in a severely jaundiced patient who has lost 30 pounds in 4 months.

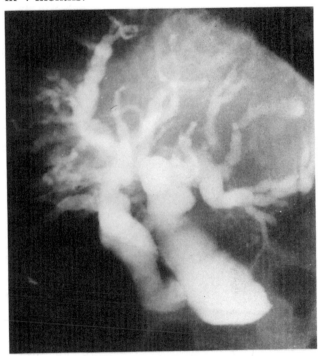

295. By what technique is such a study done

(A) oral cholangiogram
(B) ^{99m}Tc HIDA scan
(C) IV cholangiogram
(D) percutaneous transhepatic cholangiogram
(E) endoscopic retrograde cholangiopancreatography

296. The likely cause of these findings is

    (A) stone impacted in common duct
    (B) carcinoma of the pancreas
    (C) sclerosing cholangitis
    (D) unintentional surgical ligature of common bile duct
    (E) pancreatic pseudocyst

297. Treatment should be by

    (A) cholecystectomy
    (B) choledochojejunostomy
    (C) gastrojejunostomy
    (D) external permanent biliary fistula
    (E) radiation

ANSWERS AND TUTORIAL ON ITEMS 295-297

The answers are: **295-D; 296-B; 297-B**.

This patient has a very serious high grade obstruction. Without antecedent operation that would implicate surgical interruption of the common bile duct, (and it is unlikely that it would have developed slowly over the past months if that were the case), it is most probable that this is a malignant biliary obstruction. The jaundiced patient cannot undergo a contrast study in which the patient is expected to concentrate the contrast. That includes ^{99m}Tc HIDA scan, oral cholecystogram, and even IV cholangiography. The only way the contrast will appear in the biliary tree is to have it introduced there directly, and that must take place either by percutaneous delivery or by endoscopic retrograde delivery.

In this patient, ERCP would be unlikely to penetrate through to the obstructed duct on the basis of the apparent size of the mass in which the common bile duct terminates. That does not mean that ERCP should not be attempted, if not for biliary diversion, certainly it would be helpful in diagnosis and may suggest something about the resectability or palliation potential of this lesion.

In this instance, the X-ray we are examining is that of a percutaneous transhepatic cholangiogram. The termination of the duct ended in an adenocarcinoma of the head of the pancreas. With the temporary use of the percutaneous decompression of the biliary tree for several days, the patient then underwent limited exploration for choledochojejunostomy. Such an anastomosis is easy in the very dilated duct, but would be very difficult in the duct that was not previously obstructed. In this instance, the common bile duct was nearly the same caliber as the diverting jejunum which was brought up by *Roux-en-Y* loop. With this biliary bypass, his jaundice did not completely resolve, but he was more capable of consciousness for greater parts of the day for the three months that this palliation afforded.

Items 298-300

This barium enema was obtained on a first order relative of a propositus patient who has had confirmed colonic polyposis syndrome.

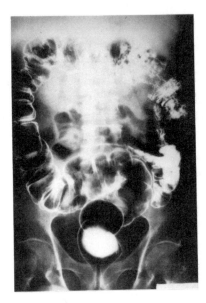

298.   The most notable and clinically significant feature of this X-ray is

(A)   diverticulosis
(B)   multiple polyposis
(C)   ulceration colitis pseudopolyps
(D)   left colon carcinoma
(E)   colovesical fistula

299.   The treatment for this disease at this stage is

(A)   left hemicolectomy
(B)   abdominoperineal resection
(C)   total proctocolectomy
(D)   left hemicolectomy and polypectomies
(E)   sleeve resection splenic flexion

300.   Advice for follow-up should include

(A)   radiotherapy
(B)   screen all family members
(C)   levamisole
(D)   5-fluorouracil adjuvant
(E)   corticosteroids

ANSWERS AND TUTORIAL ON ITEMS 298-300

The answers are: **298-D; 299-C; 300-B**.

In screening this relative of a patient with confirmed colonic polyposis, the diagnosis is confirmed in this individual as well, evident by the multiple polyposis. However, in addition, a left colon carcinoma is discovered on this barium enema, the nearly inevitable follow-up finding in a patient with the polyposis syndrome. The treatment of the syndrome is total proctocolectomy, and that would be true whether or not the colon carcinoma had already appeared, since the earliest stage of treatment is the best at reducing the death rate from dissemination of colon cancer, and the development of that colon cancer is nearly inevitable in patients with polyposis syndrome. Follow-up advice should include the screening of all first order relatives of the family for similar discoveries of potentially treatable early disease; and, in the instance of this particular familial syndrome, prophylaxis of carcinogenesis.

Items 301-303

A woman with obstipation is seen for evaluation, and after incomplete colon preparation, this barium enema is obtained.

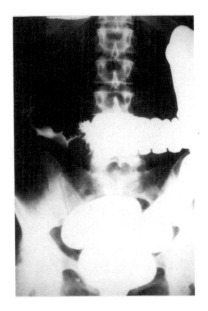

301.   The likely involvement of the tumor from the evidence seen on this X-ray is

   (A)   mucosal only
   (B)   through submucosa
   (C)   through muscularis externa
   (D)   lymphatic metastases
   (E)   hepatic metastases

302.   The chief benefit of operation is likely to be

   (A)   curative resection
   (B)   relief of impending obstruction
   (C)   decrease risk of bleeding
   (D)   to facilitate chemotherapy
   (E)   to allow radiation therapy

303.   If hepatic metastases are encountered operation should be

   (A)   terminated
   (B)   limited to resection of colonic lesion
   (C)   extended to hepatic wedge resections
   (D)   accompanied by hepatic artery ligation
   (E)   search other parts of colon for curable lesions

ANSWERS AND TUTORIAL ON ITEMS 301-303

The answers are: **301-C; 302-B; 303-B**.

This adenocarcinoma is in annular constricting configuration with impending complete bowel obstruction. The radiographic pattern of this "napkin ring" suggests that the invasion of the tumor is through muscularis externa at least, although there is no evidence from a barium enema that would suggest lymphatic metastases or hepatic metastases, the size and extension of this tumor can be expected to have high likelihood of disease extended beyond the bowel wall. If that were encountered, by some such evidence as hepatic scan, for example, that information would be irrelevant to her primary problem which is impending bowel obstruction which requires relief regardless of resectability of the tumor for cure. Should hepatic metastases be encountered, the operation would continue toward its primary focus which is the relief of the impending bowel obstruction, but there would not be an attempt at management of the oncologic problem in the liver or other parts of the colon, since her chief physiologic threat is from bowel obstruction rather than the longer term consideration of the oncologic potential.

Patients who have obstructing colon cancer typically have difficulty with bowel preparation and the operations are generally done on a semi-urgent basis rather than an elective carefully prepared bowel resection. The operations that are urgently carried out for such malignant obstructions deal principally with the obstruction. The malignancy that gave rise to the obstruction could be treated on an elective basis with adequate bowel preparation if the obstruction were not such an eminent threat.

Items 304-306

This X-ray was obtained the day following a barium enema in the post-evacuation phase of this study.

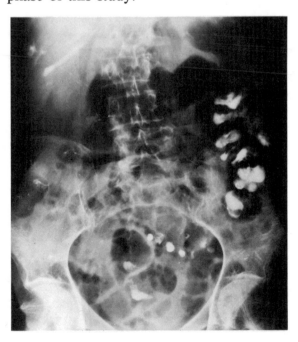

304. The X-ray reveals

(A) ileus
(B) colon obstruction
(C) ulcerative colitis
(D) granulomatous colitis
(E) diverticulosis

305. A problem clinically associated with this finding is

(A) bleeding
(B) colonic perforation
(C) toxic megacolon
(D) *pneumatosis intestinalis*
(E) fistula formation

306. The patient with such a finding would be advised to

(A) have total colectomy
(B) have sigmoid resection
(C) have twice annual colonoscopy
(D) eat a high fiber diet
(E) have CEA determinations twice yearly

ANSWERS AND TUTORIAL ON ITEMS 304-306

The answers are: **304-E; 305-A; 306-D.**

This barium enema radiograph depicts diverticulosis. There is no evidence of inflammatory disease or ileus. A clinically associated phenomenon that can be a problem with diverticulosis is bleeding. It is true that diverticulosis can lead to inflammation, and diverticulitis may be associated with perforation or fistula formation, and ulcerative colitis can

125

be associated with toxic megacolon. Bleeding is the most clinically characteristically associated problem seen with uninflamed diverticulosis. This X-ray finding represents a relatively common anatomic abnormality and should be treated by a diet high in soluble fiber. More aggressive therapy such as surgical resection would only be indicated by complications of the diverticulosis and not by the presence of diverticulosis itself.

Items 307-309

An elderly patient came to the ER from a nursing home with abdominal distension and obstipation. The first X-ray exam (A) was followed by treatment with a rectal tube (B) and a third film after the tube fell out is shown in (C).

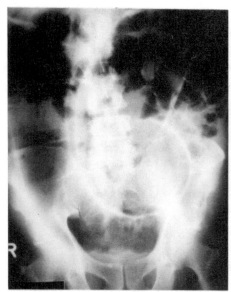 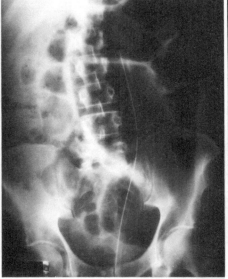 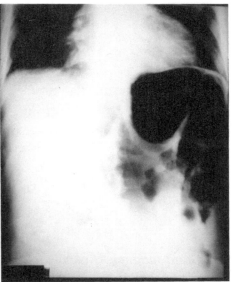

307. The diagnosis is

    (A)   acute gastric dilatation
    (B)   toxic megacolon
    (C)   cecal volvulus
    (D)   sigmoid volvulus
    (E)   ischemic colitis

308. Risk factors for this condition include all **EXCEPT**:

    (A)   advanced age
    (B)   high intake of soluble fiber
    (C)   high intake of insoluble fiber
    (D)   psychiatric institutionalization
    (E)   chronic drug use

309. Treatment of the recurrence in the condition seen in this patient is by

(A) "tacking up" the colon, fixing it to left retroperitoneum
(B) sigmoid colostomy
(C) anterior sigmoid resection
(D) rectal tube insertion daily
(E) barium enema

ANSWERS AND TUTORIAL ON ITEMS 307-309

The answers are: **307-D; 308-B; 309-C**.

This patient has a large sigmoid volvulus. Patients who experience such sigmoid volvulus are frequently psychiatric inpatients or are elderly in nursing homes. High intake of soluble fiber is a treatment recommended to reduce the likelihood of this phenomenon; whereas, some populations in which high intake of insoluble fiber occurs actually have an increased incidence of sigmoid volvulus (e.g., some populations in Afghanistan). Suspension of a sigmoid loop such as displayed here would certainly tear the retroperitoneum, and colostomy would not be advised unless there were other indications for it such as devitalization of the bowel or inability to carry out a primary bowel resection. Repeated use of the rectal tube would be dangerous in a distended colon and anterior sigmoid resection is sometimes required for recurrence of this condition to eliminate the risk of a redundant sigmoid colon loop revolvulizing.

"Good judgement comes from experience — unfortunately, experience comes from bad judgement."

Alan Gregg (1890-1957)

This 62 year-old man had a 50 year history of a bowel problem that appeared to be under control when rectal bleeding and symptoms of obstruction began. Barium enema showed the outline of his colon (A) and a focal lesion (B).

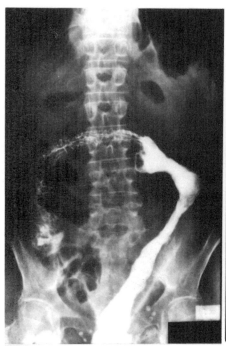 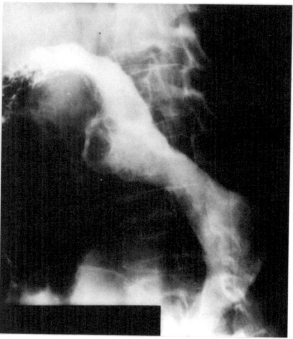

310. The bowel pattern seen is that of

(A) diverticulitis
(B) toxic megacolon
(C) contracted colon
(D) *pneumatoses intestinalis*
(E) pericolic fistulae

311. The serious consequence of this precondition is evident as

(A) carcinoma
(B) perforation
(C) bleeding
(D) fistulae
(E) abscess

312. This consequence of his underlying disease could be expected in a patient with this history in up to how many cases?

(A) 10%
(B) 25%
(C) 33%
(D) 50%
(E) 75%

ANSWERS AND TUTORIAL ON ITEMS 310-312

The answers are: **310-C; 311-A; 312-D.**

This patient has a 50 year history of chronic ulcerative colitis. It has left him with the characteristic signature of long-standing ulcerative colitis in a contracted colon, also called the "lead pipe," a shortened and fibrotic process that gives rise to this stiff, short, nonfunctional colon as it appears on the barium enema.

A problem of long-standing ulcerative colitis is the potential for malignant degeneration and carcinoma. This is evident in both X-rays showing a heaped up polypoid mucosal lesion invading the contracted lumen of the transverse colon. The incidence of this carcinoma as a consequence of ulcerative colitis appears to increase remarkably at 10 years following diagnosis, so that in a 50 year history such as this patient displayed, up to half of such patients will have developed the adenocarcinoma that he presents with in this film.

"The importance of information is inversely proportional to its probability."
Glenn W. Geelhoed

A 19 year-old had appendectomy for gangrenous appendicitis without perforation. On the third day post-operatively, he had a WBC of 20,500 cells/mm³ and a fever. A barium enema depicted here was obtained.

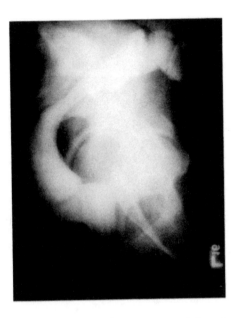

313. The finding demonstrated by the barium enema is

    (A)   proctocolitis
    (B)   ischiorectal abscess
    (C)   pelvic abscess
    (D)   hematoma
    (E)   Krukenberg tumor

314. Treatment of this condition would be by

    (A)   repeat laparotomy
    (B)   antibiotics alone
    (C)   anterior abdominal drainage
    (D)   transrectal drainage
    (E)   perineal incision and drainage

315. The method most useful for finding this complication is

(A) postoperative rectal examination
(B) CT scan
(C) gallium scan
(D) ultrasonography
(E) paracentesis

ANSWERS AND TUTORIAL ON ITEMS 313-315

The answers are: **313-C; 314-D; 315-A**.

This postoperative complication of appendectomy, particularly for perforated or gangrenous appendicitis, is an infection, but not a wound infection in the superficial abdominal layers. This is a pelvic abscess in which soilage of the peritoneal cavity has fallen to the inferior pouch in the pelvis. There it is palpable by digital rectal examination which is the most useful test for discovering it. This complication is the reason that one performs digital rectal examination in followup of a patient who returns for postoperative check following appendectomy. The position of this abscess allows transrectal drainage which is the preferred route. Repeat laparotomy is unnecessary, and contamination of tissue planes that are uninvolved as would be the case with transabdominal or perineal approaches for incision and drainage is ill-advised. The barium enema that demonstrates this pelvic abscess so nicely is also unnecessary, but its demonstration shows the relationship of the rectum to the peritoneal floor and illustrates the route of incision and drainage transrectally.

"It is that which we do know which is the great hindrance to our learning that which we do not know."

Claude Bernard (1813-1878)

Items 316-318

A 58 year-old woman had acute onset of chest pain radiating to the back with shortness of breath. No change in her position could make her comfortable. She had no previous cardiac history. Her pain increased in intensity until she could not stand it, and admission chest X-ray (A) was followed by a barium swallow (B).

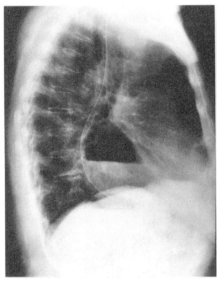 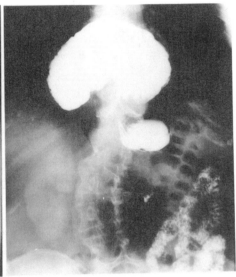

316. The most likely diagnosis is

   (A)   *angina pectoris*
   (B)   esophageal achalasia
   (C)   reflux esophagitis
   (D)   Barrett's ulcer esophagus
   (E)   incarcerated para-esophageal hernia

317. Treatment of this condition is best done by

   (A)   esophageal dilatation by bougie
   (B)   vasodilator therapy by mouth
   (C)   antacids and antihistamine
   (D)   urgent operation
   (E)   esophagoscopy and laser

318. The complication most likely to follow next if the patient is untreated would be

   (A)   hemorrhage
   (B)   perforation
   (C)   complete bowel obstruction
   (D)   myocardial infarction
   (E)   respiratory insufficiency

ANSWERS AND TUTORIAL ON ITEMS 316-318

The answers are: **316-E; 317-D; 318-A**.

   The chest X-ray in this case exhibits gas in the chest, and not either in the lung or free in the pleural space. There are no viscera containing gas aside from the lungs that should be visible on chest X-ray ordinarily, since passage of gas through the esophagus should be rapid in either direction. This might mean that viscera that should not normally be present in the chest have intruded, and that is evident on the barium swallow which opacifies the upper gastrointestinal tract. In this instance, the esophagus and an adjacent bubble containing barium are demonstrated in the radiograph (B). This represents an incarcerated para-esophageal hernia, which is an emergency, requiring urgent operation. The urgency relates to the incarceration and the likelihood that the richly vascularized gastric mucosa would ulcerate and bleed. The thick wall of the stomach makes early perforation unlikely, but hemorrhage is the most likely complication faced if treatment is delayed.

Items 319-321

A 67 year-old woman with a known ventral hernia noted obstipation, distention, and abdominal pain. On physical examination, you note a tender, irreducible protuberant abdominal mass, and order an abdominal film (A) followed by a barium enema (B).

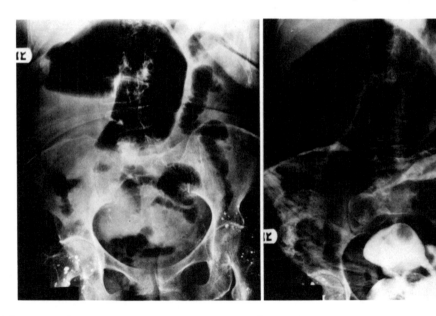

319. The most likely diagnosis is

   (A) intussusception
   (B) obstructing colon carcinoma
   (C) incarcerated transverse colon
   (D) sigmoid volvulus
   (E) acute gastric dilatation

320. The best treatment of this condition is by

   (A) oral laxative
   (B) colonoscopy
   (C) intramuscular prostigmine
   (D) urgent laparotomy
   (E) disimpaction and oil retention enema

321. The next complication most likely if the condition is untreated would be

(A) hemorrhage
(B) perforation
(C) short gut syndrome
(D) strangulation
(E) bacterial overgrowth

ANSWERS AND TUTORIAL ON ITEMS 319-321

The answers are: **319-C; 320-D; 321-B**.

In this patient with a known ventral hernia, the onset of abdominal pain, distension, and obstipation suggests acute obstruction. Herniation at the incision site of the ventral hernia has led to incarceration, and sequestered bowel gas is seen on the flat abdominal films (A). The site of the intraluminal bowel gas in the irreducible hernia is further confirmed as colon by the barium enema (B). The irreducible incarcerated transverse colon in the ventral hernia is an indication for urgent operation. Unlike the case of the prior example, in which the rich blood supply of the gastric mucosa made hemorrhage the most likely complication, here, the much thinner wall of the transverse colon makes perforation a high likelihood, giving rise to the urgency of the laparotomy indication.

"As he picks up his beautiful new tool, however, it is well for the modern biologist to remind himself how subtly and completely a fascination for gadgets can betray sound sense."
William T. Salter (1901-1952)

You are called to evaluate a newborn infant who has had a low Apgar score, and still has inadequate color on weak crying 2 hours after birth, despite suctioning and Ambulatory Mechanical Breathing Unit (AMBU) ventilation. Chest X-rays AP (A) and lateral (B) are obtained and brought to you as you listen for breath sounds in the chest.

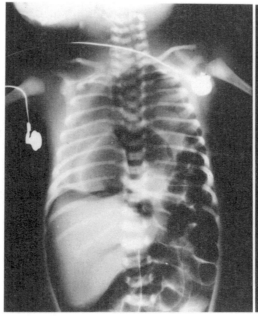 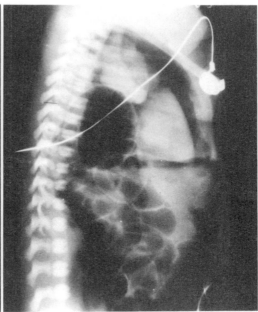

322. The likely diagnosis is

(A) pulmonary sequestration
(B) meconium aspiration
(C) tracheo-esophageal fistula
(D) diaphragmatic hernia
(E) tension pneumothorax

323. The next most likely complication to develop if this problem is untreated is

(A) hemorrhage
(B) perforation
(C) hypoxic arrest
(D) short gut syndrome
(E) organizing pneumonia

324. The rate-limiting feature that most often determines survival in such infants is

(A) time to recognition of disease
(B) degree of pulmonary agenesis
(C) adequacy of antibiotic coverage
(D) capacitance of abdominal cavity
(E) oxygen toxicity

ANSWERS AND TUTORIAL ON ITEMS 322-324

The answers are: **322-D; 323-C; 324-B**.

The chest X-rays show a newborn with a congenital diaphragmatic hernia (of Bochdalek). A large proportion of the abdominal viscera is present in the chest through the incomplete separation of the pleural and peritoneal cavities by the congenital diaphragmatic defect. The presence of the bowel in the chest decreases the ability to ventilate. Even with suctioning, positive pressure ventilation, and intubation the patient has not yet become pink and well-oxygenated. Because of the persistent hypoxia, hypoxic arrest is a likely outcome. Because the defect is large, incarceration of the abdominal viscera within the chest is not likely. Although it is true that the viscera that have become resident in the chest have "lost domain" and the peritoneal capacitance may be decreased, the rate-limiting feature of diaphragmatic hernia is the concomitant failure of pulmonary development. The degree of pulmonary agenesis is often the feature that determines survival in such infants in whom the abdominal viscera are returned to the abdomen by several surgical techniques and the diaphragmatic hernia is repaired. But the adequacy of the lungs to maintain oxygenated blood in the newborn is more a function of the pulmonary immaturity, and sometimes this may require extrapulmonary oxygenation such as with extracorporeal membrane oxygenator use.

Items 325-327

This 30 year-old man had weight loss, night sweats, elevated WBC and was found to have a right groin mass. An imaging study was employed before a surgical exploration of this mass.

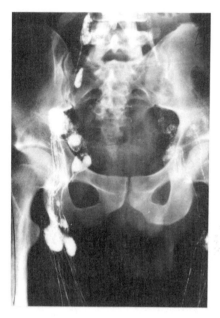

325. This study shown is a demonstration by

   (A) arteriography
   (B) venography
   (C) gallium scanning
   (D) lymphangiography
   (E) barium enema

326. The disease process shown is

   (A) localized to the superficial groin
   (B) involving only the deep groin
   (C) involving only peri-aortic tissue
   (D) systemic
   (E) benign

327. Treatment of this condition should be by

    (A) superficial groin dissection
    (B) deep groin dissection
    (C) superficial and deep groin dissection
    (D) chemotherapy
    (E) radioisotopes

ANSWERS AND TUTORIAL ON ITEMS 325-327

The answers are: **325-D; 326-D; 327-D**.

This patient is studied by a technique used less frequently in the era of noninvasive scanning, namely, lymphangiography. In this instance, the biopsy of the groin mass proved to be non-Hodgkin's lymphoma, and the lymphangiography was done as a staging procedure for determination of treatment. The lymphangiogram shows involvement in both superficial and deep groin nodes as well as peri-aortic tissue, all reflections of a systemic disease process for which chemotherapy and radiation were planned as combined treatment.

Items 328-330

A 28 year-old is brought to the emergency room after a high impact automobile collision in which he lost consciousness and broke several ribs. An aortogram is obtained after widened mediastinum was suggested on chest X-ray.

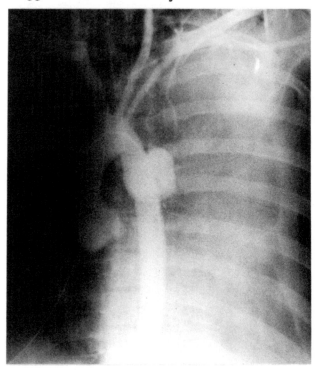

328. The X-ray shows

    (A) a luetic aneurysm
    (B) ruptured sinus of Valsalva
    (C) congenital patent ductus arteriosus
    (D) coarctation of the aorta
    (E) traumatic aortic arch aneurysm

329. The anatomic region of this defect is characteristic because

   (A) it is the center of frontal impact of the chest
   (B) the azygous vein crosses at this site
   (C) the *ligamentum arteriosum* tethers the aorta at this site
   (D) the pericardium is attenuated at this location
   (E) the aorta crosses the bony spine at this position

330. The demonstration of this lesion should be followed by

   (A) advice on avoiding hypertension
   (B) close check on renal function
   (C) analgesics for pain
   (D) vasodilators
   (E) thoracotomy

ANSWERS AND TUTORIAL ON ITEMS 328-330

The answers are: **328-E; 329-C; 330-E**.

This injury is a classic one from frontal deceleration of the "steering post collision" type. In this instance of rapid deceleration in the automobile accident, the heart literally "jumps off the aorta". The reason that this particular anatomic site is characteristically involved in this aortic disruption is that it is at this point that the *ligamentum arteriosum* tethers the aorta. When the heart and great vessels are thrown forward in the chest, it is at the site of this fixation that the tearing occurs, resulting in this aortic arch aneurysm.

Hypertension makes this lesion worse, and some control through the use of medication or otherwise would be necessary to be sure that the aortic arch aneurysm that is traumatic in origin does not dissect. However, thoracotomy is the method for treatment with a repair of this arch aneurysm probably by vascular prosthetic arch replacement.

"The seeming exactness of a mechanical device appeals much more strongly to certain minds than a process of reasoning."
   Sir James Mackenzie (1853-1925)

Items 331-333

A 46 year-old man confined to his hospital bed after an orthopedic injury in an automobile accident develops deep venous thrombosis. He has one episode of pleuritic chest pain and hemoptysis and is anticoagulated, but 2 days later develops tachypnea and this X-ray is obtained.

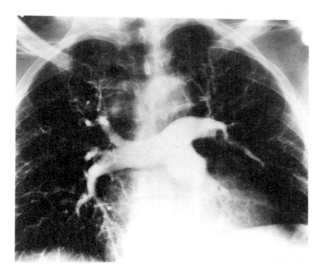

331. Indications for surgical intervention for thromboembolism include each of the following **EXCEPT**:

   (A)   pulmonary angiographic evidence
   (B)   patient having had 5,000 units heparin b.i.d.
   (C)   recurrent pulmonary emboli
   (D)   full therapeutic anticoagulation
   (E)   contraindication to full heparinization (e.g., closed head injury)

332. In the X-ray seen, the patient has

   (A)   main pulmonary arterial stenosis
   (B)   left lung defect
   (C)   right lung defect
   (D)   saddle embolus
   (E)   bilateral emboli

333. Treatment for this specific embolus might include

   (A)   transvenous umbrella
   (B)   caval clipping
   (C)   coumadin
   (D)   urokinase infusion
   (E)   heparin anticoagulation

ANSWERS AND TUTORIAL ON ITEMS 331-333

The answers are: **331-B; 332-E; 333-D**.

This pulmonary angiogram demonstrates bilateral pulmonary emboli through the cut-offs seen on the pulmonary end-arteries. Surgical means of treatment of pulmonary emboli or interruption of the next embolus before it reaches the lungs are based on *angiographic* evidence of *recurrent* pulmonary emboli on full *therapeutic* anticoagulation or in the presence of *contraindications* thereto. This means that full therapeutic anticoagulation is a necessary antecedent, and not the "mini-dose" heparin that is not anticoagulating, but does have some protective benefit in reducing the incidence of deep venous thrombosis and pulmonary emboli.

Each of the treatments for pulmonary embolus that are recommended such as transvenous umbrella, caval clipping, coumadin or heparin relate to the *next* embolus. It is urokinase infusion that relates to the embolus already present in the lung to hasten its fibrinolysis. The only directed surgical attempt at treatment of the pulmonary embolus already sustained is the so-called Trendelenburg operation in which pulmonary arteriotomy is performed and the clot is "milked" back out of the lungs in which it is lodged. This is a very major operation requiring cardiopulmonary bypass and is rarely indicated, since patients who survive to the point of getting to the operating room for such an operation are likely going to survive with full systemic heparinization and thrombolytic therapy. The majority of the patients who suffer sudden lethal pulmonary embolus have it as a saddle embolus which gives rise to rapid right heart strain and fibrillation. Such patients would be unlikely to benefit from operation which could not be mobilized in time to be of benefit.

Items 334-336

A 34 year-old man who had lived 15 years in East Africa was found to have a renal mass on sonogram (A) which was performed for suspected cholecystitis. CT scan confirms the presence of the mass (B) and its location in the kidney.

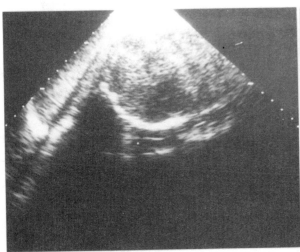 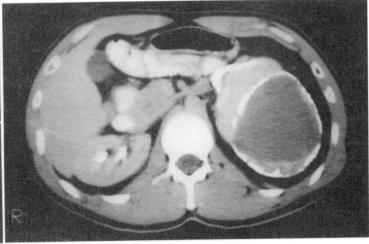

334. The cyst is likely to be of what origin?

   (A)   polycystic kidney disease
   (B)   *Echinococcus* cyst
   (C)   medullary sponge kidney
   (D)   hypernephroma with central necrosis
   (E)   organizing hematoma

335. The chief concern in operative manipulation of this mass is

   (A)   hemorrhage
   (B)   spreading the tumor
   (C)   spilling contents
   (D)   vascular invasion
   (E)   lymphatic drainage

336. A potential consequence of this mass' presence over an extended time includes each of the following **EXCEPT**:

(A) rupture
(B) anaphylaxis
(C) hypertension
(D) urinary stones
(E) bacteremia

ANSWERS AND TUTORIAL ON ITEMS 334-336

The answers are: **334-B; 335-C; 336-E.**

This patient presents with a renal mass that turns out to be an *Echinococcus* cyst. It was incidentally discovered, since it had caused him no symptoms, and the chief concern in the operative manipulation is to avoid spilling its contents. The reason to avoid this phenomenon is the probability of spreading the disease through daughter cysts from the scolices as well as anaphylaxis that may result from exposure to this antigenic material.

Items 337-339

A 51 year-old man had cough, weight loss and blood tinged sputum develop over 6 months and a chest X-ray is done. The results show a finding depicted.

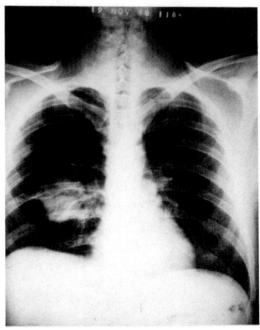

337. The next step in diagnosis is

(A) percutaneous aspiration cytology
(B) thoracentesis
(C) pulmonary function studies
(D) mediastinoscopy
(E) bronchoscopy

338. With the diagnosis of anaplastic carcinoma, the next step is

(A) pulmonary function tests
(B) thoracentesis
(C) mediastinoscopy
(D) thoracotomy
(E) chemotherapy

339. If the patient has reasonable pulmonary reserve, what determines resectability for this anaplastic carcinoma?

(A)   cell type
(B)   malignant pleural effusion
(C)   positive mediastinoscopic nodes
(D)   chest wall invasion
(E)   positive cervical nodes

ANSWERS AND TUTORIAL ON ITEMS 337-339

The answers are: **337-E; 338-E; 339-A.**

This patient has anaplastic carcinoma of the right middle lobe. Although it presents as a coin lesion, it is usually widely disseminated and unlikely to be resectable. The nonresectability of this lesion even in a patient who is operable is based on its cell type rather than any specific contraindication, since this disease is better treated with chemotherapy than by futile extensive resection. The purpose of the bronchoscopy is to establish the diagnosis, and thereafter appropriate therapy can be planned and initiated.

"Knowledge is a sacred cow, and my problem will be how we can milk her while keeping clear of her horns."

Albert Szent-Gyorgi (1893-1990)

A coal miner had been PPD skin test positive and had an interval series of chest X-rays to check for evidence of blacklung. On one such examination (A), a finding was noted that progressed in 9 months (B) and at one year (C & D).

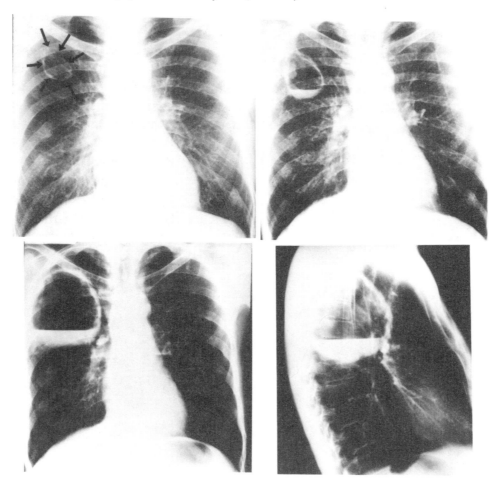

340. The next best treatment should be

   (A)   pneumonectomy
   (B)   bronchoscopy and brush biopsy
   (C)   postural drainage
   (D)   tube thoracostomy
   (E)   percutaneous aspiration

341. The likely reason for the significant change in this lesion is

   (A)   resistant mycobacteria
   (B)   malignancy
   (C)   pyogenic abscess
   (D)   fungal superinfection
   (E)   bronchopleural fistula

342. Helpful pre-operative tests of operability would include

(A) pulmonary function tests
(B) arterial P_{CO_2}
(C) thoracentesis
(D) trans-tracheal aspiration
(E) pulmonary CT

ANSWERS AND TUTORIAL ON ITEMS 340-342

The answers are: **340-B; 341-B; 342-A**.

This patient has progression of a cavitary lesion that probably began as tuberculosis. Because of the cavitation of this pulmonary abscess, and also because of the unknown nature of the lesion, bronchoscopy and brush biopsy would be recommended. The brush biopsy would give histologic evidence of the nature of the lesion as well as open up the abscess into the bronchi for the possibility of postural drainage and evacuation of the collection that is partially aerated suggesting communication with the bronchus. Although various superinfections and other problems may take place in such a lesion, the most significant one in this instance proven by the brush biopsy is a malignant degeneration.

Whether this patient can be operated on would be a determination assisted by the results of his pulmonary function tests. Abnormal arterial P_{CO_2} is a very late finding in a chronic pulmonary cripple, and the other tests listed relate largely to resectability of the tumor rather than operability of the patient.

"Achilles stabbed with his sword at the liver and dark blood came out on his tunic and the light in the eyes of Troy went out."

Homer (The Iliad)

Items 343-345

An African child was burned in a cooking fire and came for attention after the result seen in A and B. In the OR, the operation (C) is shown, with the postoperative result seen in (D).

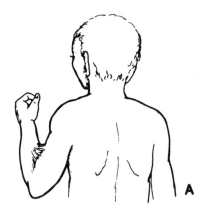
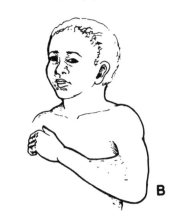

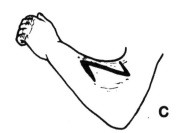
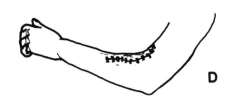

343. The operation performed was

(A) split thickness skin grafts
(B) microvascular composite grafts
(C) Z-plasty incisions
(D) tube pedicle graft
(E) tendon transfer

344. The principle purpose of the procedure is

(A) cosmetic rehabilitation
(B) prevent fused joint
(C) straighten vascular channels
(D) release of scar contracture
(E) improve sensation

345. The result is

(A) a functional upper extremity
(B) improved appearance
(C) better range of shoulder motion
(D) decreased pain
(E) increased blood flow

ANSWERS AND TUTORIAL ON ITEMS 343-345

The answers are: **343-C; 344-D; 345-A**.

This child has the disability seen with joint contracture from burns that heal by scarring with a web causing

144

immobilization of very valuable joints. In the lower extremity, such mobility can be sacrificed with less disability, but the burn contracture of the elbow leads to a useless upper extremity. Before this is allowed to persist for many years and not only cause considerable joint and other disuse atrophy in a child who would learn other compensations and accommodate this disability through never having attained skills in the use of this arm, rehabilitation by reconstruction is important.

The form that rehabilitation takes in this instance is Z-plasty scar contracture release. In this technique, an incision is made in the contracting web in the form of a "Z", and the triangular flaps interposed to disrupt the web contracture and to lengthen and make more useful the upper extremity that can be seen in extension postoperatively.

"It is impossible for any one to begin to learn what he thinks he already knows."
Epictetus (60?-120)

Each of the following techniques for employing sutures in closure of skin has indications in surgical practice.

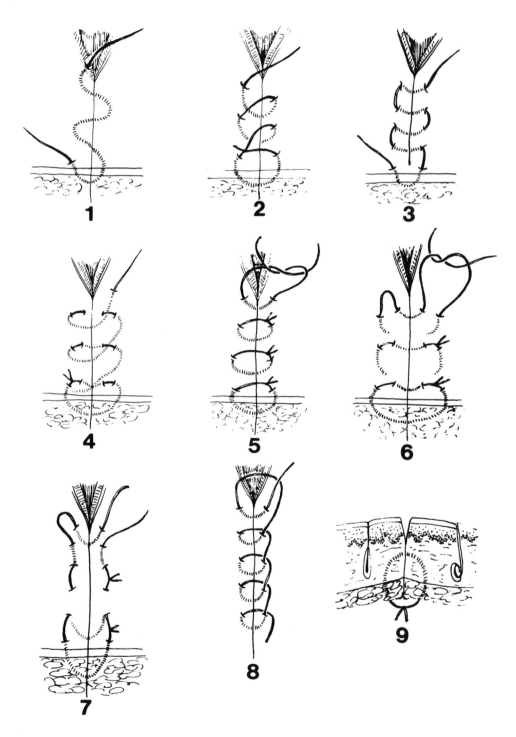

346. The interrupted stitch most like to evert skin edges

(A) 4
(B) 2
(C) 5
(D) 6
(E) 7

347. The suture **LEAST** likely to leave "stitch marks"

(A) 1
(B) 2
(C) 3
(D) 4
(E) 5

348. The suture referred to as "horizontal mattress"

(A) 4
(B) 5
(C) 6
(D) 7
(E) 8

ANSWERS AND TUTORIAL ON ITEMS 346-348

The answers are: **346-D; 347-A; 348-D**.

The suture shown in figure 6 is called the "interrupted vertical mattress". In this technique, the approximated skin edges are everted by the vertical component of the mattress. The suture that is least likely to leave "stitch marks" is one that does not come through the surface of the skin, and in this instance that would be either number 1 or number 9. The number 1 is referred to as the "subcuticular" closure that is continuous, and number 9 is that of an "interrupted buried" subcutaneous suture. The "horizontal mattress" can be either interrupted or continuous as well, but the most common use of this suture is as an interrupted stitch to maintain hemostasis and some compression of the approximated wound edges.

"Two diagnoses never made: the one you don't know about; the one you didn't think of."
Glenn W. Geelhoed

PART II
DUAL-OPTION MATCHING ITEMS

DIRECTIONS: Each set of matching items in this section consists of a list of four options followed by several numbered items. For each numbered item, select the **ONE** lettered option that is most closely associated with it. In the interest of efficiency in addressing matching sets with large numbers of options, it is generally advisable to begin each set by reading the list of options. Then, for each item in the set, try to generate the correct answer and locate it in the option list, rather than evaluating each option individually. Each lettered option may be selected once, more than once, or not at all.

Items 349-352

(A)	Cholecystitis
(B)	Cholangitis
(C)	Both
(D)	Neither

349. jaundice

350. stones

351. mortality

352. sphincteroplasty

ANSWERS AND TUTORIAL ON ITEMS 349-352

The answers are: **349-B; 350-C; 351-B; 352-B**.

Cholecystitis is a disease of significant morbidity; cholangitis is associated with high mortality. Both may be associated with gall stones and usually are. Frequently gall stones previously associated with cholecystitis may pass into the common duct producing obstruction and cholangitis. It is this obstructive component of cholangitis that produces the jaundice, which should not be associated with cholecystitis unless cholangitis is involved.

Sphincteroplasty is a method to increase flow and reduce pressure in the common duct, and this release of obstruction of the common duct should relieve cholangitis, but should have nothing to do with the gall bladder, which has its own distal resistance in the spiral valve in the cystic duct at the junction with the common duct. Sphincteroplasty should not relieve cholecystitis, although it is a method of managing cholangitis. Sphincteroplasty can also allow reflux from the duodenum or pancreatic juices into the common duct, and may therefore be associated with cholangitis as an etiology, but this should be a much more benign condition following sphincteroplasty than that which could occur in its absence in which the inflammation under pressure in the obstructed duct would have a much greater likelihood of going on to septicemia in the patient with obstructed cholangitis.

Items 353-356

(A) Acalculous cholecystitis
(B) Gallstones
(C) Both
(D) Neither

353. total parenteral nutrition

354. hereditary spherocytosis

355. cholecystectomy

356. cholecystolithotomy

ANSWERS AND TUTORIAL ON ITEMS 353-356

The answers are: **353-A; 354-B; 355-C; 356-D**.

Acalculous cholecystitis is associated with total parental nutrition over an extended period, when it is presumed that bile stasis in the gall bladder and lack of motility in emptying is the mechanism of the initiation of inflammation. With an insufficient time course over the period that total parenteral nutrition is usually administered, gall stones would not develop that are a later complication of cholecystitis. The reason for the gall bladder atony is the gut rest without the duodenal stimulation that would release the cholecystokinin to activate gall bladder contraction.

Gallstones may be formed by pigment breakdown products from hemolysis, and gall stones at an early age are seen in patients with hematologic abnormalities, pigmented stones being the usual source of the cholecystitis. Cholecystectomy is the treatment for cholecystitis whether associated with gallstones or not. Cholecystolithotomy, a potential procedure in which the gall bladder is opened, the stones removed, and the gall bladder closed (much as would be the treatment for common bile duct stones) is *not* performed. The reason is that the gallstones' presence is *prima facie* evidence of cholecystitis, and — as just stated — the treatment of cholecystitis is cholecystectomy. Removing the inflammatory tissue with which the gallstones are associated is preferable to allowing cholecystitis to persist because new stones would be formed later, if only the gallstones were removed without addressing the underlying cholecytitis.

Items 357-360

(A) Superficial thrombophlebitis
(B) Deep venous thrombosis
(C) Both
(D) Neither

357. pulmonary embolus

358. occult visceral malignancy

359. heparin therapy

360. early ambulation reduces likelihood

ANSWERS AND TUTORIAL ON ITEMS 357-360

The answers are: **357-B; 358-A; 359-C; 360-B**.

The biggest threat from deep venous thrombosis is dislodging and embolizing the clot which may migrate to the lungs. This would be unlikely to occur with superficial thrombophlebitis, which is above the fascia through which perforating veins carry superficial venous return to the deep venous system or through the saphenous collecting system. Migratory superficial thrombophlebitis that is otherwise unexplained may be a harbinger of malignancy, particularly in neoplasms that are associated with a hypercoaguable state.

Heparin therapy is useful in both. Low dose heparin is used for prevention and therapeutic anticoagulation levels for treatment, which do not so much dissolve the clots as prevent coagulation and any propagation as the thrombolytic system works on clot lysis. Early ambulation enlists the assistance of muscular contraction to minimize stasis, pumping blood up to the next higher venous valve enroute to the heart. The superficial venous system is external to the fascia enveloping the muscles, and would not experience compression from muscular exertion. Locally applied heat might increase blood flow through the superficial venous system, but muscular pumping would be on the opposite side of the fascial barrier, and if the perforating veins have competent valves, that pressure would not be translated to the superficial venous system.

Items 361-364

    (A)   Ureteral colic
    (B)   Appendicitis
    (C)   Both
    (D)   Neither

361.   acute abdomen

362.   retroperitoneal signs occur often

363.   uneven geographic distribution

364.   hyperparathyroidism

ANSWERS AND TUTORIAL ON ITEMS 361-364

The answers are: **361-C; 362-C; 363-C; 364-A**.

Both ureteral colic and appendicitis are parts of the differential diagnosis of an acute abdomen. Although peritoneal signs are more frequently seen with appendicitis, both may exhibit retroperitoneal signs in the referral of the pain, with appendiceal location occasionally being entirely retroperitoneal. Both the reference pain and physical examination (e.g., by rectal examination) may lateralize in the retroperitoneum for each condition.

There is a strong association with Western lifestyle for appendicitis which is very uncommon in developing world environments and highly prevalent in the West. There is a maldistribution of urinary calculi, also, which are not distributed in the same pattern as appendicitis. There are "stone belts" across various geographic regions, often associated with hot, dry climate, but there are additional unknown factors besides the obvious association with potential dehydration that are involved with this peculiar geographic distribution. Some groups of patients can be associated with a higher risk of urinary calculi, such as those with high urate excretion (gout, leukemia) or those with unusually high calcium clearance. Hyperparathyroidism is found to be an associated factor in from one to two percent of patients whose first presentation is calcium oxalate urinary stones.

Items 365-368

(A) Undescended testis
(B) Torsion of testis
(C) Both
(D) Neither

365. testicular malignancy

366. infertility

367. acute emergency

368. operation by scrotal approach

ANSWERS AND TUTORIAL ON ITEMS 365-368

The answers are: **365-A; 366-C; 367-B; 368-D.**

An undescended testis is infertile, since the lower body temperature of the scrotum is necessary for spermatogenesis. The undescended testis, if left in its high inguinal position for a prolonged period, has successively higher risks of later associated malignancy. This malignant

threat is not a component of torsion of the testis, which is an acute emergency presentation. If torsion of the testis results in infarction, sperm production may be reduced, but fertility should not be impaired unless both testes were involved. That is true also for the undescended testis, and infertility results from both conditions if it is bilateral. The operation for both conditions is carried out by a groin incision, as a scrotal approach should not be employed for most operations on the testis.

Items 369-372

(A) Open pneumothorax
(B) Tension pneumothorax
(C) Both
(D) Neither

369. interferes with airflow in opposite lung

370. survivable in absence of emergency treatment

371. impairs cardiac output

372. dyspnea

ANSWERS AND TUTORIAL ON ITEMS 369-372

The answers are: **369-B; 370-A; 371-B; 372-C.**

Open pneumothorax interferes with airflow in the lung on the affected side due to the portion of lung that has collapsed, but does not appreciably interfere with ventilation of the opposite side. Because of the shift in the mediastinum from the air trapped in the pleural space under tension, tension pneumothorax compromises the ventilatory function of the opposite lung as well. This pressure of accumulated intra-thoracic air also interferes with venous return, and impairs cardiac output, an effect only minimally possible with open pneumothorax which should have no additional effect beyond the loss of negative intrathoracic pressure that may help in venous return in the closed chest.

Dyspnea is a feature of both conditions, with the sucking sound of an open pneumothorax creating high anxiety in the patient so afflicted. However, since tension pneumothorax is not survivable without emergency treatment and open pneumothorax is, an emergency method of management would be to convert the tension pneumothorax into an open one, and that is the definitive medical treatment as well when that open pneumothorax is controlled by tube thoracostomy to a waterseal.

Items 373-376

    (A)   Acute appendicitis
    (B)   Tubo-ovarian abscess
    (C)   Both
    (D)   Neither

373.   cervical tenderness

374.   can rupture

375.   treated medically

376.   can lead to sterility

ANSWERS AND TUTORIAL ON ITEMS 373-376

The answers are: **373-B; 374-C; 375-D; 376-C**.

Both acute appendicitis and tubo-ovarian abscess are acute abdominal emergencies and require operation. Medical treatment of both conditions is inappropriate alone, since each can rupture and lead to extensive intra-abdominal sepsis. Acute appendicitis is typically not associated with cervical tenderness unless it has involved adjacent structures or caused an intrapelvic abscess following rupture. The extensive inflammation of both conditions can cause scarring of the infundibulum and these adhesions can impair fertility from each of these origins of peritonitis.

Items 377-380

    (A)   Hepatitis
    (B)   Hepatoma
    (C)   Both
    (D)   Neither

377.   B viral antigen

378.   cirrhosis

379.   aflatoxin

380.   most probably lethal

ANSWERS AND TUTORIAL ON ITEMS 377-380

The answers are: **377-C; 378-C; 379-B; 380-B.**

Hepatitis B is clearly associated with hepatitis B viral antigen, but so is hepatoma which is the most common lethal visceral cancer in the world, distributed with highest incidence in the regions where the highest serum antibody positivity to the hepatitis B antigen prevails. There is a study in the railway workers in Taiwan that have been followed over twenty years, and it has been found that there may be benefit to hepatitis B vaccination not only in preventing the inflammatory component of hepatitis, but also reducing the incidence of hepatoma which appears to be a late complication of hepatitis.

Cirrhosis is associated with both hepatitis and hepatoma, since nearly all hepatomas arise in cirrhotic livers, most of which are in the context of hepatitis B seropositivity and having had hepatitis. There have been allegations that aflatoxin is associated with hepatoma, not yet disproved, but overshadowed by the much more powerful evidence of hepatitis B viral etiology for hepatoma as well as hepatitis. It remains a brutal fact that the most common visceral cancer occurs in the parts of the world where the expensive and highly intensive surgical care would be most needed but is least likely to be obtained. It is an even more sobering fact that the surgical treatment is most likely ineffective in either development setting.

Items 381-384

(A) Chronic pancreatitis
(B) Pancreatic cancer
(C) Both
(D) Neither

381. jaundice

382. surgical cure

383. alcoholism

384. normal serum amylase likely

ANSWERS AND TUTORIAL ON ITEMS 381-384

The answers are: **381-C; 382-D; 383-A; 384-C.**

Both chronic pancreatitis and pancreatic cancer may produce jaundice, and do so with about even likelihood. The classic pancreatic adenocarcinoma that presents with obstruction to the bile duct in the head of the pancreas may represent the only fortunate early presentation because of the location of the disease in the peri-ampullary area. Chronic pancreatitis with peri-ampullary inflammation, alkaline reflux ("common channel") and pseudocyst formation may give rise to obstruction and jaundice with the same frequency as pancreatic cancer arising anywhere in the pancreas does, including those few that obstruct early in the peri-ampullary area.

Alcoholism is a nearly invariable association of chronic pancreatitis but is not remarkable for pancreatic cancer. In both instances the serum amylase is likely to be normal. There may be a higher urinary amylase clearance with pancreatitis, but many of the pancreatic cancers are associated with pancreatic ductal obstruction and some degree of regional pancreatitis, and have as high a likelihood of showing elevations of amylase. In both instances, the most probable serum amylase would be within normal range.

In nearly all instances in which it is employed, surgical therapy is palliative for both conditions. The objective of surgical treatment is typically management of pain, diversion of obstruction of gastric outlet or bile flow, and minimizing disruption of gastrointestinal function. That does not mean that radical operations are not undertaken with intent to cure, but the somber fact remains that the majority of those curative attempts are futile and proven so with distressingly frequent failed postoperative results.

Items 385-388

    (A)   Benign gastric ulcer
    (B)   Malignant gastric ulcer
    (C)   Both
    (D)   Neither

385.   treatment with H_2-receptor antagonists

386.   associated microorganism

387.   pernicious anemia

388.   elevated gastrin

ANSWERS AND TUTORIAL ON ITEMS 385-388

The answers are: **385-A; 386-A; 387-B; 388-A.**

Gastric ulcers have a difference in distribution in the stomach and differing etiologies. With peptic ulceration, there is a bacterium (*Helicobacter pylori*) implicated in loose association with some suggestion that benign peptic ulcer could be an infectious disease. This organism is associated with peptic ulceration so that it would be the benign gastric ulcer. Gastric malignancy is associated with hypochlorhydria. This hypochlorhydria and atrophic gastritis are often features of pernicious anemia. Because malignant gastric ulcers already occur in a state of decreased gastric acidity, H_2-receptor antagonists would not be appropriate as treatment. Whereas the cephalic phase of gastric acid stimulation is very prominent in duodenal ulcer, gastrin elevation is a principle stimulus to HCl production in benign gastric ulcer with its associated high acidity, not the response seen in the event of the low acidity of the malignant gastric ulcer.

Items 389-392

    (A)   Duodenal ulcer
    (B)   Gastric ulcer
    (C)   Both
    (D)   Neither

389.   malignancy

390.   blood group O

391.   perforation

392.   bleeding

ANSWERS AND TUTORIAL ON ITEMS 389-392

The answers are: **389-B; 390-A; 391-A; 392-C**.

Duodenal ulcers are almost never malignant. Gastric ulcers have the possibility of being either malignant or benign given the circumstances of their clinical context. There is a Blood Group O association of duodenal ulcers, particularly those that secrete the antigen in mucosa; but this is true for *duodenal* ulcer. The duodenum in chronic inflammation can develop significant deep ulceration and the thin wall of the duodenum makes perforation possible if that ulceration is anterior in the duodenal bulb. The thicker gastric wall makes perforation much less likely, and there are gastric mucosal protective factors to keep the autodigestive processes controlled in the stomach. Protective factors are not as prominent in the duodenum. Both gastric and duodenal ulcers are sources of upper GI bleeding, and this differential diagnosis of source of bleeding is attempted because the clinical implications that depend on ulceration in gastric or duodenal sources make treatment and follow-up different.

Items 393-396

    (A)   Parietal cell vagotomy
    (B)   Truncal vagotomy
    (C)   Both
    (D)   Neither

393.   gastric drainage required

394.   diarrhea and dumping

395.   acid reduction but with recurrence risk

396.   not accompanied by bowel anastomosis

ANSWERS AND TUTORIAL ON ITEMS 393-396

The answers are: **393-B; 394-B; 395-C; 396-A**.

The objective of vagotomy, both truncal and parietal cell, is to denervate the cephalic phase of gastric acid stimulation. The highly selective parietal cell vagotomy attempts to do so without denervating the motor function of the stomach, so it is *not* accompanied by a bowel anastomosis. Truncal vagotomy requires a gastric drainage procedure.

One of the advantages of parietal cell vagotomy at the outset is that no entry into the bowel is necessary. Therefore, no leaking anastomosis or complications inherent in resection are part of the process. Truncal vagotomy, however, is often aimed at reducing acid production in combination with other procedures, such as subtotal gastrectomy. Since enterotomy and anastomosis will be required for gastric drainage, resection of the antrum, for example, reduces a second stimulus to acid production in reducing gastrin. Both parietal cell and truncal vagotomy reduce acid, but both have an associated recurrence rate, since peptic ulcer is not only a product of the cephalic phase acid stimulation.

The early concerns about parietal cell vagotomy were that there would be a higher failure rate, since it is a technically more demanding operation in identifying and denervating entirely the acid secreting cells of the stomach by meticulous dissection along the lesser curvature, attempting to identify and preserve the motor nerves to the antrum. If they were sacrificed, then, like truncal vagotomy, a drainage procedure would be required and many of the advantages of parietal cell vagotomy would be lost. The principle disadvantage of accompanying the operation with a drainage procedure is that obliteration of the pyloric function and truncal vagotomy may lead to the dumping syndrome, and this disadvantage of truncal vagotomy is theoretically abolished in the parietal cell vagotomy as intended.

Items 397-400

    (A)   Esophageal varices
    (B)   Duodenal ulcer
    (C)   Both
    (D)   Neither

397.   exsanguinating hemorrhage a risk

398.   sclerotherapy effective as first therapy

399.   compression balloon

400.   portal hypertension

ANSWERS AND TUTORIAL ON ITEMS 397-400

The answers are: **397-C; 398-A; 399-A; 400-A**.

Patients with alcoholism and cirrhosis may have portal hypertension. One of the risk factors for development of duodenal ulcer is alcoholism, but portal hypertension is not invariably present, as it is as a rule in esophageal varices. The mechanism of bleeding is quite different, but both can lead to exsanguinating hemorrhage. This may be treated by a compression balloon in the stomach and esophagus, as it is sometimes used in control of bleeding varices, but this is for the control of elevated portal venous pressure, and would be ineffective in arterial hemorrhage, which is the dominant source of worrisome bleeding in duodenal ulcer. Endoscopic sclerotherapy is a preferred treatment in the control of esophageal varices. This procedure is not successful as primary treatment of duodenal ulcer.

Items 401-404

    (A)   Anterior duodenal ulcer
    (B)   Posterior duodenal ulcer
    (C)   Both
    (D)   Neither

401.   perforation

402.   exsanguinating hemorrhage

403.   pancreatitis

404.   duodenal stenosis

ANSWERS AND TUTORIAL ON ITEMS 401-404

The answers are: **401-A; 402-B; 403-B; 404-C.**

Both anterior and posterior duodenal ulcers may give some upper GI bleeding, but the life-threatening exsanguinating type of hemorrhage is seen with posterior ulcers. The large caliber of blood vessels supplying the duodenum and pancreas in this position, and the posterior penetration into the pancreas releasing lytic enzymes, make large caliber arterial hemorrhage the biggest threat to life from a posterior ulcer. Pancreatitis is associated with posterior penetration, and not typically with anterior ulceration.

The anterior duodenal ulcer perforates, and can give rise to an acute, board-like, rigid abdomen as an emergency, even in patients who have no history or clue of a

pre-existing ulcer. If duodenal ulcer is recurrent or prolonged, the duodenum may be scarred down from either anterior or posterior primary duodenal ulcer positions. This scarring can give rise to gastric outlet obstruction in either cause.

Items 405-408

    (A)   Cephalic phase acid stimulation
    (B)   Gastric phase acid stimulation
    (C)   Both
    (D)   Neither

405.   blocked by H_2-receptor antagonists

406.   abolished by vagotomy

407.   prominent in recurrent ulceration and duodenal stenosis

408.   produces erosive gastritis

ANSWERS AND TUTORIAL ON ITEMS 405-408

The answers are: **405-C; 406-A; 407-B; 408-C.**

The cephalic phase of gastric acid secretion is triggered by the vagus nerve, and abolished by vagotomy. However, both cephalic and gastric phases of acid stimulation are ultimately mediated by histamine. H_2-receptor antagonists can block both at the parietal cell. In the event of chronic ulceration and duodenal scarring, duodenal stenosis may cause gastric distention and antral release of excess gastrin. Gastrin is the primary mediator of the gastric phase of acid secretion, and therefore it would be the prominent stimulus to acid production in the event of gastric dilatation. For that reason, peptic ulceration of the duodenum can often be combined with and followed by gastric ulceration or recurrence from increased acid production even after vagotomy. Erosive gastritis is a peptic hyperacidity response, and occurs with both stimuli.

Items 409-412

    (A)   Sliding hiatal hernia
    (B)   Para-esophageal hiatal hernia
    (C)   Both
    (D)   Neither

409.   medical therapy is primary

410.   high risk of hemorrhagic infarct

411.   sclerosing esophagitis

412.   treated by H_2-receptor antagonists

ANSWERS AND TUTORIAL ON ITEMS 409-412

The answers are: **409-A; 410-B; 411-A; 412-A**.

The treatment of sliding hiatal hernia is primarily medical. Surgery is indicated only for complications of the hiatal hernia and not its presence. This is not the case for a para-esophageal hernia, in which strangulation and infarction lead to a high risk of associated hemorrhage. The presence of the hernia in the para-esophageal position is the indication for its repair.

The sliding esophageal hernia is complicated by reflux esophagitis. This sclerosing esophagitis may lead to stenosis, a very significant complication of hiatal hernia. Among the medical means of treatment are included: methods to reduce intra-abdominal pressure which would be appropriate for both forms; reduction of acid production would help decrease the damage from reflux even if the reflux continued. For sliding hiatal hernia, H_2-receptor antagonists are frequently employed in medical management.

Items 413-416

    (A)   Esophagitis
    (B)   Esophageal cancer
    (C)   Both
    (D)   Neither

413.   stricture prominent

414.   perforation a significant concern

415.   surgical cure

416.   colonic interposition

ANSWERS AND TUTORIAL ON ITEMS 413-416

The answers are: **413-C; 414-C; 415-A; 416-C**.

Esophagitis and esophageal carcinoma both have esophageal stricture as a prominent part of their presentation and this represents a continuing patient management problem. Perforation is a very prominent possibility for both, especially since each is diagnosed, biopsied, and observed with semi-rigid endoscopes. Both consist of friable tissue and neither have any serosa to contain any mucosal penetration that erodes muscle. Therefore, for both conditions, perforation is a significant concern.

Surgical treatment is employed for each of these conditions, although medical therapy is primarily indicated for esophagitis. Surgical treatment may be indicated if medical therapy does not control the disease. The esophageal carcinoma is not treated medically, but surgical attention is directed toward relief of obstruction, and only in rare instances is resection for curative rather than palliative intent appropriate. Whereas there are many procedures to correct reflux esophagitis, and many of them have the satisfying result of surgical cure, most prominent among these surgical procedures being the Nissen fundoplication, surgical cure is a fatuous hope for the vast majority of patients with esophageal carcinoma of the stage it typically is at presentation. Surgical treatment has such a high probability of failure in curative intent that it should principally concentrate on its palliative role. In contrast, there is a significant probability that the patient with esophagitis might be cured if antireflux operations are performed.

Colonic interposition replacement of the esophagus is necessary in some instances when very high resection of the esophagus is necessary for esophageal carcinoma and the more common procedure of the pull-up of the stomach into the chest is thought inappropriate. Colonic interposition is also indicated for some forms of esophagitis, especially following multiple complicated and recurrent procedures for esophageal stenosis of significant segmental length, and many of those that involve lye ingestion and the extensive destruction of the esophagus that this form of esophagitis entails.

Items 417-420

(A) ABO blood typing
(B) HLA tissue typing
(C) Both
(D) Neither

417. necessary before transplantation

418. type specific matching is required

419. incorrect typing leads immediately to renal shutdown

420. if the patient does not have the antigen, he has the antibody against it

ANSWERS AND TUTORIAL ON ITEMS 417-420

The answers are: **417-C; 418-D; 419-D; 420-D**.

A recipient does not receive a kidney from a patient if that patient could not also serve as his or her blood donor. ABO blood grouping and HLA tissue typing are performed similarly, with known antisera to identify tissue types. Matching of donor and recipient is done to align the types according to major compatibilities, but the typing is less important than the cross match, because the cross match identifies preformed antibodies against any of the donor antigens. Therefore, full type specific matching is not required for either transfusion or transplantation.

It is intuitive that minimizing compatibility differences would make a "take" in recipient function more likely, and further compromise future potential transfusion or transplantation less by not sensitizing the recipient to the donor's antigens not shared by the recipient. This is especially true in women who are or could become pregnant with intimate connection between circulations of antigenically different individuals.

A mistake in *crossmatch* would lead to immediate or hyperacute rejection of a kidney or hemolysis of a transfusion and consequent renal shutdown. It is not likely that immediate rejection would occur in the event of a mistake in typing, but it is likely that there would be an incidence of sensitization over time if the typing error submitted the recipient to antigens not shared. It is true that the patient is potentially likely to develop antibodies against antigens that are not "self", but that is a potential and not realized possibility. It is only likely that the patient would have preformed antibodies if he had had prior experience to the foreign antigen that the donor organ or unit of blood contains, and such prior experience can come from infection with similar antigens, prior

transfusion, pregnancy, or a previous transplant. In that event, antibodies against the foreign antigens may be preformed, and should result in a positive crossmatch which would eliminate the transfusion or transplantation however close the antigen typing compatibility might have been.

Items 421-424

(A) Diverticulitis
(B) Diverticulosis
(C) Both
(D) Neither

421. life-threatening hemorrhage

422. perforation associated

423. acute abdomen

424. high fiber diet preventive

ANSWERS AND TUTORIAL ON ITEMS 421-424

The answers are: **421-B; 422-A; 423-A; 424-C.**

To use a mnemonic that may be helpful: "'osis bleeds; 'itis perfs". Diverticulosis may be associated with life-threatening bleeding, since the diverticulum that is acquired in the patients who get older with a predilection for forming this disorder have atherosclerotic vessels at the site where the mucosa herniates out through the muscular wall of the colon. The close association of the diverticulum and the blood vessel makes hemorrhage, including arterial bleeding from athero-sclerotic nonretracting vessels possible. Bleeding diverticulosis must be considered in any massive lower GI hemorrhage. In contrast, diverticulitis typically does not bleed since the inflammatory fibrous proliferative reaction scar entraps the area of the vessel and also frequently scleroses down the opening. This is why it acts as an obstructed appendix like a "bayou off the main channel" with bacterial over-growth, obstruction and distention possible in the diverticulum. When the pressure of distention exceeds the pressure of the mucosal "wind sock" of the mucosa that has extended outside of the confines of the muscular bowel wall, perforation is possible, and much more likely in diver-ticulitis than it would be in diverticulosis. Acute abdomen is more often associated, therefore, with diverticulitis, since diverticulosis without the inflammation would have no peritoneal presentation.

A high fiber diet is helpful in reducing intracolonic pressures and also causes microfloral changes. Thus the incidence of both diverticulosis and diverticulitis might be reduced in patients on a high fiber diet. Those patients who already have the established diagnosis of either condition might reduce the incidence of com-plications when placed on a high fiber diet. There is also the question of malignant association, and there is none with either diverticulosis or diverticulitis preferentially, but both are associated with the Western lifestyle that also seems to have a prominent incidence of malignancy. In the instance of diverticulitis, however, the fibrous scarring that results and shows annular constriction on barium enema may sometimes be confused with similar patterns seen with infiltrating adeno-carcinoma, so that diverticulitis may be similar to but not causative of colon carcinoma.

Items 425-428

    (A)   Ulcerative colitis
    (B)   (Crohn's) granulomatous colitis
    (C)   Both
    (D)   Neither

425.   proven premalignant

426.   "skip areas" on barium enema

427.   pseudopolyps

428.   transmural inflammation

ANSWERS AND TUTORIAL ON ITEMS 425-428

The answers are: **425-A; 426-B; 427-A; 428-B.**

Differentiation of Crohn's colitis from ulcerative colitis in the end-stage is not clinically significant, since each requires similar management when colon function has been progressively destroyed for each. Ulcerative colitis begins as a mucosal disease, and granulomatous disease has earlier transmural involvement with patchy areas that are seen on barium enema as "skip areas" with earlier and more frequent involvement of proximal colon. Pseudo-polyps are a prominent feature of ulcerative colitis, and are in essence islands of mucosa with ulceration around them, recalling that ulcerative colitis is principally a mucosal disease characterized by ulcers through that mucosa. Late stage ulcerative colitis has a proven tendency for malignant degeneration. That is about one per cent per year after ten years of the established ulcerative colitis. This has been suggested for Crohn's colitis, but is not proven, since the population of patients in whom these diseases develop typically are members of populations with high risk factors for colon cancer without the inflammatory diseases to confound them, and there is no substantial proof for oncologic potential from Crohn's disease as there is for ulcerative colitis.

Items 429-432

(A) Hypovolemic shock
(B) Septic shock
(C) Both
(D) Neither

429. renal impairment

430. cold, pale, constricted extremities

431. treated with high volume infusion

432. increased cardiac output

ANSWERS AND TUTORIAL ON ITEMS 429-432

The answers are: **429-C; 430-A; 431-C; 432-B**.

Hypovolemic and septic shock are both types of inadequate nutrient flow, and the one sensitive vascular perfusion bed that recognizes this and loses function is the kidney. In both forms of shock, the kidneys are a sensitive indicator of shock. The classic signs of increased vaso-constriction in the periphery, in order to preserve the decreased volume for circulation through the core, are classically apparent in hypovolemic shock. However, warm, pink and well-perfused extremities and nail beds are evident in septic shock, since in this instance the cardiac output is increased. The increased cardiac output is principally a function of decreased peripheral vascular resistance, but there would be a relative insufficiency of nutrient flow to the core because of this shunting. Therefore, both hypovolemic shock and septic shock are treated with high volume infusion. It is sometimes difficult for the observer to appreciate that a patient with warm extremities and a bounding pulse is in shock, but cerebral function, renal output, and an impending acidosis reflect that this is a status of anaerobic tissue metabolism, and that whatever flow is being delivered is not adequately sustaining aerobic metabolism.

(A) Hemorrhoids
(B) *Fistula-in-ano*
(C) Both
(D) Neither

433. portal hypertension

434. inflammatory bowel disease

435. treated with frequent Sitz baths

436. treatment by sphincter muscle divisions

ANSWERS AND TUTORIAL ON ITEMS 433-436

The answers are: **433-A; 434-B; 435-C; 436-D**.

Hemorrhoids are venous varices connected to the portal venous system and can be prominent in circumstances of portal hypertension. They may also be present without portal hypertension if there is some factor of increased pressure in the colon or rectum that is translated to hemorrhoidal venous hypertension. They are not necessarily related to inflammatory bowel disease, although the factors of increased intraluminal pressure may include inflammatory bowel disease as one of the associated features, whereas *fistula-in-ano* is very regularly a feature, particularly of Crohn's disease, but also of other inflammatory GI pathology.

The law of the fistula states that most fistulae in the gastrointestinal tract should close unless there is distal obstruction. The distal obstruction in the case of *fistula-in-ano* is the anal sphincter. Because it is not a good idea to relieve this obstruction (that is, produce incontinence) the purpose of therapy of the *fistula-in-ano* is to cause inflammatory scarring that would obliterate the fistula, as well as identify the factors that gave rise to the inflammatory process to begin with and treat them as appropriate. This might mean anti-inflammatory drugs for Crohn's disease, treatment of specific infections such as tuberculosis, or recognition of the inflammation subsequent to radiation. In order to induce the scarring to obliterate the fistula, the distal obstruction (i.e., the anal sphincter) might have to be cut, but in *only one sector*. In this way, the sphincter fibers could scar together and continence be maintained so long as there is a circular constrictor muscle that can still function by pulling against its scar union. If the sphincter is cut in more than one place, the circular muscle would not contract effectively and the patient would be incontinent. The serious problems that would follow are much worse than the *fistula-in-ano*.

The fistula usually originates in cryptitis. If this can be identified and the origin of the fistula from the inside identified, a gradual way of performing the sphincterotomy without loosing sphincter function during the excision is to insert a seton, a foreign body such as a wire, or suture, that could be gradually moved through the sphincter so that the scarring process that closes the muscle in a healed union behind it would similarly obliterate the fistula. This is like moving a string through butter, and this management of a *fistula-in-ano* is a gradual interruption of this sphincter without total loss of sphincter function as it heals behind the advancing edge. Both hemorrhoids and *fistula-in-ano* are treated with frequent Sitz baths, largely to encourage circulation and relax constrictive tone for shrinking the dilated varix of the hemorrhoid, and to maintain clean granulation as the *fistula-in-ano* is excised.

Items 437-440

(A)   Internal hemorrhoids
(B)   External hemorrhoids
(C)   Both
(D)   Neither

437.   requires anesthesia for excision

438.   thrombosis and bleeding are frequent features

439.   surgery is the primary treatment choice

440.   rubber band ligation for prolapse

ANSWERS AND TUTORIAL ON ITEMS 437-440

The answers are: **437-B; 438-A; 439-D; 440-A**.

Internal hemorrhoids are covered by mucosa, and are not innervated with cutaneous sensation as are external hemorrhoids. Therefore, rubber band ligation and excision without anesthesia would be possible for the mucosal internal hemorrhoids, but not for the external ones which are covered with skin which has somatic sensory fibers.

The external hemorrhoids are, already, external — therefore, they do not prolapse. Prolapse into the constrictive sphincter may cause venous stasis in the prolapsed internal hemorrhoid. Thrombosis and bleeding are frequent features associated with internal hemorrhoids. It is not primarily a feature of the hemorrhoid but the complication that results from its prolapse, and its venous hypertension or ulceration in being present in the anal canal during defecation. For neither internal nor external hemorrhoids is surgery the primary treatment choice. Both of these should be treated medically, since each has a tendency to resolve on high fiber diet, perineal hygiene, and methods for symptomatic relief.

Items 441-444

(A)   Wound healing by primary intention
(B)   Wound healing by secondary intention
(C)   Both
(D)   Neither

441.   less scarring

442.   contraction is prominent

443.   inflammation is involved in the process

444.   accelerated by steroids

ANSWERS AND TUTORIAL ON ITEMS 441-444

The answers are: **441-A; 442-B; 443-C; 444-D**.

A wound is an injury that resolves through inflammation, so wound healing by either intention involves inflammatory processes. If that inflammation is controlled, and if linear apposition of the tissue to be scarred is made surgically contiguous, there is less scarring, which is what the intent of primary intention wound healing is. Wound healing by second intention occurs if a tissue defect is left that must be filled from the lateral sides, not only by re-epithelialization possible directly, but by granulation before epithelial overgrowth can cover the granulation. This takes longer, producing more scarring. Contraction is a prominent process as granulation precedes epithelialization, and the resultant closure is smaller than the original wound which has shrunk over the course of that progress.

There are any number of things that can interfere with the resolution of the inflammatory process and a healed wound, but few things that accelerate it, and none of them that can improve over the basic process of primary intention healing. Chief among the inhibitors of wound healing is infection, but foreign body reaction, tension and mobility, and some drugs are prominent as well. Corticosteroids, being anti-inflammatory, actually inhibit the healing process rather than contribute to it, and that is true for both primary and secondary intention healing.

Items 445-448

(A)   Acute pancreatitis
(B)   Chronic pancreatitis
(C)   Both
(D)   Neither

445.   hemorrhage is *not* a prominent feature

446.   saponification of retroperitoneal fat

447.   diabetes mellitus

448.   calcified pseudocystojejunostomy

ANSWERS AND TUTORIAL ON ITEMS 445-448

The answers are: **445-B; 446-A; 447-C; 448-B**.

Acute pancreatitis is a life-threatening emergency with hemorrhage a prominent part of the retroperitoneal phlegmon which also includes saponification of retroperitoneal fat. This process actually decreases serum calcium, and is a feature characteristic of acute pancreatitis which may have a fulminant and malignant behavior. Chronic pancreatitis is a more mature inflammation with a greater fibrous component, and may even reach the stage of calcification. Depending on the degree of destruction of pancreatic parenchyma, the islet cells may be destroyed in either acute or chronic pancreatitis. Some degree of impairment in glucose metabolism happens with inflammation of the whole organ whether acute or chronic, so diabetes is a feature that can often develop in both.

A pseudocyst is the mark of a maturing pancreatitis, and acute pseudocyst may resolve along with the other more fluid transudative inflammatory processes in the retroperitoneum. Only when the pseudocyst has matured to a fibrous capsule capable of holding sutures is diversion into the gastrointestinal tract surgically feasible, and the more thickened the fibrous and even calcified capsule around the pseudocyst interior, the better likelihood for success in internal surgical drainage. Therefore, pseudocystojejunostomy would be carried out only for this later complication of chronic pancreatitis.

Items 449-452

    (A)   Gastrinoma
    (B)   Insulinoma
    (C)   Both
    (D)   Neither

449.   malignant

450.   solitary

451.   angiographically demonstrable in most cases

452.   sensitive to somatostatin analog octreotide

ANSWERS AND TUTORIAL ON ITEMS 449-452

The answers are: **449-A; 450-B; 451-B; 452-C.**

Insulinomas are typically solitary, benign and resectable for cure. Gastrinomas are typically multiple, malignant, and metastatic when first encountered. Because of this multifocal status for gastrinoma, angiographic demonstration is unsatisfying; whereas, the vast majority of insulinomas can be localized through angiography. Since somatostatin analog is a peptide inhibitor, whether the peptide is gastrin or insulin, its use in both insulinoma and gastrinoma has been successful in decreasing both the peptide secretion and the symptoms associated with either insulin or gastrin excess.

Items 453-456

    (A)   Nasogastric tube (Levin)
    (B)   Naso-intestinal tube (Miller-Abbot)
    (C)   Both
    (D)   Neither

453.   differentiates secretory diarrhea of gastrinoma from VIPoma

454.   metabolic acidosis

455.   aspiration pneumonitis

456.   may be used for enteral feeding

ANSWERS AND TUTORIAL ON ITEMS 453-456

The answers are: **453-A; 454-D; 455-C; 456-C.**

In the postoperative patient "the scaphoid abdomen" (as stated by Dr. Francis Moore) "is a desideratum." Since postoperative patients frequently have ileus or may have been brought to the operating room by an obstructive problem, distention of the stomach and lower GI tract are frequently a problem, and according to Starling's law, the bowel decompensates during distention after a certain fibril distraction occurs, much as cardiac decompensation occurs with congestive failure. To restore adequate motility, and to decompress the bowel to relieve the edematous state so the bowel can resume its absorption function, intubation of the gut is important in many surgical treatments.

Tubes, placed through the nose into the stomach or beyond, each have the problem of passing through the hypopharynx and esophagus, where they may act as capillary for a return of gastric contents that may be aspirated into the airway, since the presence of the tube as foreign body makes hypopharyngeal seal incompetent. Therefore, aspiration pneumonitis is common to each tube.

Aspiration of the gastric contents would produce metabolic alkalosis. However, when the stomach juices are mixed with the intestine, and together these are aspirated by an intestinal tube, the neutralized fluid loss would not result in either metabolic acidosis or alkalosis, so neither tube should be implicated in an acidosis if it should develop in the patient so treated.

Since the watery diarrhea in case of a VIPoma originates entirely from intestinal secretion distal to the ligament of Treitz, and the acid diarrhea that comes from the excess gastric secretion in gastrinoma is all secreted proximal to the pylorus, a

nasogastric tube can differentiate these two, since it will abolish diarrhea in the gastrinoma syndrome. This simple technique is far more discriminating, immediate and cheaper than quite a number of assays that may not be as definitive. Both nasogastric and intestinal tubes may be used for enteral feeding. The nutrient put through those tubes will be different if the tip is in the stomach or in the jejunum, but enteral nutrition is a very natural route of alimentation, and if the gut works, it should be used in preference to total parenteral nutrition, and both nasogastric and intestinal tubes may be used to serve this nutrient purpose.

Items 457-460

    (A)   Ileus
    (B)   Small bowel obstruction
    (C)   Both
    (D)   Neither

457.   gas in small bowel

458.   gas in colon

459.   edematous bowel

460.   high-pitched bowel sounds

ANSWERS AND TUTORIAL ON ITEMS 457-460

The answers are: **457-C; 458-A; 459-C; 460-B**.

Both ileus and bowel obstruction are problems in which fluid does not move through the gastrointestinal tract, in the former because of a motor problem, and in the latter because of a resistance impediment. The end-stage of bowel obstruction is the decompensation of the bowel and, once bowel distention passes the limit of Starling's curve, proximal bowel is atonic. The end-stage of any bowel obstruction, therefore, would be ileus from lack of propulsive activity in the decompensated paralyzed bowel.

There are ways to differentiate these two problems, since one is a surgically urgent condition and the other requires time and decompression for return of bowel motility. In both instances, intraluminal pressures increase and bowel edema occurs as lymphatic pressures rise and absorption fails. Gas is usually transported rapidly through the small bowel, and would be blurred on X-ray film because of the prolonged exposure. It is often seen in the colon, since there is less rapid motility, and it is present long enough to be recognized on a prolonged exposure in a flat plate film. If there is no propulsive force or if the propulsion isn't capable of passing the air, this air shows up on X-ray. Air is typically in both small bowel and colon in paralytic ileus, and is not in colon but distributed with differential levels in small bowel if there is a resistance between them ("step ladder" air fluid levels).

Bowel sounds are present, vigorous, tinkling and crescendo in timbre early in bowel obstruction. As the obstruction develops proximal distension and dilatation, the contractile force gets stronger and the rushes get louder and higher in pitch on the rising slope of Starling's curve. As the distention and further distraction of the smooth muscle fibers progresses, bowel motility "falls off

the crest" of Starling's curve, and bowel sounds decrease as atony takes over later in the obstructive course when the bowel begins to not only lose function, but undergoes anatomic changes of congestion and ischemia as well.

Items 461-464

    (A)   Right colon cancer
    (B)   Left colon cancer
    (C)   Both
    (D)   Neither

461.   polypoid tumor

462.   occult blood loss

463.   obstructing

464.   early presentation

ANSWERS AND TUTORIAL ON ITEMS 461-464

The answers are: **461-A; 462-C; 463-B; 464-B.**

Right colon cancers differ from left colon cancers in their anatomy largely because of the bowel function at the site in which they arise. The classic right large bowel carcinoma as described in the cecum is a polypoid fungating tumor with frond-like projection from the bowel wall into the lumen. As such, it can grow to some considerable size without symptoms of obstruction, but often gives occult bleeding.

In moving further down the colon to the left side, the more annular pattern of the colon cancers is related to the propulsive musculature of the left colon and its thicker wall with submucosal lymphatics arranged to favor the "napkin ring" configuration. There is considerable overlap in these morphologies. However, both can give rise to bleeding, and this bleeding is typically occult. Only at lower rectal levels is the bleeding recognized as bright red blood, and that intermittently. Therefore, occult blood tests are useful in identifying patients that should undergo screening to find the origin of occult blood loss.

Because there is the added dimension of obstruction to flow in left colon cancers these obstructive symptoms may bring patients to the attention of physicians before they are aware of other symptoms. Occult blood detection may lead to the diagnostic work-up for either side of the colon. For a right colon cancer to be obstructing, it would have to be larger than a similar obstructing lesion occurring on the left side. Therefore, the tumors typically present earlier with respect to tumor size, and not necessarily with respect to stage.

Items 465-468

(A) Familial colonic polyposis
(B) Juvenile colonic polyp
(C) Both
(D) Neither

465. malignancy potential

466. inflammatory

467. colectomy

468. occurs in teenagers

ANSWERS AND TUTORIAL ON ITEMS 465-468

The answers are: **465-A; 466-B; 467-A; 468-C.**

The juvenile colonic polyp is an inflammatory excrudesence. It is frequently sloughed and passed with bleeding being the chief sign. Juvenile lower GI bleeding should include juvenile colonic polyp and bleeding Meckel's diverticulum among the differential diagnosis. As an inflammatory polyp, it is very self-limited, and does not have any potential to develop into long-term problems such as ulcerative colitis which is distinguished by the pseudopolyp, essentially an island of mucosa with circumferential ulceration, nor any particular association with later disease potential.

That is in distinct contrast to familial colonic polyposis, although both conditions may occur in teenagers. One is a transient and self-limited event, and the other is a genetic defect that will continuously recur, and invariably lead to the development of colon cancer, even at very young ages. For that reason, total proctocolectomy is the treatment for familial colonic polyposis. In distinct contrast, not only is such radical extirpative therapy not necessary for a juvenile colonic polyp, but it needs neither treatment nor special follow-up after its diagnosis, other than principally to distinguish it from other more significant patient problems.

Items 469-472

(A) Squamous cell carcinoma
(B) Basal cell carcinoma
(C) Both
(D) Neither

469. metastatic to lymph nodes

470. locally recurring

471. Moh's chemosurgery

472. radiation therapy

ANSWERS AND TUTORIAL ON ITEMS 469-472

The answers are: **469-A; 470-C; 471-B; 472-A**.

Squamous cell and basal cell carcinomas of the head and neck are often in sun-exposed areas, and are differentiated because of their difference in potential threat to the patient as well as management difference. Squamous cell carcinoma may

be aggressive and invasive locally, a trait not shared typically by basal cell carcinoma, but it also can be metastatic to lymph nodes. For that reason, resection of invasive cancer involves operation to include regional lymph nodes or their inclusion in a field of radiotherapy, since squamous cell carcinoma can be treated with radiation therapy as well. However, basal cell carcinoma does not require inclusion of lymphatic resection, but is a very stubborn lesion that can recur locally unless completely excised. This excision can take place by means of surgical excision, but is also done with Moh's chemosurgery, studying the margins to see when the "rodent ulcer" has been completely eradicated.

Both of these lesions are locally occurring. The squamous cell carcinoma extends to distant recurrence as well. For that reason, there is more attempt to get complete control of it in its regional spread without such concern for basal cell carcinoma. However, basal cell carcinoma has a similar concern in its treatment for complete eradication locally because of its high propensity to recur. There is a second possible association, and that is that squamous cell carcinoma may result from radiation therapy, and it may be the tumor that occurs in radiation portals after therapeutic radiation is delivered for other purposes and may constitute a second malignancy in someone who has been treated for a first with primary radiotherapy.

(A) Wilms' tumor
(B) Neuroblastoma
(C) Both
(D) Neither

473. the younger, from newborn to 2 years old, the higher the incidence

474. catecholamine secretion

475. combination chemotherapy effective

476. benign transformation with growth occasionally occurs

ANSWERS AND TUTORIAL ON ITEMS 473-476

The answers are: **473-B; 474-B; 475-A; 476-B**.

Neuroblastoma is the commonest malignant extracranial tumor in children. The higher incidences are in the younger ages. In fact, many premature stillbirths can be found with the tumor, many more than are seen in incidence after live birth. This should lead to the inference that the tumor goes away with growth and development of the newborn. And, it rarely does. The very encouraging inference drawn from the high incidence of neuroblastoma in premature still births, the lower incidence in live births at term and the decreasing incidence with the child's age advancing toward two years of age and the very rare cases of maturation of the undifferentiated neuroblastoma toward the benign ganglioneuroma — all give a window into the potential reversal of carcinogenesis; however, this is not translated into very hopeful therapy for these tumors.

Surgical treatment is the mainstay for neuroblastoma resection. Screening for this tumor can include catecholamine secretion which is variably present, secreting different species of catecholamines depending on the stage and grade of the tumor at the child's age. After surgical treatment, however, the last bright hope for cure has passed, since highly aggressive therapy including combination chemotherapy has not been effective in contrast to Wilms' tumor where even subtotal resection has had prolonged survival with combination chemotherapy protocols used as adjunct to operation.

(A) Epidural hematoma
(B) Subdural hematoma
(C) Both
(D) Neither

477. chronic

478. bridging veins

479. lucid interval

480. concussion

ANSWERS AND TUTORIAL ON ITEMS 477-480

The answers are: **477-B; 478-B; 479-A; 480-C**.

The principle difference between epidural hematoma and subdural hematoma besides their obvious anatomic location above or beneath the dura is that the former is from *arterial* bleeding accumulating very rapidly under arterial pressure, and the latter is from venous bleeding which originates from torn bridging *veins* with the corresponding venous pressure limiting the hematoma's rate of accumulation. This difference immediately suggests that subdural hematoma may be chronic and may even be diagnosed at some distance in time after the closed head injury during which it was sustained. Epidural hematoma is an emergency.

Both are most often accompanied by concussion, and both are injuries that typically come from deceleration blows on the head, although, particularly in older individuals, the trauma may be minimal enough to have been forgotten by the time a late subdural hematoma diagnosis is made. That is rarely the case with epidural hematoma which not only is associated with a concussion, but is often accompanied by skull fracture, and peculiarly the fracture through the temporal area that entraps the middle meningeal artery, one of the most frequent sources of arterial hemorrhage into the head subsequent to trauma to the skull. Because a concussion occurs at the time of the blow, but it clears readily, the patient may be normal in cerebral function for a period of time until arterial pressure has caused considerable collection of blood and the patient loses consciousness for a second time after this lucid interval.

Treatment of both types of bleeding into the cranium involve decompression and hemostasis, but the epidural is a true neurosurgical emergency that should be recognizable and treatable by most physicians with surgical experience because of the very short time interval from the second loss of consciousness to the likelihood of "coning" — herniation at the foramen compressing the brainstem which would stop the vegetative functions of respiration and control of heart rate.

Items 481-484

    (A)   Meningioma
    (B)   Glioblastoma
    (C)   Both
    (D)   Neither

481.   benign

482.   rarely cured

483.   intracerebral

484.   encapsulated

ANSWERS AND TUTORIAL ON ITEMS 481-484

The answers are: **481-A; 482-B; 483-B; 484-A.**

Meningiomas are tumors of the dura. Consequently they have compressed dura that may encapsulate them. They are benign, and although not always resectable, they have a high success rate for surgical resection depending on their location and size. They can even be re-operated on if there is recurrence after subtotal resection.

Glioblastomas, however, are not from dural origin but from glial origin and as such do not encapsulate as much as spread by finger-like projections in the brain parenchyma. Both because of their malignant dedifferentiation and because of their growth pattern, surgical cure is rare. Most palliative therapy would be directed toward decreasing intracranial pressure as the mass expands, but there is some strategic question as to whether that would extend to removing the craniectomy skull plate to allow continuous expansion of the tumor with potential complications of draining, sepsis and discomfort from cerebral protrusion through the cranium. Prolonging functional survival might include medication for cerebral edema and occasionally radiotherapy for a period of consciousness, and then a merciful coma when elevated intracranial pressure is not relieved by these measures treated in a closed cranium.

Items 485-488

(A) Proximal fibula
(B) Proximal tibia
(C) Both
(D) Neither

485. associated with treatment of compartment syndromes

486. healing fracture requires more than three months without weight bearing

487. bone graft donor site

488. internal fixation for alignment

ANSWERS AND TUTORIAL ON

174

The answers are: **485-A; 486-B; 487-A; 488-D.**

The proximal fibula is expendable. It does not contribute significantly to the stability of the knee as it does indispensably to stability of the ankle at the lateral malleolus. In fact, the proximal fibula is sometimes taken as a donor bone graft for implantation elsewhere, and is excised and simply discarded in a patient who has a compartment syndrome, as in the case of postischemia reperfusion or crush injury of the legs.

In contrast, the proximal tibia is not only the articular surface of the knee, but also the sole source of support to weight bearing on the leg. Alignment to take this weight bearing stress is important, but that is typically achieved through external fixation and a prolonged period of healing with immobilization excluding weight bearing for three months or more to prevent malunion. The proximal fibula is not fixed at all, and the tibia generally aligns without the need for internal fixation.

Items 489-492

(A) Bone fracture
(B) Ligament sprain
(C) Both
(D) Neither

489. trimalleolar fracture

490. more common in children

491. very often requires casting

492. screw fixation

ANSWERS AND TUTORIAL ON ITEMS 489-492

The answers are: **489-C; 490-A; 491-C; 492-A.**

With a proportionate amount of joint trauma, the child would be more likely to break bone and the adult tear ligaments as a general rule. The ligament itself may avulse the bone in some instances, particularly around joints with considerable leverage such as the ankle, knee or elbow. When the ligament holds and bone is avulsed, frequently screw fixation can fix the bone which has failed before the ligament did. It is not the case that a fracture is more serious than a ligament injury, and both very often require immobilization in a cast. The mechanics of a blow that would disrupt the mortise of the ankle to give a trimalleolar fracture has likely done ligamentous injury as well, and this ankle will likely be significantly damaged and may be unstable despite closed and/or open fixation.

Items 493-496

(A) Split thickness skin graft
(B) Full thickness skin graft
(C) Both
(D) Neither

493. requires granulation recipient bed

494. contracture prominent

495. color and texture are determinants of donor site

496. expandable

ANSWERS AND TUTORIAL ON ITEMS 493-496

The answers are: **493-D; 494-A; 495-B; 496-A.**

A clean granulation bed is often described as "hungry for a graft", but this surface is not required for implantation, and both split and full thickness skin grafts can be placed on fresh wounds without second intention granulation. Their purpose in being so grafted would be to achieve primary intention re-epithelization. So, neither require granulation in the recipient bed for successful engraftment.

A split thickness skin graft is often chosen to cover a wound that one would wish to have become smaller, since contracture is a prominent feature that may proceed under a split graft without a dermis. It is also the case that it may be expanded through mesh extension, which is not the case with a full thickness graft which cannot be stretched beyond its elastic limit. Frequently the donor sites of full thickness skin grafts are selected according to the color and texture of the skin of the donor site that would be an appropriate match to the surrounding tissue in the recipient site, since these will persist as features where a full thickness skin graft is implanted. In contrast, the split thickness graft contracts and further changes in texture and color.

Items 497-500

(A) Femur fracture in child
(B) Femur fracture in elderly
(C) Both
(D) Neither

497. hip contracture common

498. internal fixation is the rule

499. immobilization advisable

500. traction is a preferred treatment

ANSWERS AND TUTORIAL ON ITEMS 497-500

The answers are: **497-B; 498-B; 499-A; 500-A.**

As anyone who has tried to restrain a child into an unwanted position knows, the young are very limber and nimble. Immobilization of a limb in which a fracture lies between joints rarely results in any contracture of those joints in a child;

whereas, it would be common in an older individual to have contracture. This is particularly true in the hip which contracts in flexion. Immobilization, then, is advisable for the femur fracture in the child either by the preferred traction method or by some form of hip spica immobilization. This would be a disservice in the older person who has such disability secondary to immobilization that early ambulation is the rule, which is why internal fixation becomes the first choice of treatment for femur fracture in the adult.

Items 501-504

(A) Gastroschisis
(B) Omphalocoele
(C) Both
(D) Neither

501. peritoneal sac

502. postoperative respiratory insufficiency

503. staged repair

504. worse prognosis

ANSWERS AND TUTORIAL ON ITEMS 501-504

The answers are: **501-B; 502-C; 503-C; 504-A.**

Omphalocoele is a congenital defect in which the midline abdomen has a defect in which viscera are protruding in a peritoneal sac. The sac may be ruptured, either at birth or thereafter, but the bowel has been covered for at least the period of time up to diagnosis. Gastroschisis is also a midline upper abdominal defect, but does not have a sac lining, and the bowel is therefore often desiccated from exposure or contaminated, with inflammation and edema sometime to the point of devitalization.

Since the portion of the gut that has been outside the abdominal cavity has not been accommodated during the period of intrauterine growth, there is no room for it in that there is no potential space that it has left behind in migrating outside the abdominal wall, since it did not develop inside the confines of that wall. For that reason, it must be returned gradually into the abdominal cavity which must expand to accommodate it. This is frequently done with prosthetic mesh material which is constricted in the form of a "chimney" to contain and preserve the bowel in a large prosthetic ventral hernia as gradual progressive staged procedures plicate more of this prosthesis and return more of the viscera to intra-abdominal position. If this were done rapidly, the diaphragm would be pushed up with respiratory insufficiency resulting, which remains a problem for both conditions. Because of the better state of the viscera at the time of the repair if the sac remains intact and protective for the omphalocoele, gastroschisis has a worse prognosis than does omphalocoele and the outlook for accomplishing the reduction of viable bowel into the abdominal cavity is worse. Once repair has been accomplished, prognosis is good for both conditions.

Items 505-508

    (A)   Resectability
    (B)   Operability
    (C)   Both
    (D)   Neither

505.   sometimes improved by radiotherapy

506.   contraindication criteria for operation

507.   most dependent on host factors

508.   determines that operation *should* be done

ANSWERS AND TUTORIAL ON ITEMS 505-508

The answers are: **505-A; 506-C; 507-B; 508-D**.

Operability is a function of the patient's condition, and resectability is a feature of the extent of the tumor and the surgical skill and equipment at hand. Either/and/or both of these features are criteria for contraindicating operation. For example, a resectable tumor in an inoperable patient or an unresectable tumor in an operable patient both are contraindications for proceeding. Occasionally radiotherapy and more rarely chemotherapy can convert resectability if the margins of the tumor are brought away from vital organs, for example. By the same token, a patient may be inoperable but after a period of "buffing" through use of cardiotonic agents, nutritional support, and conditioning, the patient operability may have improved, and — it is hoped — the resectability of the tumor has not changed.

That a patient is operable and the tumor resectable do not automatically indicate operation, since neither determines that an operation *should* be done. Such an example is a prostate cancer limited to the confines of one lobe in an otherwise healthy 95 year-old man. Factors that go into clinical judgment as to whether a tumor should be resected when it is agreed that it can be in a patient who can tolerate the operation should extend to whether direct benefit will outweigh the risk, discomfort, cost and time invested in this imperfect process. If the tumor just mentioned, for example, is not giving debilitating obstruction or threatened loss of productive life expectancy, the very presence of the tumor and willingness of the patient to undergo a treatment that can be performed with anticipated success does not mean that the operation should proceed. Clinical judgment, therefore, must include tumor resectability and patient operability, each of which are factors necessary, but not sufficient, for recommendation of operation.

Items 509-512

    (A)   Lobectomy
    (B)   Pneumonectomy
    (C)   Both
    (D)   Neither

509.   occasionally used in tuberculosis treatment

510.   operable patient can climb only two flights pre-operatively

511.   required for stage IV lung carcinoma

512.   chest tube not necessary

ANSWERS AND TUTORIAL ON ITEMS 509-512

The answers are: **509-A; 510-A; 511-D; 512-B.**

Pulmonary resection is an operation based on recommendations of resectability and operability with a view to improved postoperative function. The rule of thumb has been that a patient who can walk one flight of stairs without stopping can undergo thoracotomy, two flights of stairs lobectomy, and three flights of stairs pneumonectomy. This simple rule of thumb is as close an approximation to quick and inexpensive pulmonary function testing as can be obtained in practical circumstances. So, a patient who cannot climb (based on pulmonary insufficiency) a third flight of stairs is inoperable if the lesion requires pneumonectomy for resection. A tumor, therefore, resectable by pneumonectomy in this inoperable patient would mean that such an operation should not be undertaken, since the patient would be a pulmonary cripple who could not survive without ventilator therapy even if that brief survival were tumor free. Neither lobectomy nor pneumonectomy would be adequate resection for stage IV lung cancer, and would not be recommended, let alone required.

Lobectomy is occasionally used for the cavitary destruction of a lobe which has not collapsed with the encouragement of endoscopic drainage. Tuberculosis, it is granted, is not an anatomically confined disease but may be spread more widely through the lungs, bilaterally at that. But the surgical treatment is not that of tuberculosis but of a complication of tuberculosis, since it is presumed that the tuberculosis is treated with chemotherapy and the architectural unresolved problem in the lobe may be resected. Because tuberculosis is a pneumonia, it usually leaves some degree of impairment in pulmonary function in the scarred healing process. It is unlikely, therefore, that pneumonectomy would be a treatment for a complication of tuberculosis, since the opposite lung that would have to support the patient would have some degree of disease if the tuberculous complication that is present in one side of the chest is so extensive as to require total pneumonectomy.

When total pneumonectomy is performed, a chest tube is not required, whereas it is for lobectomy, in which evacuation of the pleural air is performed in order to allow expansion of the lung that remains to fill the pleural space. Since there is no lung remaining after total pneumonectomy, fibrothorax is anticipated, and the fluid and air in the pleural space

left at the time of closure are not evacuated.

Items 513-516

(A) Coarctation of aorta
(B) Aneurysm of abdominal aorta
(C) Both
(D) Neither

513. congenital

514. acute dissection

515. antihypertensive therapy

516. cardiopulmonary bypass

ANSWERS AND TUTORIAL ON ITEMS 513-516

The answers are: **513-A; 514-B; 515-C; 516-D.**

Coarctation is a constriction of the aorta and is congenital; aneurysm is a dilatation of the aorta and is usually acquired. Both are associated with hypertension, the former because coarctation is a cause of hypertension. The latter often has hypertension associated with it, and antihypertensive therapy is often used in management of aneurysm, particularly in conservative follow-up of those aneurysms that have not reached size thought to be a threat for dissection. When expansion or dissection occurs, antihypertensive treatment can be employed as an emergency, lowering the pressure head on the dissecting aorta which might recanalize into a "double barrel", and if there is no compromise to visceral organ function (particularly the kidneys or gut) elective aneurysm resection can be carried out rather than an emergency operation for the dissection. Cardiopulmonary bypass would be needed for neither instance of operation on the abdominal aorta. Thoracic arch aneurysm resection has a different clinical disease pattern, and it may be repaired, frequently employing cardiopulmonary bypass for repair of aortic arch aneurysm.

Items 517-520

(A) Hypercalcemia
(B) Hypocalcemia
(C) Both
(D) Neither

517. tetany

518. cardiac systolic arrest

519. cardiac hyperirritability arrhythmia

520. acidosis improves

ANSWERS AND TUTORIAL ON ITEMS 517-520

The answers are: **517-B; 518-A; 519-B; 520-B.**

Ionized calcium is a very important component of extracellular fluid and is carefully maintained at a level and ionized state through buffering and disassociation from readily available reserves. Since it is one of the most zealously guarded elements in the body with respect to a narrow range in which its biologic functions are optimum, disorders on either side give considerable symptoms and compensatory efforts toward correction. Hypocalcemia gives irritability and lower threshold for excitation in both neural and muscular conduction and contraction. This is noted by the patient with distressing symptoms of tetany, and the clinician worries about the cardiac arrhythmias that are also reflections of this hyperexcitability.

Because hydrogen ion and calcium compete for binding sites on serum albumin, an increase in hydrogen ion concentration off-loads ionized calcium increasing the amount of biologically active calcium in the serum in the presence of acidosis. This is the rationale behind rebreathing to increase CO_2 retention and a respiratory acidosis to help compensate for the acute deficiency in ionized serum calcium. Cardiac abnormalities are also present in hypercalcemia, such as that seen in the rare situation referred to as "parathyroid poisoning". In this instance, however, with excess calcium there is failure to relax following muscle contraction. This is reflected in the unusual cardiac manifestation of systolic arrest, which is a terminal event of hypercalcemic crisis.

     (A)   General anesthesia
     (B)   Regional anesthesia
     (C)   Both
     (D)   Neither

521.   can cause hypotension

522.   muscle relaxation

523.   requires intravenous access

524.   patient can often hear and remember

ANSWERS AND TUTORIAL ON ITEMS 521-524

The answers are: **521-C; 522-A; 523-C; 524-C.**

The choice of regional versus general anesthesia is sometimes made on the assumption that regional anesthesia is somehow less invasive and disturbs the patient's physiology less, so that the patient can be left alone as far as ventilation and circulation are concerned when only "one leg is put to sleep." Apart from the consequences of a high spinal and its respiratory consequences, spinal anesthesia causes a major change in circulation, with paralysis of the capacitance reservoirs allowing peripheral pooling of blood. General anesthesia can also cause peripheral pooling by vasodilatation, so both may lead to hypotension without careful fluid support of circulation. Neither should be attempted without intravenous access.

It is also thought that with regional anesthesia such as axillary block, intravenous lidocaine with tourniquet, spinal or epidural anesthesia, a patient can hear and remember events in the operation even if some supplementary neuroleptic agent is given. This is true. But it is also true for general anesthesia in which the patient may have lost consciousness at induction but certainly has lost ability to express what he hears or feels when paralyzed and intubated. It is often the case that patients can relate vividly details of the events that have occurred, particularly toward arousal from anesthesia, and often express less fear than alarm and offense at apparently callous behavior and remarks. Protection of the operative team is not an indication for the choice of anesthetic! In this instance, behavior modification would be more appropriate to continually consider each patient as you would yourself, monitoring the activity of each.

Items 525-528

     (A)   Hypoxemia
     (B)   Hypercarbia
     (C)   Both
     (D)   Neither

525.   agitation

526.   anesthesia at significant levels

527.   respiratory drive

528.   dangerous in neurosurgery

ANSWERS AND TUTORIAL ON ITEMS 525-528

The answers are: **525-A; 526-C; 527-C; 528-C.**

The patient who is agitated and difficult to quiet must never be assured, sedated or dismissed until hypoxemia is ruled out! One does not sleep or "rest comfortably" when one's adrenals are squeezed in a survival response, and hypoxemia is a serious fixable etiology for restlessness and complaints disturbing the nursing staff. If the clinician should give orders for sedation to the patient who is combative, pulling tubes and smashing bottles, hypoxemia can be converted to anoxia with lethal consequence. Hypoxemia must first be ruled out before any management method that might not resolve it or make it worse.

Hypercarbia has the opposite effect, and at higher levels of CO_2 tension, carbon dioxide is anesthetic. The combination of hypercarbia and hypoxia are a highly effective anesthetic with no margin of safety between anesthesia and death. This maxim has been proven with a practice to be discouraged in which dental procedures or other short operations were performed following ninety seconds of pure nitrous oxide ventilation. This was intended to produce what was euphemistically called "nitrous cyanosis" which meant that the effective anesthesia under which the tooth was pulled was hypercarbic anoxia. No one should require closer experience with death in a dental chair than by this observation to take necessary preventive precautions.

Both hypoxemia and hypercarbia are respiratory drives. Over time, the patient who loses sensitivity to hypercarbia through CO_2 retention in chronic lung disease survives almost exclusively on the hypoxic drive which is why a short course of inhalation oxygen can stop such a patient breathing when the anesthetic role of hypercarbia takes over.

Hypercarbia is dangerous in patients with head injury, since cerebral blood flow is sensitive to CO_2 tension. Hyperventilation of the patient with a closed head injury can prevent rapid and progressive cerebral edema, and a continuous maintenance of appropriate oxygen tensions is the only way to maintain vitality in the brain — since there are no oxygen stores, no readily available alternate metabolic pathways other than aerobic metabolism, and no energy stores for glycolysis in this vital organ dependant on minute to minute delivery of oxygen.

Items 529-532

    (A)   Ketoacidosis
    (B)   Insulin shock
    (C)   Both
    (D)   Neither

529.   50 ml 50% glucose push IV is harmful

530.   coma

531.   potassium therapy

532.   Kussmaul respirations

ANSWERS AND TUTORIAL ON ITEMS 529-532

The answers are: **529-D; 530-C; 531-C; 532-A.**

In a diabetic patient who presents in coma, either too little or too much insulin may have resulted in too much or too little blood sugar. Kussmaul respiration is indicative of diabetic coma and the aroma of ketones being hyperventilated may be helpful. However, a blood sugar determination may be drawn, but results not awaited before a simple differentiation by a therapeutic test.

It would be very dangerous to inject insulin to see if that would help differentiate the two sources of coma in the diabetic, and the results would be neither immediate nor definitive. However, this is not the case with the obverse. An IV push of 50 ml of 50% glucose abruptly awakens the patient in the event of hypoglycemic coma and will not significantly harm the patient if this diagnostic test turns out not to be correct. This is one of the simplest, most dramatic and commonest of the instances in which the therapy for disease precedes diagnosis or is its equivalent.

Potassium therapy should accompany treatment for either condition, since administration of insulin will drive both sugar and potassium into the cell and might result in dangerous hypokalemia. The two extremes of coma in the diabetic can be safely differentiated by a trial pulse of glucose which will dramatically help in one instance confirming the diagnosis and will not harm the patient if the coma is due to the alternate problem of too little insulin effect.

Items 533-536

(A) Adrenal cortical adenoma
(B) Bilateral adrenocortical hyperplasia
(C) Both
(D) Neither

533. treated by subtotal bilateral adrenalectomy

534. invariably due to primary drive outside the adrenal

535. hypertension

536. malignant hypertension

ANSWERS AND TUTORIAL ON ITEMS 533-536

The answers are: **533-D; 534-D; 535-C; 536-D.**

Adrenal cortical adenoma can give rise to primary aldosteronism, Cushing's syndrome, and — much more rarely due to a benign adenoma — virilizing or masculinizing syndromes, depending on the principle cell type in which the adenoma arose: zona glomerulosa, fasiculata, and reticularis respectively. The same features, however, can be produced by the same secretions based not in a benign adenoma but bilateral (micronodular) hyperplasia. In the instance of Cushing's disease, this hyperplasia is due to the stimulation of ACTH from pituitary or ectopic para-endocrine source of peptide secretion. Therefore for Cushing's syndrome, adrenocortical hyperplasia is secondary and only extremely rarely has hyperplasia been a primary autonomous adrenal source of Cushing's syndrome.

This is *not* the case for aldosteronism. In secondary aldosteronism there is an excess secretion from both adrenals secondary to renin and angiotensin-driven stimulation, but there is also a not infrequent syndrome of primary aldosteronism based in bilateral micronodular cortical hyperplasia. In this case, this hyperplasia is not invariably due to a primary drive outside the adrenal gland, since this aldosteronism is primary.

Whether due to an outside peptide stimulus or due to a primary autonomous hyperfunction, bilateral cortical hyperplasia should *not* be treated by subtotal bilateral adrenalectomy. The reason for this is that it will inevitably recur whether or not it is responding to an external drive. Bilateral micronodular hyperplasia in primary aldosteronism is not successfully treated by bilateral subtotal adrenalectomy. In addition, bilateral total adrenalectomy carries the very high disadvantage of requiring corticosteroid replacement therapy, a price too high to pay for a disease that can be managed by medication that is less dangerous with a higher margin of safety. Both primary aldosteronism and Cushing's syndrome have associated hypertension. In neither case is this hypertension a malignant hypertension, and each is relatively easily managed without desperate complications based in hypertension.

Items 537-540

(A) Parotid gland tumor
(B) Submandibular gland tumor
(C) Both
(D) Neither

537. sialolithiasis

538. 80% benign

539. high recurrence rate

540. "commando" composite resection

ANSWERS AND TUTORIAL ON ITEMS 537-540

The answers are: **537-C; 538-A; 539-C; 540-B.**

Parotid gland tumors are usually benign, may grow huge, and are resectable for cure, but with a high recurrence rate. Submandibular gland tumors are almost always malignant, have a high recurrence rate, and require extensive composite surgical resection such as the "commando" mandibulectomy/floor of the mouth excision with radical neck dissection. Both of the salivary glands may have ductal stones, but these are more frequently associated with inflammatory conditions than malignant ones. Calcification may be seen on X-ray that may be part of the sialolithiasis, inflammatory salivary gland changes or benign or malignant tumors in each location.

(A)   Papillary thyroid cancer
(B)   Follicular thyroid cancer
(C)   Both
(D)   Neither

541.   increasing incidence

542.   high cure rate

543.   hematogenous spread

544.   external beam radiation therapy

ANSWERS AND TUTORIAL ON ITEMS 541-544

The answers are: **541-A; 542-C; 543-B; 544-D**.

At the same time follicular thyroid cancer is decreasing in incidence as iodine deficiency and associated problems linked to it decrease, papillary thyroid carcinoma is increasing. Both tumors, however, have a high cure rate experienced with primary surgical therapy, particularly when adjunctive radioiodine therapy is added in follow-up for clinically significant thyroid cancer. This term refers to a presumed higher potential for malignant behavior, largely based on the patient's age, gender, tumor size and degree of differentiation.

Follicular carcinoma does not primarily spread by means of lymphatic metastases, but hematogenous spread is most common for follicular thyroid cancer. This is not the case for papillary thyroid cancer. For neither of them is external beam radiation therapy a part of primary treatment. In

selective instances of bony metastases for which thyroid cancer has a predilection, radiotherapy can be attempted, but only after a much more rational targeted source of ionizing radiation, i.e., radioiodine which can be taken up in the thyroid cells, particularly when enhanced with TSH by external administration or endogenous elevation from hypothyroidism that follows withholding thyroid replacement for a period of weeks.

(A)   Tension pneumothorax
(B)   Pericardial tamponade
(C)   Both
(D)   Neither

545.   interferes with venous return to the heart

546.   jugular venous distension

547.   survival likely if untreated

548.   needle aspiration both diagnostic and therapeutic

ANSWERS AND TUTORIAL ON ITEMS 545-548

The answers are: **545-C; 546-C; 547-D; 548-C**.

Tension pneumothorax and pericardial tamponade are both collections of fluid under pressure that interfere with a normal fluid flow in and out of thoracic cavities. In the case of tension pneumothorax, the fluid trapped under pressure is air and the principle disturbance is to the flow of air in and out of not only the affected lung, but also the opposite side. In the case of pericardial tamponade, the fluid trapped outside the circulation is blood and it is in the pericardium rather than the air in the pleura, with an interference in venous return that compromises cardiac output.

However, both "tensions" also interfere with blood flow, impeding venous return to the heart by abolishing the changes in intrathoracic pressure that is negative on the inspiratory cycle of normal respiration. Therefore, jugular venous distension occurs in both and cardiac output impairment occurs with both. Needle aspiration of the pleura and the pericardium is both diagnostic and therapeutic in each. It is also necessary, since survival in each circumstance is very unlikely if untreated, and each is an emergency that should be managed immediately once recognized.

"Apollo was held the god of physic and sender of diseases. Both were originally the same trade, and still continue."
Jonathon Swift (1667-1745)

Items 549-552

(A) Peptic ulcer
(B) Cholecystitis
(C) Both
(D) neither

549. pain resolves with eating

550. pancreatitis may be a complication

551. truncal vagotomy improves

552. may produce peritoneal signs

ANSWERS AND TUTORIAL ON ITEMS 549-552

The answers are: **549-A; 550-C; 551-A; 552-C.**

The presentation of epigastric pain is frequent and requires differentiation since these two major sources of upper abdominal pain have a different etiology and management strategy. The timing of pain in relation to meals is intuitive, since acid neutralization occurs with food and peptic ulcer is improved after eating. This is not typically the case with cholecystitis which usually is prodded into exacerbation by food intake, particularly fatty foods which induce gall bladder contraction. Pancreatitis may be a complication of both conditions, since cholecystitis may lead to pancreatitis and vice versa through common channel reflux, and gall stones may impact in the ampulla inciting pancreatitis. Peptic ulcers, particularly posterior penetrating ulcers, may erode into the pancreas and set up pancreatitis.

Truncal vagotomy is used as a treatment for peptic ulcer, if combined with a drainage or resection procedure, but truncal vagotomy does not improve, and some say may cause cholecystitis by denervation of the vagal branches that run to the gall bladder. The principle control of the gall bladder contractility, however, is humoral (cholecystokinin) rather than neural, and until further evidence, we might limit ourselves to acknowledging that peptic ulcer would be improved and cholecystitis would not.

If the inflamed gall bladder fundus contacts the parietal peritoneum on inspiration under the examiner's hand, peritoneal signs are elicited (Murphy's sign). Peptic ulcer also can give duodenitis close to the porta and peritoneal signs may also be present, but less frequently localized in the anterior parietes.

"He would have been known in the world as a Patriot, had he not been known as something greater — a Physician."

Inscription on the statue of Dr W. E. D. Davis
Birmingham, AL, unveiled 1904

PART III
SIMPLE AND EXTENDED MATCHING ITEMS

DIRECTIONS: Each set of matching items that follows consists of a list of four or more lettered options followed by several numbered items. For each numbered item, select the **ONE** lettered option that is most closely associated with it. To avoid spending too much time on matching sets with large numbers of options, it is generally advisable to begin each set by reading the list of options. Then for each item in the set, try to generate the correct answer and locate it in the option list rather than evaluating each option individually. Each lettered option may be selected once, more than once, or not at all.

Items 553-557

(A) Intraductal papilloma
(B) Fibroadenoma
(C) Breast abscess
(D) Paget's disease
(E) Fibrocystic disease
(F) Bilateral inflammatory breast carcinoma
(G) Infiltrating intraductal adenocarcinoma
(H) Lobular *in situ* adenocarcinoma

553. A 16 year-old is found to have firm mobile nodules in both left upper and right lower breast quadrants.

554. The most common lethal condition of women in the prime of life.

555. A 28 year-old woman who has breast pain and fever with onset during her second month of nursing.

556. A benign condition that can give a bloody nipple discharge.

557. A scaly nipple rash associated with underlying malignancy requiring further investigation.

ANSWERS AND TUTORIAL ON ITEMS 553-557

The answers are: **553-B; 554-G; 555-C; 556-A; 557-D**.

The distinction of benign from malignant is the most important diagnostic feature of breast disease. Characteristic clinical patterns make the probability more or less likely in any given list of characteristics, but it is important to remember that breast cancer is not only the leading nonskin cancer in women, it is the overall most likely cause of death in women in the Western world in the prime of life. It is for that reason that cancer's early recognition should be distinguished from among the other benign breast problems that outnumber it.

Dominant nodules are often the earliest presenting feature of breast cancer, but in a teenager, they most often represent a firm and rubbery kind of tumor known as fibroadenoma, particularly if multiple.

A bloody nipple discharge can be a presenting sign of cancer, but it is also characteristic of a benign condition known as intraductal papilloma from which it must be distinguished. One of the harbinger signs of breast cancer is a peculiar scaly nipple rash known as Paget's disease, and it is not so much a diagnosis as a mandatory indication for further investigation. In the context of lactation, a focal tender breast mass in the region of the areola is likely to be a breast abscess. These benign conditions are treated differently from breast cancer; however, the most important step in that treatment is their differentiation to rule out a malignant tumor which may sometimes co-exist.

Items 558-562

(A)   Fine needle aspiration
(B)   Needle localization biopsy with specimen mammography
(C)   Incision and drainage
(D)   Excisional biopsy
(E)   Quadrant subtotal mastectomy
(F)   Total mastectomy
(G)   Modified radical mastectomy
(H)   Extended radical mastectomy
(I)   Radiation therapy
(J)   Anti-estrogen therapy
(K)   Prosthetic breast reconstruction
(L)   Combination chemotherapy

558.   Treatment for non-palpable stippled calcification seen on screening mammogram.

559.   Appropriate therapy for a 92 year-old woman with congestive heart failure found to have an ulcerating 6 cm left breast mass.

560.   Appropriate outpatient management of a patient with bilateral upper outer quadrant breast nodularity with one nodule firmer and larger than the surrounding tissues.

561.   The best adjunctive treatment to be used following modified radical mastectomy for estrogen receptor-negative, poorly differentiated Stage II carcinoma in a premenopausal woman.

562.   The most frequent operation performed in the US in the last five years for treatment of Stage I breast cancer in premenopausal women also treated by radiation therapy.

ANSWERS AND TUTORIAL ON ITEMS 558-562

The answers are: **558-B; 559-F; 560-A; 561-L; 562-E**.

The invasive procedure for definitive diagnosis of breast cancer depends on whether the lesion is palpable or whether it is a screening finding on mammography. If not palpable, its precise targeting is difficult without radiographic assistance. Marking it with needle insertion with the assistance of mammography gives needle localization technique a chance to sample the very specific tissue identified as suspicious by mammography, and to confirm that it has been excised for biopsy with specimen mammography. In a woman who has findings in several fields of the breast that may resemble fibrocystic changes, but with one dominant nodule, invasive diagnosis is still required for that dominant nodule. Out-patient management would include fine needle aspiration of the suspicious component.

For the majority of women with Stage I carcinoma at premenopausal ages in the US, quadrant sub-total mastectomy is combined with lymph node sampling for staging and primary radiotherapy is administered with the breast conserving procedure. An alternative is mastectomy with immediate reconstruction, which is a somewhat more invasive undertaking. Neither condition results in a normal postoperative breast appearance, but in each instance women may look nearly normal in clothes. If the disease turns out to be Stage II, particularly if undifferentiated, adjunctive chemotherapy administered in combination drug regimens is recommended. For an elderly patient with compromised cardiac reserve, who presents with an enlarged ulcerating breast mass, the principle threat to life is the cardiac rather than the oncologic problem. Breast tumors in such individuals are frequently indolent, but can cause local disfiguring and socially unpleasant problems, and this morbidity can be reduced by what is referred to as "toilet mastectomy" which rids the principle problem related to the large breast tumor — namely, the ulceration and soilage. For the great majority of women with breast cancer; however, therapy is tailored toward that which gives the highest probability of prolonged disease-free survival, and secondarily to morbidity reduction related to the treatment, particularly the loss of the breast.

Items 563-567

    (A)   Melanoma
    (B)   Dermatofibroma
    (C)   Erysipelas
    (D)   Neurofibroma
    (E)   Rodent ulcer
    (F)   Junctional nevus
    (G)   Actinic keratosis

563.   *Streptococcus* is an etiologic factor.

564.   May occur in families with other features of a recognized syndrome.

565.   A pigmented mole with premalignant potential.

566.   Squamous cell cancer is a consequence.

567.   Characteristically spreads to lymph nodes.

ANSWERS AND TUTORIAL ON ITEMS 563-567

The answers are: **563-C; 564-D; 565-F; 566-G; 567-A**.

Erysipelas is a superficial cellulitis that spreads with the rapidity of streptococcal infections and the associated enzymes that prevent the body from walling off and containing them. It is a lesion that is inflammatory and infectious, and distinct from the other acquired lumps or moles in this list in that it has a clinically recognizable pattern that is treatable by antibiotic and local therapy. Two of these skin lumps have fibroma as a component of their names, but the one is of neurofibroma origin and may occur in a familial syndrome with other abnormalities known as von Recklinghausen syndrome.

There are some lesions here that are malignant and some that are premalignant, and actinic keratosis is one that is cutaneous in exposed areas of the body in which sunlight or X-irradiation has been a chronic stimulus, and squamous cell carcinoma is the malignant consequence of actinic keratosis. There are two pigmented mole lesions, the one being junctional nevus, and it has a premalignant potential in the junctional component of the mole. When it becomes malignant, it degenerates to melanoma (a threat distinctly absent in the other pigmented mole with which it can be confused, compound nevus) and the characteristic dissemination of melanoma is through lymphatic metastases.

Items 568-572

(A) Hepatitis
(B) Cirrhosis
(C) Cholecystitis
(D) Peri-hepatitis (Curtis-Fitzhugh)
(E) Cholangitis
(F) Portal vein thrombosis
(G) Hepatoma
(H) Hypersplenism

568. *Gonococcus* is an etiologic factor.

569. Obstructive jaundice often associated.

570. Associated with abrupt onset of varices.

571. Three-fold elevation in alpha-fetoprotein (AFP).

572. *Salmonella* carrier state.

ANSWERS AND TUTORIAL ON ITEMS 568-572

The answers are: **568-D; 569-E; 570-F; 571-G; 572-C**.

Pain over the liver may not be due to a problem originating in the liver. That is the case with pelvic inflammatory disease, which can give pericapsular adhesions which are related to the same pelvic inflammatory process and its etiologic agents. The early causes of pelvic inflammatory disease include *Gonococcus*, but later, a variety of organisms may be responsible for the Curtis-Fitzhugh syndrome, particularly if the origin is from chronically scarred adnexae with repeated antibiotic therapy changing the flora.

Cholecystitis is a condition of some morbidity, but may be asymptomatic, and resident parasites may be lodged in the gall bladder in the chronic carrier state for such patients as can spread typhoid. *Salmonella* has a propensity for the biliary tract as a residence in the carrier state. In contrast to cholecystitis morbidity, cholangitis is a disease of high mortality, and that risk is often related to not only the sepsis associated with it, but also the obstruction potential in which the bile necessary for both liver excretion and secretion cannot achieve access to the gut. Therefore, inflammation in the biliary tree, as distinct from the parenchymal hepatocytes, with jaundice, suggests obstruction of the common bile duct rather than simply the cystic duct.

Cirrhosis can give rise to esophageal varices, but that typically takes place over a prolonged period of time, and may be infrequently abrupt in onset or at least recognition. However, a source of acute portal hypertension is portal vein thrombosis. This may be secondary to extension from the mesenteric venous drainage of the gut, and that may be due to inflammatory processes or obstructive phenomena within the GI tract. In cirrhosis and hepatitis there is occasionally an elevation in the AFP, but when that elevation becomes quite significantly greater than normal, hepatoma is a likely source of excess values in these three-fold ranges.

Items 573-577

(A)　　Hypovolemic shock
(B)　　Cardiogenic shock
(C)　　Peripheral pooling
(D)　　Endotoxic shock

573.　　High fluid volume and transfusion harmful.

574.　　Seen after spinal anesthesia.

575.　　A cellular defect in metabolism.

576.　　Pericardial tamponade.

577.　　Warm pink extremities with bounding pulse.

ANSWERS AND TUTORIAL ON ITEMS 573-577

The answers are: **573-B; 574-C; 575-D; 576-B; 577-D**.

Shock is a state of insufficient nutrient flow, and adequate nutrient flow is necessary for aerobic metabolism. The markers of insufficiency or non-nutrient flow include the products of anaerobic metabolism and incomplete glucose breakdown — hydrogen ion, lactate and pyruvate. Each of these conditions, to be called "shock", share the common feature of insufficient nutrient flow, and all are marked by the anaerobic metabolic features.

Hypovolemic shock may be among the most common (and was the first type recognized and treated), but it is not the only form of shock, and if all shock is treated as hypovolemia, volume therapy is actually harmful to cardiogenic shock in which the volume is not insufficient but the capability of delivering that volume is. Another form of cardiogenic shock is the interference in venous return that may occur with pericardial tamponade, making the insufficiency not so much a form of inadequate cardiac contraction but of inadequate ventricular volume to be propelled.

Spinal anesthesia may paralyze the capacitance venous reservoirs that dilate and make for an effective subtraction in the circulating volume. A similar phenomenon occurs with neurogenic shock, sequestering volume that would otherwise be in circulation. Endotoxic shock is a form of cellular defect in which the cells are not using the nutrients delivered to them because of a cytochrome inactivation such as some poisons (cyanide, endotoxin) or an inability to get either glucose or oxygen inside the cell (diabetes, carbon monoxide poisoning). This is a form of shock for which recognition is counterintuitive, since the extremities may be warm and pink with the nailbeds apparently well perfused and bounding pulses palpable in the extremities. Despite the high cardiac output from the low peripheral vascular resistance, the cells are in shock and reflect this with an accumulating hydrogen ion burden that generally causes this high cardiac output to decrease when acidosis neutralizes the catecholamine compensation.

Items 578-582

(A) Femoral hernia
(B) Indirect inguinal hernia
(C) Direct inguinal hernia
(D) Umbilical hernia
(E) Para-esophageal hernia
(F) Incisional hernia
(G) Richter's hernia
(H) Sliding hiatal hernia

578. Medical treatment indicated.

579. No treatment is typically recommended.

580. An incarceration.

581. High potential for hemorrhage.

582. More common in girls than in boys.

ANSWERS AND TUTORIAL ON ITEMS 578-582

The answers are: **578-H; 579-D; 580-G; 581-E; 582-A**.

A sliding hiatus hernia is treated medically, not so much treatment directed to the hernia as to minimize the damage that may occur with esophageal reflux. In contrast, the other hernia at the hiatus is the para-esophageal hernia, which has high potential for hemorrhage in entrapment of the richly vascularized gastric wall. The presence of a para-esophageal hernia is indication for operation. For the umbilical hernia, particularly in the infant and toddler stage in which it is most often seen, no treatment is typically recommended. Should umbilical hernia persist or recur later in life under circumstances of increased intra-abdominal pressure such as pregnancy, it may then become symptomatic, and this may indicate its repair. Of the hernias listed, the Richter's hernia is an incarceration of partial circumference of the bowel wall. Of the inguinal hernias, indirect inguinal hernia is the most common hernia in young girls, even more common in young boys. However, girls have femoral hernias more often than do boys, even though femoral hernias represents a minority fraction of the groin hernias for both genders.

Items 583-587

    (A)   Chronic bronchitis
    (B)   Emphysema
    (C)   Asthma
    (D)   Tuberculosis
    (E)   Pneumoconiosis
    (F)   Cystic fibrosis

583.   Treatment with epinephrine.

584.   Most common cause of fixed "barrel chest".

585.   Pneumothorax once was used for treatment.

586.   Silo fillers may experience one type of this condition.

587.   Decreased reproductive potential.

ANSWERS AND TUTORIAL ON ITEMS 583-587

The answers are: **583-C; 584-B; 585-D; 586-E; 587-F.**

Of the chronic lung diseases listed, asthma is primarily of the broncho-constrictive variety and treatment with epinephrine infusion is appropriate for asthma and not for the other conditions. Hyperinflation and difficulty with incomplete exhalation is characteristic of emphysema, and over time, the hyper-inflated chest expansion becomes fixed in the "barrel chest" deformity. Of the inflammatory lung diseases that leads to fibrosis, one is a peculiar occupational hazard related to inhalation of oxides of nitrogen in the process of silage decomposition. Inhalation of these oxides can result in acid injury to the lungs, and this silo fillers' disease is one form of pneumoconiosis.

Pneumothorax, not as complication, but as treatment, was employed at one time for tuberculosis. This took the form of phrenic nerve crush, or stuffing the chest with masses that could deflate the lung such as ping-pong balls; eventually this pneumothorax has given way to thoracoplasty in which the lung is not collapsed within the chest as much as the chest is brought down to the lung. These forms of late-stage tuberculosis treatment, fortunately, are now rare with better antimicrobial chemotherapy, but with the emerging resistance in high risk patient groups, it may be too early to describe these forms of therapy as obsolete.

Cystic fibrosis is described also by another name mucoviscidosis. Not only is this a disease of pulmonary secretory epithelium, but it also effects secretory epithelium everywhere giving rise to problems in the gut, pancreas, and in germ cell production as well. Reproductive potential is impaired in this epithelial defect.

Items 588-592

(A) Mitral stenosis
(B) Mitral insufficiency
(C) Aortic stenosis
(D) Coronary insufficiency

588. Most common chronic cardiac consequence of rheumatic fever.

589. Source of migratory pulmonary abscesses in addicts.

590. (Stokes-Adams) syncopal attacks.

591. Characteristic jugular venous pulsation.

592. Lowering diastolic blood pressure may result in symptoms.

ANSWERS AND TUTORIAL ON ITEMS 588-592

The answers are: **588-A; 589-A; 590-C; 591-B; 592-D.**

Mitral stenosis is a common cardiac consequence of rheumatic fever, and with the decrease in rheumatic fever (presumably because of the reduction in streptococcal valvular disease from the ubiquitous administration of penicillin in childhood) rheumatic mitral stenosis has been decreasing in the United States. If acute valvulitis occurs as may be the case with illicit drug and excipient debris injected into the venous circulation, right heart vegetations can give rise to migratory pulmonary abscesses, which is radiographic evidence of IV drug abuse. Insufficiency of

the mitral valve would give venous regurgitation, being evident on clinical exam in jugular venous pulses.

At the level of the aortic valve, stenosis may give rise to transient attacks of ischemia in the carotid circulation, and these acute ischemic episodes give syncopal or Stokes-Adams attacks. This is a very dangerous threat to neurologic function. The aorta has as its first branches from the sinuses beyond the aortic valve the coronary artery ostia. The coronaries are perfused with diastolic blood pressure, since the maximum blood flow occurs when the aortic valve is closed and the coronary ostia are open to perfusion at maximum flows. Therefore, lowering the diastolic blood pressure may result in symptomatic coronary insufficiency.

Items 593-597

(A) Acute appendicitis
(B) Sigmoid diverticulitis
(C) Torsion ovarian cyst
(D) Pelvic inflammatory disease
(E) Mesenteric adenitis
(F) Inflammatory bowel disease

593. May show calcific dental pattern in abdomen or pelvis on X-ray.

594. Not a primary pre-operative diagnosis.

595. Immunosuppressive therapy.

596. May occur in absence of prior inflammation.

597. More prominent in children than teenagers.

196

ANSWERS AND TUTORIAL ON ITEMS 593-597

The answers are: **593-C; 594-E; 595-F; 596-C; 597-E**.

Each of the listed causes of acute abdominal pain may be present in a pre-operative differential diagnosis; however, if mesenteric adenitis were primarily diagnosed, operation would not follow, since it is not an operative indication. One of these abnormalities may exist without a preceding inflammatory process, and the teratoma of the ovary that may twist and give rise to an acute abdomen may sometimes be diagnosed by recognizing calcific patterns of teeth or other structures within the teratoma in a characteristic radiographic pattern that would be diagnostic because of the unusual location of these dental structures.

Mesenteric adenitis is more common in children than it is in teenagers, but that does not mean that the more threatening diagnosis of appendicitis should be displaced by a pre-operative diagnosis of mesenteric adenitis and operation deferred in this age group. Only one of these conditions is treated by immuno-suppression therapy, and that is the inflammatory bowel disease, which is thought by many to have an autoimmune etiology. Therefore, a decrease in the inflammatory process with immuno-suppression is the rationale for therapy.

Items 598-602

GI bleeding from:

    (A)   Esophageal varices
    (B)   Esophagitis
    (C)   Barrett's ulcer
    (D)   Mallory-Weiss tear
    (E)   Esophageal cancer
    (F)   Gastric ulcer
    (G)   Erosive gastritis
    (H)   Gastric cancer
    (I)   Duodenal ulcer
    (J)   Hemobilia
    (K)   Bleeding Meckel's diverticulum
    (L)   Enteritis
    (M)   Diverticulosis
    (N)   Ulcerative colitis
    (O)   Colon cancer
    (P)   *Fissure-in-ano*
    (Q)   A-V malformations
    (R)   Angiodysplasia
    (S)   Fistula from arterial prosthetic graft

598.   Associated with deceleration liver trauma.

599.   Tenesmus.

600.   Prolonged vomiting.

601.   Most common source of occult blood loss in 65 year-olds in the United States.

602.   Balloon compression therapy.

ANSWERS AND TUTORIAL ON ITEMS 598-602

The answers are: **598-J; 599-P; 600-D; 601-O; 602-A.**

Each of the sources listed is a potential site of gastrointestinal tract bleeding. One is peculiar to liver injury, in particular of the kind that leaves a large intrahepatic hematoma, and that is blood decompression into the biliary tree, or "hemobilia". One is characteristically associated with prolonged vomiting, although any may cause vomiting from the irritation of blood in the gastrointestinal tract. However, the one that is associated with prolonged vomiting as an etiologic agent is the Mallory-Weiss tear in the upper gastrointestinal tract.

Esophageal varices, and to a lesser extent those in the epigastric cardia, are treated by tamponade with a compression balloon since the pressure within the varices that is the driving force of the hemorrhage through the ulcerated surface is an elevated portal venous pressure. The balloon would be much less effective if it were designed to stop arterial pressure, since it would not only be unlikely to accomplish that, but if it did it would cause necrosis of the epithelium and further hemorrhage. The one form of lower anorectal bleeding that is highly symptomatic is that of *fissure-in-ano*, which can occasionally give the involuntary spasm of the voluntary muscles known as tenesmus, a highly symptomatic condition. In terms of occult blood loss into the gastrointestinal tract, it is important to remember that benign conditions are less significant than malignancy, and colo-rectal cancer remains the most likely origin of occult blood loss into the gastrointestinal tract in older people in the United States.

Items 603-607

Hemostasis by:

(A) Lavage
(B) Arteriographic pressor or embolus
(C) Tamponade (e.g., packing balloon)
(D) Sclerotherapy
(E) Diathermy
(F) Laser
(G) Actual (hot) cautery
(H) Topical pharmacology (e.g., collagen constrictors)
(I) Ligation
(J) Expectant therapy

603. Control of accessible artery by operative exposure.

604. Retinal hemorrhage.

605. Recommended for split thickness skin graft donor site.

606. Injection technique via endoscopy.

607. Management method for crush fracture pelvis.

ANSWERS AND TUTORIAL ON ITEMS 603-607

The answers are: **603-I; 604-F; 605-C; 606-D; 607-B.**

The method of control of bleeding is determined by the type of vessel bleeding and the exposure to it for application of energy via various techniques. For example, a retinal hemorrhage has really only recently had pinpoint precision control through laser photocoagulation. For a bleeding artery that is accessible by means of surgical exposure, ligature remains the most secure and reliable method of hemostasis. If the bleeding site can be seen and the pressure propelling the hemorrhage is less than full systolic arterial pressure, sclerotherapy may be successful in such positions as the esophagus or lower GI tract via endoscopic technique. Direct pressure application is often sufficient for end vessel bleeding as occurs with the donor site of a split thickness skin graft. Although various dressings have been promoted that have some pharmacologic agent or collagen or other clot promoter impregnated in them, the active ingredient is the application of topical pressure for hemostasis.

A very vexing problem of multiple trauma is the hemorrhage that is experienced with pelvic fractures from crush injury. One of the more successful techniques to date for this combined venous and arterial bleeding from the efferent side that cannot be exposed or controlled is the use of arteriographic therapy, infusing constrictors or occasionally even embolizing the feeding arterial vessel to decrease the perfusion pressure associated with the fracture site bleeding.

Items 608-612

(A)   Stress ulcer
(B)   Cushing's ulcer
(C)   Curling's ulcer
(D)   Steroid ulcer

608.   Infected ulcers.

609.   Closed head injury.

610.   Highest mortality.

611.   Ablated by vagotomy.

612.   Prevented in the ICU by strict neutralization of gastric acid.

ANSWERS AND TUTORIAL ON ITEMS 608-612

The answers are: **608-C; 609-B; 610-A; 611-B; 612-A**.

Secondary ulceration of the upper gastrointestinal tract has been associated with several kinds of critical illness. One of these kinds was described by Curling in patients with severe burns. These patients who have burns and developed upper GI bleeding are found to have peptic ulcer, but only if the patients are infected, as most of the patients with major burns inevitably are. The very ulcers themselves are infected with the same agent that can be cultured from the blood of the burn patient.

The ulcer described by Harvey Cushing is related to an increase in intracranial pressure, which occasioned severe upper gastrointestinal bleeding in a sequential series of sixteen patients. He made the pre-operative diagnosis in the next one in this long series of patients who had undergone intracranial operations with increasing intracranial pressure as the common feature. This is due to strong vagal stimulation which increases acid output, and is therefore interruptable by vagotomy. Since the cephalic phase can be blocked pharmacologically now through antihistamine interception, this would constitute the equivalent of a medical vagotomy with respect to inhibition of gastric acid stimulation.

Stress ulceration is seen with a variety of causes that lead to multiple sequential organ failure, sepsis prominent among them. This is a reflection of the low flow state and an erosion with serpentiginous undermining of the mucosa and diffuse bleeding. Because of the underlying circumstances that give rise to the disease, the mortality is highest among patients with stress ulcer, but the ulceration itself can be minimized by compulsive attention to gastric juice and its neutralization. This can be done by a nasogastric tube with continual titration of the pH to maintain it in excess of 7, or, by a less labor-intensive method, an antihistamine can be given that would block the H_2 receptors and maintain a gastric juice in neutral range with either buffers or receptor blockade.

Items 613-617

Pressures:

(A) Arterial
(B) Venous
(C) Lymphatic
(D) Gut luminal

613. Primarily responsible for perforation.

614. First mural vessel to have elevated pressure in bowel obstruction.

615. Increasing pressure does *not* lead to stasis.

616. Blue congestion macroscopically, diapedesis microscopically.

617. Primarily responsible for edema.

ANSWERS AND TUTORIAL ON ITEMS 613-617

The answers are: **613-D; 614-C; 615-A; 616-B; 617-C**.

In mechanical or functional bowel obstruction, the intraluminal pressure in the gut rises from both secretions entering it and the propulsion of those secretions along its length. It is the luminal pressure that first rises and is ultimately responsible for perforation of the gastrointestinal tract, usually at a point weakened by necrosis after all other vascular pressures within the bowel wall have been elevated to the intraluminal pressure. The first of these mural vessels to experience increased pressure is the lymphatic system. It is the lymphatic pressure increase that is primarily responsible for edema, with transudation of plasma evident in a boggy pale and thickened bowel. The next pressure elevation in the next lowest system of intraluminal vessel pressures is the vein, and when venous hypertension sets in translated through from the greater resistance imparted by the edematous bowel from lymphatic pressure rise, blood cells now pass through the vessel walls as well as the plasma "weeping" that had started earlier with the lymphatic and early venous pressure rise. This makes the bowel blue and congested in appearance macroscopically. In microscopic appearance, the passage of red cells through the wall is recognized as diapedesis. Stasis occurs stopping all blood flow when venous pressure rises to arterial pressure, and since the arterial perfusion is the highest pressure system, a further rise in its pressure is the only rise that would not contribute to stasis of perfusion.

Items 618-622

Deficiencies in:

- (A)   Factor VIII
- (B)   Factor IX
- (C)   Factor XIII
- (D)   Calcium
- (E)   Silk ligature

618.   Deficiency that is the most frequent cause of postoperative hemorrhage

619.   Chelation is anticoagulant

620.   Christmas disease

621.   von Willebrand's disease

622.   Classic hemophilia

ANSWERS AND TUTORIAL ON ITEMS 618-622

The answers are: **618-E; 619-D; 620-B; 621-C; 622-A.**

Calcium is a necessary factor in the clotting cascade, and it is by chelating calcium that most donated blood is able to be stored in refrigerated bags without clotting. The anticoagulant in most donated blood, therefore, carries this ability to continue binding calcium, and multiple unit transfusions should consider the possibility that calcium deficiency would result after the equivalent of the fifth unit of banked blood with its citrate anticoagulant binding calcium. Factor VIII deficiency causes classic hemophilia, and infusions of this factor can prevent the spontaneous hemorrhage with minimal trauma such as that seen in joints of the hemophiliac patient.

Factor IX deficiency gives an atypical hemophilia referred to as Christmas disease named after the family in which it was first isolated, and Factor IX therapy is corrective for this deficiency. Factor XIII deficiency is referred to as von Willebrand's disease, and has more to do with vascular fragility than with a missing protocoagulant.

Of all the sources of bleeding encountered postoperatively, the deficiency most commonly responsible for the bleeding is "acute silk deficiency" — that is, failure to effectively achieve ligation of bleeding vessels.

(A)   Insufficient clotting
(B)   Ineffective clotting
(C)   Excess clotting
(D)   Excessive fibrinolysis
(E)   Platelet abnormalities
(F)   Circulating anticoagulants

623.   Therapy with aminocaproic acid.

624.   Disseminated intravascular coagulation.

625.   Amniotic fluid embolus hypo-fibrinogenemia.

626.   Prolonged partial thromboplastin tissue.

627.   Prolonged prothrombin time.

ANSWERS AND TUTORIAL ON ITEMS 623-627

The answers are: **623-D; 624-C; 625-A; 626-F; 627-A.**

The list of options includes most sources of uncontrolled postoperative bleeding. If there are inadequate pro-thrombin factors (such as by consumption of these labile factors or because of deficiency in their production because of hepatic insufficiency or coumadin poisoning of their production), clotting will be insufficient. That is also true if there is inadequate fibrinogen, and that may occur from such sources as rapid consumption in the event of infusion of amniotic fluid in peripartum amniotic embolus. In each of these events and in one more generalized one called disseminated intravascular coagulation, the reserve supply of labile clotting factors is consumed, and bleeding thereafter is uncontrolled by effective clotting in a quantity sufficient to maintain control after securing bleeding vessels.

In order to allow restoration of these clotting factors to the level where they can sustain effective clotting in sufficient quantity, some bleeding patients are paradoxically treated with anti-coagulation to reduce the consumption until an additional means of local control is added and the anticoagulation stopped or reversed so that the clotting cascade can resume.

The other sources of excessive bleeding include circulating anticoagulant, and that would give rise to a partial thromboplastin time that was prolonged as evidence that it might be one origin of the bleeding problem. An additional factor might be the premature dissolution of clots by excessive plasminogen activator activity. To slow down clot dissolution by plasminogen activator, aminocaproic acid can be used therapeutically to prolong the life of fibrin clot. It is important to state again that each of these maneuvers are considered after local surgical control has been achieved or has failed after a thorough attempt because of some systemic problem, but focal bleeding from an open vessel is not treated by factor therapy.

Items 628-632

(A)   Oral erythromycin base and neomycin

(B)   Oral penicillin

(C)   Oral chloramphenicol

(D)   Intravenous cefoxitin

(E)   Intravenous cefazolin

(F)   Intravenous imipenem

(G)   Topical sulfamylon

(H)   Topical iodophores (Betadine)

(I)   Irrigation with dilute (Dakan's) hypochlorite

(J)   None of the above

628.   Associated with aplastic anemia.

629.   Induces brisk catharsis.

630.   Appropriate systemic prophylaxis for elective colon resection.

631.   Appropriate prophylaxis initiated in the postoperative recovery room.

632.   Preferred treatment following full thickness burn escharectomy.

ANSWERS AND TUTORIAL ON ITEMS 628-632

The answers are: **628-C; 629-A; 630-D; 631-J; 632-G.**

Oral erythromycin base and neomycin are considered "pipe cleaners", i.e., minimally absorbable antibiotics, that largely exert their affect in the colon where floral populations are highest. One of the effective means of colon preparation stemming from the use of these antibiotics is that they induce a brisk mechanical bowel purging from their cathartic effect. Another oral antibiotic that would be effective against the principle flora of the colon (the predominant *Bacteroides* and other anaerobic gram-negative species) would be oral chloramphenicol. However, this antibiotic is absorbable, and has been associated with the catastrophe of aplastic anemia that is rare but lethal. The same antibiotic injected by vein does not seem to give rise to this complication as often, therefore the utility of chloramphenicol in the hospitalized patient should be limited to non-oral use.

Topical therapy can be employed for reducing inoculum in large denuded surfaces, such as that which occurs in burn patients following excision of devitalized tissue and eschar. Sulfamylon is appropriate therapy for such denudation since it has good local flora control on surface contamination with less significant effects of absorption than other topical agents that have also been employed.

Prophylaxis is mandated in procedures in which the inoculum cannot be adequately prevented or there is high risk such as prosthetic implantation in patients undergoing elective operation. Surface and intracavitary decontamination is attempted, but in the colon the flora are so numerous that intravenous antibiotic prophylaxis is appropriate, particularly selecting an agent that would be active against the flora most likely to be encountered. Intravenous cefoxitin fulfills these requirements, and is appropriate as prophylaxis for elective colon resection.

Although intravenous imipenem might have a broad spectrum and high effectiveness, it should never be used in prophylaxis to guard its utility as a highly effective antibiotic monotherapy in seriously ill patients. If widely used in such instances as prophylaxis, when patient benefit is marginal, its effectiveness as an antibiotic might be compromised by generating bacterial resistance.

By definition, prophylaxis is that antibiotic that is circulating before the inoculum, and therefore, there is no prophylaxis claim that can justify the use of an antibiotic first employed post-operatively. To be employed following operation, an antibiotic must be justified on a therapeutic claim, and this would require clinical evidence, (fever chart, urinalysis, chest X-ray, white blood count elevation) or microbiologic evidence (Gram stain, culture and sensitivity). Prophylaxis is prospective, and there is a contradiction in terms in the use of prophylaxis in the context of trauma or post-operative events. Unless the antimicrobial employed is circulating before the inoculum that cannot be prevented, its use fails the definition of prophylaxis.

"Everywhere the old order changes and happy they who can change with it."
Sir William Osler (1849-1919)

Items 633-637

(A)	Whole blood	
(B)	Packed red cells	
(C)	Fresh frozen single donor plasma	
(D)	Human serum albumin	
(E)	Plasmanate	
(F)	D_5/Ringer's lactate	
(G)	D_5/W	
(H)	Normal saline	
(I)	Platelet pack concentrate	

633. Treatment of anemia.

634. Rapid sequestration in hypersplenism.

635. Inappropriate resuscitation fluid for recent trauma victim.

636. Most frequently used infusion for trauma.

637. Can produce seizures in head injured patient.

ANSWERS AND TUTORIAL ON ITEMS 633-637

The answers are: **633-B; 634-I; 635-C; 636-F; 637-G**.

Each of these infusion or trans-fusion fluids is used in resuscitation selected on the basis of the predominant utility of crystalloid, colloid, or red cell mass. The treatment of anemia requires hemoglobin, and the most efficient way that is distributed is in red cells. Whole blood should be used extremely rarely, since it has more functional utility when divided into components and the component is selected for a patient deficit in that function. Of the several colloids, fresh frozen single donor plasma may have abundant labile coagulating factors contained within it, but should not be used as resuscitation for a recent trauma victim who has no demonstrated deficit in any of these factors as yet.

The most frequently used fluid for trauma victims is crystalloid solution such as Ringer's Lactate. One of the types of trauma that may be encountered is closed head trauma which may exhibit the unusual affect of retaining water excessively and dilutional hyponatremia. This is especially true in the unusual syndrome that may follow some forms of intracranial injury called "the syndrome of inappropriate diuretic hormone" (SIADH). Moreover, an excess water volume will lead to cerebral edema, and free water clearance ought to be encouraged in these patients, most generally by fluid restriction.

Platelet pack concentrate is a highly specialized infusion of fresh platelets from several donors after separation from the plasma which can be employed for multiple other factor extractions and then pooled colloid content. In a patient who has platelet deficit, this may help raise platelets to adequate clotting level, but will not relieve the patient of the source of thrombocytopenia to begin with. In the event that the patient continues to have hypersplenism as platelets are administered, those platelets will be rapidly sequestered in the spleen and will drop off rapidly unless a platelet transfusion is a component part of surgical therapy or at least medical suppression of the hypersplenic activity.

Items 638-642

   (A)   Sickle cell disease
   (B)   Sickle-thalassemia
   (C)   Hereditary spherocytosis
   (D)   Falciparum malaria

638.   Lethal thromboembolism is a high risk.

639.   Cortical brain infarcts are a major problem.

640.   Chronically enlarged spleen long term.

641.   Abdominal crises frequent.

642.   High oxygen saturation beneficial.

ANSWERS AND TUTORIAL ON ITEMS 638-642

The answers are: **638-B; 639-D; 640-C; 641-A; 642-A**.

In sickle cell disease, sickling occurs as red blood cell deformation in circumstances of falling oxygen tension and acidosis from ischemic tissue. This creates more ischemic tissue by plugging end vessels, and this form of micro-infarction can give rise to acute abdominal crises. Maintaining high oxygen saturation is a way of preventing these crises of ischemia and infarction. If the sickle cell gene is combined with thalassemia, sickle-thalassemia hemoglobin carries a very high risk of lethal thromboembolism.

Protozoan parasites in the blood can also cause distal arteriolar plugging, and in the central nervous system this can be evident as cerebral malaria from falciparum malaria. This is a particularly lethal form of malaria, and is associated with *Plasmodium falciparum*. Each of these conditions that can give rise to deformations in blood cells can cause splenic enlargement as the spleen removes the deformed cells from the circulation. Over time, however, the spleen also undergoes multiple infarctions, and it may fibrose down in the process of "autosplenectomy" as an end-stage of sickling and other causes of splenic infarction. The one form of cellular deformation that gives rise to splenomegaly but does not give rise to splenic infarctions and subsequent fibrosis is hereditary spherocytosis. In this form of spleno-megaly, the enlargement of the spleen and its hyperfunction are chronic and sustainable over prolonged periods.

Items 643-647

(A)   Incisional biopsy
(B)   Fine needle aspiration cytology
(C)   Thyroid scan
(D)   Laryngoscopy

643.   A young man with recently acquired hoarseness and a thyroid mass.

644.   An asymptomatic 58 year-old man with left posterior triangle neck mass discovered on examination.

645.   A 62 year-old alcoholic woman with an ulcer in the retromolar trigone.

646.   A neck mass in a 44 year-old smoker with dysphagia and grossly normal exam except for the supraclavicular nodule.

647.   A solitary 2 cm firm left lateral lobe thyroid mass in a 26 year-old woman.

ANSWERS AND TUTORIAL ON ITEMS 643-647

The answers are: **643-D; 644-B; 645-A; 646-B; 647-B**.

To use a clinical maxim attributed to Dr. George Crile, "the presence of a solitary solid mass in the thyroid of a male is an indication for its removal." This clinical pearl suggested that there is a much higher malignancy rate among nodules in males than in females. Although females have the same incidence of thyroid cancer as do males, they have a much higher incidence of benign thyroid nodularity, and this much greater frequency dilutes the finding of thyroid cancer in females. Dr. Crile did not have aspiration cytology technique available to him to help in this discrimination, but it is a useful starting point to recognize that there will be a much higher index of suspicion with respect to the thyroid mass in a male than there would be in a female, and few of those in a male would be managed by temporizing; whereas, many more of the female patients with thyroid nodules can be observed over time with the additional help of aspiration cytology which would select out those with positive cytology for operation.

A worrisome sign associated with a thyroid mass is vocal cord paralysis. In fact, a negative aspiration cytology would not keep one from operating on such a patient if in fact the cord showed a paralysis suggestive of recurrent laryngeal nerve involvement. Since the cytology, if negative, would not preclude the operation, the operation will be a much more inclusive sampling of the thyroid tissue than would the aspiration. The finding of the limited sampling in cytology that is negative would not keep the patient from operation, and the cord paralysis "trumps" cytologic finding in any event. There would be no need for the fine needle aspiration but patients should proceed directly to thyroid exploration. Therefore, laryngoscopy to confirm the hoarseness as based in recurrent laryngeal nerve paralysis is the next procedure that need be performed for the young man, both as confirmation of the worrisome diagnostic suggestion of thyroid cancer, and also as pre-operative baseline for postoperative repeated laryngoscopy.

The fine needle aspiration would be appropriate management of the woman with a solitary mass since not only does she not have more worrisome signs, but also being a young woman has a much higher likelihood of having a benign thyroid nodule than malignant one, and the negative cytology would encourage follow-up on the basis of clinical findings. A positive cytology would immediately recommend a change in this policy of observation. It is helpful to think of cytology as yielding information when positive, and not negative information but *noninformation* when it is negative — that is, as though the study were not done — and that allows one to return to any clinical findings upon which one would base a judgement in the absence of the cytologic test.

The focus has been on the thyroid as the source of pathology in the younger individuals, whereas epidermoid malignant abnormalities are likely in the older patients, particularly those with associated risk factors. Aspiration cytology would be quite helpful in these instances, since the neck mass represents the only evident disease in two of those patients, so aspiration cytology would be the best technique at the only targetable lesion. For the patient with an intra-oral ulcer, likelihood of malignancy is high, and incisional biopsy would yield tissue adequate for confident diagnosis whereas cytologic means would be insufficient for secure exclusion of malignancy in the superficial ulcer with the probability of many inflammatory cells among the few that would be obtained for examination with cytology compared to the full thickness and greater quantity that would be obtained with incisional biopsy.

    (A)   Oral cholecystogram
    (B)   Ultrasound
    (C)   Harrey-technetium-99m iminodiacetic acid (^{99m}Tc HIDA) scan
    (D)   CT scan
    (E)   Hepatic arteriogram
    (F)   Spleno-portography
    (G)   Percutaneous transhepatic cholangiogram
    (H)   Endoscopic retrograde pancreatic cholangiography

648.   Acute right upper quadrant pain in a 42 year-old obese woman who has had abrupt pain onset 2 hours after eating.

649.   A jaundiced 58 year-old man with pre-operative elevated pancreatic and hepatic enzymes who has failed earlier CT demonstration of abdominal pathology except to show dilated ducts and a portal fullness.

650.   An 18 year-old member of a spherocytosis family has had episodes of colicky pain and splenectomy has been considered for persistent anemia.

651.   A patient with known cirrhosis and CT-demonstrated large liver tumor is being evaluated as a candidate for operation.

652.   A woman with painless jaundice who had a vague fullness found by CT in the peri-ampullary area is being evaluated as a candidate for operation.

ANSWERS AND TUTORIAL ON ITEMS 648-652

The answers are: **648-B; 649-G; 650-C; 651-E; 652-H**.

The typical candidate for acute cholecystitis might have the first study be the last one if ultrasound shows a "halo" of edema around the gall bladder which may be distended and as a bonus, shows gall stones. These gall stones are unlikely to be radio-opaque, so there would be no benefit in getting a flat abdominal film for this relative unlikelihood, whereas the ultrasound has a very high likelihood of achieving a diagnosis sufficient for recommendation of therapy. The ultrasound would also not be limited by a certain level of bilirubin for function, as would both oral cholecystogram and ^{99m}Tc HIDA scan. The ^{99m}Tc HIDA scan would be helpful in the definition of the abdominal pain in the young man with spherocytosis, since the pigment stones are often associated with the gall bladder with enough absorption capacity to still give visualization, and it is faster and more reliable than the oral cholecystogram. A reasonable question might be whether any diagnostic testing was necessary, since the gall bladder might be removed on the basis of the high likelihood that cholecystitis is present and would be, given his underlying hereditary disease, and the likelihood that chole-cystectomy could be performed as accessory to an operation already being considered in abdominal exploration.

The other three patients have longer standing liver disease, two of whom have jaundice ruling out tests sensitive to a functioning liver and absorbent gall bladder (oral cholecystogram and ^{99m}Tc HIDA scan). CT scan has already been performed in each of the three which was sensitive to the degree that CT discrimination would be higher than that of ultrasound, but no definite localization of a mass was obtained. In one instance, because of the obstructive jaundice and dilated ducts, the patient is anticipating an operation, and pre-operative percutaneous cholangiography may not only help demonstrate the site of the lesion, but allow pre-operative drainage for better anesthestic and postoperative management in this patient.

In the woman with painless jaundice, peri-ampullary malignancy is anticipated, and an effective way to study this would be with an endoscopic retrograde pancreatic cholangiography. This might not only identify the site of obstruction, but also retrieve tissue for its diagnosis to compare with that seen on the imaging. The imaging studies may indicate operation because of the location of this obstruction (which would include planning both palliative and curative operation) or on the basis of demonstrated extension of the disease that would contraindicate curative resection and recommend limiting the operative strategy to palliation.

One patient already has CT demonstration of a large liver tumor, and at this point, the diagnosis is not the question but the extent of the resection that would be necessary to encompass the tumor and still leave viable amounts of liver. Because there is parenchymal damage from an underlying cirrhosis, it is important to see if this tumor can be resected without the loss of a large majority of the liver or interference with its arterial supply — which is the same thing. If more than 20 to 25% of the liver can be anticipated to be residual with an intact arterial supply not

encased by the hepatoma, then curative operation is possible. These studies not only may contribute to diagnosis, but also define resectability and even in some instances help in the determination of operability.

Items 653-657

(A) Upper GI barium swallow
(B) Esophageal gastroduodenoscopy
(C) CT scan
(D) Arteriography

653. A woman suspected of bleeding varices has which primary diagnostic/treatment method of first choosing?

654. After failed sclerotherapy, bleeding rate increases; the next step before operation might be?

655. Which of these tests might still be likely to find the bleeding point if the vessel were bleeding 5 ml/10 min?

656. Which of these tests might demonstrate a small leak in an esophageal anastomosis?

657. Which of these studies may be useful to decrease portal perfusion pressure?

ANSWERS AND TUTORIAL ON ITEMS 653-657

The answers are: **653-B; 654-D; 655-B; 656-A; 657-D**.

Upper gastrointestinal endoscopy is highly specific in diagnosis, and sometimes can be extended to therapy through such means as sclerotherapy in the case of bleeding varices. If the sclerotherapy fails, even when repeated, and if the bleeding rate increases, the next therapeutic step might be arteriography, since pharmaco-therapy can be infused through the arteriography catheter to diminish portal pressure through decreasing splanchnic blood flow. When blood flow is minimal, arteriography is not very helpful as a localization method, but minimal blood loss can be detected by endoscopy, even in finding areas where bleeding had been issuing but now was no longer actively bleeding from identification of the ulcerated site.

Both arteriography and CT would not be very helpful in finding the site of a leak, which can often be missed on endoscopy as well. Further, in a fresh anastomosis, there would be no enthusiasm for inserting a fiber-optic tube into a recently postoperative patient, since the anastomotic perforation might be found by causing it. Contrast swallow might be the best way to determine a leak in an esophageal suture line. It is preferred that this be with water-soluble contrast if it is anticipated that it might find its way into the mediastinum, but a recent anastomosis will likely still have chest tubes available, and probably would require re-operation if it were substantial, so a higher definition possible with the greater opacity of barium may be preferable.

(A)   H$_2$-receptor antagonist (cimetidine, ranitidine, famotidine)
(B)   H$_1$-receptor antagonist (Probantheline)
(C)   Sucralfate
(D)   Proton pump inhibitor (omeprazole)
(E)   Milk and antacids

658.   Appropriate therapy for atrophic gastritis.

659.   May be helpful in relieving gas bloating symptoms.

660.   Reduces hydrogen ion secretion dramatically.

661.   Probably safe for prolonged therapy.

662.   Most frequently employed pre-scription medication for gastro-intestinal disorders.

ANSWERS AND TUTORIAL ON ITEMS 658-662

The answers are: **658-C; 659-B; 660-D; 661-E; 662-A**.

Atrophic gastritis frequently is associated with hypoacidity, so antacids would be less effective in this instance. Some form of therapy that might assist in mucosal healing, such as sucralfate or an experimental use of prostaglandins may be beneficial. Both H$_1$ and H$_2$-receptor blocking antihistamines are employed in relief of gastrointestinal symptoms: probantheline is frequently used for relief of gas bloating distress, and H_2-receptor antagonists are the most frequently employed prescription medications for gastrointestinal disorders (and, for that matter, the most frequent prescription medication in the US and have been for a period of time, vying closely with tranquilizers for outpatients and antibiotics for inpatients).

The use of the proton pump inhibitor omeprazole is a potent inhibitor of gastric acid production. The use of this agent for prolonged periods of time is not indicated, as it has some potential for unforeseen side effects, such as later association with gastric carcinoid or other malignancies. One could look upon the widespread use of acid reduction medications for prolonged periods of time (omeprazole and H_2-receptor antagonists) as producing an entire generation of pernicious anemic patients, with the associated malignancy potential that they experience. For that reason, prolonged antacid therapy with milk, cream and antacids is probably the safest recommendation. Whatever the affects on atherosclerosis of the high milk lipid diet might be, it appears that milk-alkali syndrome is not a real or frequently experienced complication of prolonged antacid therapy, and is the safest of the options listed.

Items 663-667

(A) Gram-positive aerobes
(B) Gram-negative aerobes
(C) Gram-negative anaerobes
(D) Protozoa
(E) Viruses

663. Cellulitis and superficial abscess.

664. Endotoxemia.

665. Late intra-abdominal abscess.

666. Pneumonia in HIV positive patients.

667. Commonest skin flora.

ANSWERS AND TUTORIAL ON ITEMS 663-667

The answers are: **663-A; 664-B; 665-C; 666-D; 667-A.**

Gram-positive aerobic agents (*Staphylococci* and *Streptococci*) are among the commonest of the skin flora, and are responsible for cellulitis and superficial abscess formation in any break in the first line of defense and exposure of the interior milieu to these skin flora. In contrast, gram-negative aerobes are the flora associated with endotoxin release and the high mortality of endotoxemia in contrast with the morbidity of skin flora in causing cellulitis and abscess.

Late in the mixed inoculum, intra-abdominal abscess is predominately a factor of anaerobic proliferation, since the more numerous anaerobes gradually outgrow the aerobes. The mixed aerobic and anaerobic flora are synergistic, since micro-aerophilic circumstances later in an abscess favor a higher number of anaerobes that survive from the original mixed inoculum.

One protozoan organism, *Pneumocystis carinii* has a predilection for patients with immunocompromise, which includes those with HIV infection. The HIV is not responsible for the pneumonia, but for the immunosuppressed status that allows the protozoan pneumonia to become established.

Items 668-672

(A) *Staphylococcus aureus*
(B) β-hemolytic *Streptococcus*
(C) *Hemophilus influenza*
(D) *Escherichia coli*
(E) *Proteus mirabilis*
(F) *Pseudomonas aeruginosa*
(G) *Clostridium perfringens*
(H) *Clostridium difficil*
(I) *Bacteroides fragilis*

668. Earliest widespread infecting organism of spreading cellulitis.

669. Associated with pseudomembranous colitis.

670. Organism frequently found in humidifiers of ventilators.

671. Most numerous species by weight in colon contents.

672. Most common organism cultured from urinary tract infections.

ANSWERS AND TUTORIAL ON ITEMS 668-672

The answers are: **668-B; 669-H; 670-F; 671-I; 672-D.**

Cellulitis due to β-hemolytic streptococci spreads because of the enzymatic activity of this organism, and the inability of the host to wall it off as frequently occurs with staphylococcal infections that can be limited to abscesses. Of the gram-negative anaerobes, *Bacteroides* are the most numerous, constituting the majority of the dry weight of colon contents. Clostridia are also present in this class of gram-negative anaerobes, and *Clostridium difficil* secretes an exotoxin which is associated with pseudomembranous colitis. One of the organisms found in the damp environments of ventilators, particularly in the humidifiers, is *Pseudomonas aeruginosa*. It is particularly hard to eradicate without sterilizing this equipment by complete disassembly between patients.

The urinary tract is not an anaerobic environment. In essence, one does not need to concern oneself about the likelihood of upper urinary tract infection with any species other than the gram-negative aerobe. The lower urinary tract has the likelihood of skin flora invasion, which is what happens frequently with indwelling catheters, as a channel between the flora of the skin conducted into the mucosal environment of peri-urethritis.

That the mixed flora of the gut is mainly anaerobic and the pathogens responsible for urinary tract infections are principally coliforms means that therapy can be tailored to avoid impact on the most numerous species of the gut so as to minimize GI flora disturbance in such anaerobe sparing therapy as quinolone treatment. For example, norfloxacin might be given with minimal gastrointestinal flora upset and cover the majority of risks to urinary tract colonizing organisms.

Items 673-677

(A) IVP excretory urogram
(B) Voiding cysto urethrogram
(C) Retrograde pyelography
(D) Renal perfusion scan
(E) Renal arteriogram
(F) Computed tomography (CT)
(G) Ultrasound
(H) KUB flat plate (kidney, urinary bladder)

673. Sometimes treats as well as diagnoses ureteral calculi.

674. First screening test for kidney stones.

675. Indicated in male trauma patient with blood at external urethral meatus.

676. May be an early sign of acute rejection episode.

677. May define extension of hypernephroma and be useful in reducing its size pre-operatively.

ANSWERS AND TUTORIAL ON ITEMS 673-677

The answers are: **673-A; 674-H; 675-B; 676-D; 677-E.**

Excretory urography uses an intravenous bolus of contrast material that acts as an osmotic diuretic. Not only does it opacify the urinary collecting system, the osmotic effect causes a diuresis and dilatation proximal to the obstructing lesion that might be diagnosed by IVP and simultaneously may clear by the dilatation and peristalsis of diuresis facilitating stone passage. A first screening test for presence of kidney stones is the flat plate abdominal film known as KUB, for encompassing the region of the kidney and urinary bladder with the ureter in between. If there is an opaque stone (as the majority of calcium oxalate — the most frequent calculi — are, with the exception of urate stones) it is frequently visible in the urinary tract distribution if other extensive calcification or opacity such as barium does not obscure it.

An IVP would not be the first study for a patient who has a drop of blood at the urethral meatus, in which disruption of the urethra or distal urinary tract outlet from bladder down would be more likely than a higher urinary tract lesion, and voiding cystourethrography would be recommended to define the area of potential disruption.

Since rejection is an early vascular phenomenon and usually is accompanied by a rise in vascular resistance to perfusion, a renal perfusion scan is frequently the sensitive early indicator of acute rejection episodes in a transplanted kidney. Renal arteriography is a very useful study in hypernephroma to define the extent and extension of the tumor and its frequent site of capsular or intravenous invasion. In addition, through the same arteriography catheter, an obstruction can be introduced into the artery through a spring coil with Dacron wool. This will shrink the size of the tumor when employed immediately pre-operatively and facilitate the resection.

Items 678-682

    (A)   Morphine
    (B)   Nitrous oxide
    (C)   Epidural tetracaine
    (D)   Spinal anesthetic
    (E)   Local infiltration lidocaine/epinephrine
    (F)   Axillary block regional
    (G)   Alcohol nerve block
    (H)   Sympathectomy

678.   May be useful for plastic surgery procedure in hemostasis.

679.   May temporarily increase marginal blood flow to a limb threatened by small vessel disease.

680.   Reversed by naloxone.

681.   May be useful for 72 hours post-operative analgesia with minimum respiratory depression.

682.   May be helpful in long-term control of chronic cancer pain.

ANSWERS AND TUTORIAL ON ITEMS 678-682

The answers are: **678-E; 679-H; 680-A; 681-C; 682-G.**

Anesthesia and analgesia are tailored to the indication, duration, and procedure. In some plastic surgical procedures, anesthesia by infiltration injection by the surgeon performing the procedure is actually preferred, since the injection of lidocaine may give local anesthesia, but the combination with epinephrine may actually reduce skin bleeding and facilitate primary closure. It is important that this use of vaso-constriction be employed only in tissues that would not be impaired by it to the degree that they might suffer ischemia and infarction if they are supplied by end vessels; this would include those on tip of the nose, and cartilaginous portions of the ear or flaps with marginal and compromised blood flow.

Regional nerve block may be done by a temporary method using reversible pharmacology, or may actually attempt destruction of the nerve for a longer term relief of pain. Injection of alcohol in sensory nerve block after demonstration of its effect using short-term anesthetic agents may be useful in long-term control of intractable cancer pain. Similarly, by either surgical sympathectomy or pharmacologic ablation using similar techniques as that for cancer pain control in sensory nerves, sympathectomy may allow — at least for a period of months — an increased blood flow to a marginally supplied extremity in threatened limb loss.

Morphine, with its excellent analgesic properties, carries with it some risk of respiratory depression as well as associated nausea and some properties such as histamine release or stimulation of sphincter spasm at pancreatic or biliary outlet. For that reason, on some occasions, morphine analgesia may not be just inappropriate, but there may be therapeutic benefit to reversing it with naloxone as an opioid antagonist. In order to achieve analgesia over a prolonged period of time without the respiratory hazard particularly observed with the use of morphine and its associated obtundation, an epidural catheter can be placed and infused with a dilute analgesic for a period of time indwelling in the epidural space. Since the catheter might constitute a channel for skin flora to contaminate this space in which an abscess would be very hazardous, it is not suggested that such an indwelling epidural catheter remain over a very extensive period, but usually this is satisfactory for the period of most intense postoperative pain when respiratory suppression would be most hazardous, and the catheter can be pulled and this form of analgesic sub-stituted for by systemic analgesia when the patient is ambulating and at less risk for various consequences of respiratory suppression.

Items 683-687

(A) Repeat serum calcium
(B) Urinary calcium
(C) Serum parathormone
(D) Thallium-technetium substraction scan
(E) Ultrasound
(F) Thyroid scan
(G) Arteriogram
(H) Venous sampling
(I) CT scan
(J) Surgical exploration

683. Next step for asymptomatic patient with diagnosed primary hyper-parathyroidism with serum calcium 12.5 mg/dl.

684. Next step in hypercalcemic patient with unsuccessful parathyroid operation whose brother is now reported to have had the same result from the procedure.

685. A preferred procedure for a patient with suspected mediastinal parathyroid tumor who would like to avoid re-operation.

686. A study which can lateralize hypersecretion in the absence of an imaged mass.

687. A patient has had two calcium determinations one of 11.0 which caused a look back to records 3 years ago when it was 10.0. The next step should be

ANSWERS AND TUTORIAL ON ITEMS 683-687

The answers are: **683-J; 684-B; 685-G; 686-H; 687-A**.

The patient with the established diagnosis of primary hyperparathyroidism requires no more localization than to locate an experienced parathyroid surgeon! The next step is surgical exploration, since it is this study that is both the most sensitive diagnostic localizing test as well as therapeutic in the vast majority of instances.

In contrast, the patient who has had a failed primary cervical exploration and then only in retrospect is it found that a close relative has the same process, before localization studies should have a recheck of the primary diagnosis. Since the patient is documented hypercalcemic, a urinary calcium determination would be an appropriate test to determine whether there was a familial component based in hypocalciuria. The other possibility is that the patient is part of an endocrinologic kindred, and multiple endocrine adenopathy hyperparathyroidism is always based in multiple gland disease. The most common source of failure in primary cervical operations that do not correct primary hyperparathyroidism is the failure to appreciate multiple gland disease and to correct it. If a patient has had a prior failed operation that does not find the focal source of the hyperparathyroidism and it is suspected in the mediastinum, if that mediastinal tumor is from the inferior thyroid arterial supply, a re-operation that is limited to the cervical approach can tease it back up into the cervicotomy incision along with the thymic extension. However, if the arterial supply is from the internal mammary artery, internal mammary arteriography can be carried out with staining of the tumor with hyper-osmotic contrast material. This osmotic shock has destroyed the hyperfunction of parathyroid adenoma and has maintained successful control of hyperparathyroidism when followed for many years thereafter. This percutaneous procedure is an attractive alternative to sternotomy and those patients in whom that operation would otherwise be indicated.

An invasive lateralizing procedure that is helpful since it correlates form and function is venous sampling. That can be true even in the absence of an imaged mass. For example, if CT or arteriography had shown no evidence of a suspicious lesion in a postoperative patient's neck, venous sampling might be able to lateralize an elevated N-terminal parathormone

secretion step-up on one side or the other of the neck, and exploration could begin with the site of the elevated parathormone.

A patient who has had an evident hypercalcemia requires that this be confirmed and that it is shown to be based in primary hyperparathyroidism. With respect to the one patient who is asymptomatic but had a calcium of 12.5 mg%, there is very little likelihood that he would remain asymptomatic for a prolonged period of time, and this operation should be restorative in sparing tissue that might suffer metastatic calcification as well as bone demin-eralization. In the patient with a calcium of 11 mg%, the course of such an asympto-matic patient might be observed if that were the preference, but first the diagnosis has to be confirmed. If the prior serum calcium was 10, and that (with the appropriate correction for albumin and judged against phosphate) is normal, the appropriate next step would be to repeat the serum calcium. If there were a steady trend upward, and the hypercalcemia on this occasion was proven not to be a fluke of random variation, then further determ-ination could be made based in the other information from the SMA-12 determ-ination (phosphate, chloride and albumin) and a parathormone ordered if appropriate based on these data.

(A)   Radiolabeled ^{131}I fibrinogen
(B)   Venogram
(C)   Plethysmography
(D)   Doppler flow scan
(E)   Pulmonary arteriogram

688.   The definitive accurate test of deep venous thrombosis.

689.   Required before surgical treatment of thromboembolism is considered.

690.   Can localize future blood clot but not those that have already been formed.

691.   A noninvasive test that does not require complete obstruction for detection of clot.

692.   The test with the highest risk of communicable disease transmission.

ANSWERS AND TUTORIAL ON ITEMS 688-692

The answers are: **688-B; 689-E; 690-A; 691-A; 692-A.**

The "gold standard" of deep venous thrombosis diagnosis is venography. However, it is invasive to the degree that it causes some degree of venous inflammation that may even lead to deep venous thrombosis if none were present before the test. Therefore, alternatives to this best study are sought, and several noninvasive methods are proposed. Fibrinogen that is radiolabeled can determine clot formation without complete obstruction. However, it only localizes blood clot prospectively and does not identify that which has already been formed. It also has a disadvantage in that it is the test of those listed with the highest risk of transmission of communicable disease, since it is a plasma-derived product.

Before surgical treatment of thromboembolism is considered, pulmonary angiographic evidence of recurrent pulmonary embolism on adequate anti-coagulation therapy or with major contraindications thereto must be confirmed. Medical treatment of thrombo-embolism does not have these require-ments, and it is the primary therapy of thromboembolism, not limited to recurrent disease that is not only present in the deep veins of the lower extremities but has also migrated by angiographic proof to the lungs.

"Never use malignant treatment for benign disease."

Glenn W. Geelhoed

217

Items 693-697

(A) Low dose heparin
(B) High dose heparin anticoagulation
(C) Caval filtration umbrella
(D) Operative caval clip application
(E) Ligation inferior vena cava
(F) Ligation left ovarian vein
(G) Venous thrombectomy
(H) Pulmonary embolectomy (Trendelenburg procedure)

693. A widely applicable method of thromboembolism prevention.

694. An operation for risk reduction that has no application outside the iliac area.

695. A percutaneous means of preventing the next thromboembolism.

696. Adequate therapy for most patients with deep venous thrombosis.

697. A last salvage procedure after recurrent pulmonary embolism in patients who have been on full anticoagulation.

ANSWERS AND TUTORIAL ON ITEMS 693-697

The answers are: **693-A; 694-G; 695-C; 696-B; 697-H**.

Low dose heparin (5000 Units subcutaneously q 12 hours) is widely applicable, since it can be employed in patients who are unable to ambulate or cooperate in the other measures of thromboembolism prevention. It does not require monitoring, since this dose of heparin therapy is not anticoagulating. Venous thrombectomy should in theory be appropriate as a procedure to reduce thromboembolism risk by removing the thrombus. However, it has no role in any area outside the iliac veins where it is quite limited in application as well. The better means of removing thrombus would be by thrombolytic process, and that occurs without invasion of the vein and the potential for suture line or other endothelial interruption and new clot formation on the nidus of local inflammation.

Most surgical therapy of thromboembolism is directed at the prevention of the next thromboemboli migrating to the lung, and intercepting them in the cava. A percutaneous method of accomplishing this is by the introduction of caval filters (Mobin-Uddin, Greenfield). This same means is applied, frequently as accessory to operation in which the caval area is already exposed, through application of a clip or other compartmentalization procedure. Most patients who have deep venous thrombosis are adequately treated by full anticoagulation high dose heparin therapy. This allows the natural process of clot lysis to occur while preventing the formation of new thrombus.

The final salvage procedure in some patients might be those who have suffered recurrent pulmonary embolism that has used up the last of their marginal reserves and put them into acute right heart failure despite full anticoagulation therapy. This is the Trendelenburg procedure which requires full cardiopulmonary bypass in its performance and is a very major undertaking with very low probability of survival in most patients who would be most in need of it.

Items 698-702

GI bleeding clinical characteristics:

    (A)   Exsanguinating hemorrhage - patient comes to ER in shock, after 3 units rapid transfusion, patient remains in shock

    (B)   Severe - the patient comes to the ER in shock, after 3 units of rapid transfusion is no longer in shock, but still actively bleeding

    (C)   Moderate - patient comes in to ER with evident bleeding, not in shock, but is treated for the bleeding and the bleeding stops, but then restarts, often repeatedly

    (D)   Occult - evidence of blood loss is an incidental finding, sometime on incidental stool guaiac performed on rectal exam specimen

698.   Presenting feature is usually anemia.

699.   Bleeding colonic diverticulosis's usual pattern.

700.   Requires treatment *before* diagnostic procedures such as X-ray or endoscopy.

701.   Upper GI endoscopy preferred diagnostic method.

702.   Barium enema is appropriate primary diagnostic procedure.

ANSWERS AND TUTORIAL ON ITEMS 698-702

The answers are: **698-D; 699-C; 700-A; 701-B; 702-D**.

The patient who is experiencing exsanguinating hemorrhage needs therapy, and quickly. This means that there will be no trip to the X-ray suite, nor time for refined diagnostic localization when the patient needs to be resuscitated from shock. This means the patient goes directly from the emergency room to the operating room while intensive support continues in order to achieve stable perfusion. There are only one or two sites of massive blood loss into the GI tract that are compatible with this clinical scenario. The most usual is the posterior penetrating duodenal ulcer with erosion of the gastroduodenal or inferior pancreaticoduodenal artery. It would be an appropriate step in treatment to continue infusion and transfusion of patient in the operating room, and if the patient remains in shock to open the abdomen and go immediately to the duodenum for control and ligation of the large caliber bleeding vessel if that is what is open in the base of the ulcer. If it is not, aortic compression can help in the resuscitation process while a source of blood loss is estimated by the position of the maximum bleeding rapidly entering the gut. This is sometimes the case at the erosion of a vascular prosthesis into the GI tract, and that might be suggested by any pre-operative history or scar.

In the patient who enters in shock and is briefly resuscitated from it, continuing to actively bleed, a single diagnostic study might be performed, and the highest yield procedure with the safest rapid process toward therapy would be endoscopy.

Endoscopy is useful because it might be helpful in one form of initial therapy if the source of bleeding was from portal hypertension through bleeding esophageal varices. If upper GI endoscopy revealed the source to be duodenal, an emergency operation can then be expeditiously carried out with that ulcer bleeding site targeted. It is important to recognize that the indication for operation is the bleeding, and not the ulcer diathesis. Ulcer disease can be treated medically, or can be treated surgically by a later elective procedure. Vagotomy and gastric resection would be appropriate treatment for the ulcer diathesis, but not for a bleeding duodenal ulcer in a patient who had entered in shock.

The usual bleeding pattern of colonic diverticulosis is that of moderate hemorrhage in which the patient "stutter stops". This bleeding is annoying since it is significant blood loss requiring transfusion up to half or more of the blood volume in 24 hours, but just at the time a diagnostic localization procedure is carried out, the blood flow rate seems to decrease below the sensitivity of the method to find it. Arteriography is useful here since it can not only find the source of bleeding, it may be useful through that catheter to administer pharmacologic therapy to slow visceral flow. Arteriography or endoscopy might be appropriate to localize this flow, but it is unlikely that barium study will be helpful, and should be avoided in the patient with moderate or greater bleeding rates.

For the patient who has occult blood loss the presenting feature is usually anemia and whatever high output cardiac consequences result from it. A barium enema is an appropriate primary diagnostic procedure in this event; arteriography plays a role, and endoscopy may be appropriate, but less for discovery of the bleeding site than for identification of a primary pathology or tumor, which is more likely than a primary ulcer.

Items 703-707

(A)   Mesenteric venous thrombosis
(B)   Mesenteric arterial embolus
(C)   Ischemic colitis
(D)   Desmoplastic fibrous adhesions

703.   A complication of abdominal aortic aneurysm resection.

704.   Post-infarction intracardiac thrombosis.

705.   A feature characteristic of extensive carcinoid tumor.

706.   Most common vascular catastrophe of the gut.

707.   May lead to portal venous thrombosis.

ANSWERS AND TUTORIAL ON ITEMS 703-707

The answers are: **703-C; 704-B; 705-D; 706-A; 707-A.**

The most common vascular catastrophe in the gut is mesenteric venous thrombosis. The term for a gut vascular crisis is often used parallel to "CVA" using a stroke analogy. However, arterial vascular crises in the abdomen are rare, and are usually associated with arterial disease elsewhere. For example, an intracardiac thrombus against a mural infarction may flip into the arterial tree and give rise to a gut infarction, but the more frequent mesenteric vascular problem is one of a primary gut compromise as in, for example, obstruction, and the resultant rise in venous pressure gives stasis and thrombosis which then raises venous pressure to arterial levels and infarction occurs when the two pressures equilibrate.

Ischemic colitis can also result from operative sacrifice of arterial blood supply as happens when the inferior mesenteric artery is ligated in aortic aneurysm resection. This ischemic colitis may be the more prominent consequence than infarction, since usually the marginal artery of Drummond gives sufficient collateral blood supply to make the bowel's survival probable but its function impaired, at least until some compensation can occur. If the venous mesenteric thrombosis occurs, this propagates back, not into the systemic venous circulation up the vena cava, but into the superior mesenteric vein which joins the splenic vein to become the portal. This means that mesenteric venous thrombosis can also give rise to a problem in the portal distribution as well as in vascular compromise to the bowel, and portal venous thrombosis is a serious consequence of mesenteric venous thrombosis.

An external inflammatory process that affects the bowel seems peculiar to the carcinoid tumor that has extended into areas adjacent to the bowel. Without having metastatic tumor causing adhesion from one loop of bowel to another, there seems to be elicited a desmoplastic reaction which yields very thick and matting adhesions with a plastic adherence of bowel loops that give evidence of bowel obstruction, not so much from the tumor as the adhesive fibrous reaction that it has induced.

In ischemic disease of the gut, the old clinical axiom is that one should direct attention to treating the heart and not the gut. However, when that ischemia becomes infarction and the ischemia is complicated by the primary probable obstruction, then the bowel problem must be addressed even if the heart has been compromised in its function as well. Since patients aren't dependent for minute to minute function on the gut, but there is a substitute for nutrient absorption function of the GI tract in total parental nutrition, rapid resolution of the GI problem such as by external diversion proximal to any devitalized section of the gut and simple excision of the infarcted segment would be appropriate, while primary therapy is addressed at improving cardiac function with probable need for anticoagulation because of the evident hypercoagulability that gave rise to the first intravascular thrombosis.

(A) Medical therapy
(B) Extracorporeal shock wave lithotripsy
(C) Laparoscopic excision
(D) Exploratory laparotomy

708. painless jaundice with palpable gall bladder

709. asymptomatic stones in gall bladder, incidentally discovered by sonography

710. acalculous cholecystitis associated with total parenteral nutrition

ANSWERS AND TUTORIAL ON ITEMS 708-710

The answers are: **708-D; 709-C; 710-A**.

Intervention in biliary tract disease may take the form of medical therapy, some external form of lithotriptic energy transmission, minimally invasive surgery through laparoscopy, or open exploratory surgery.

Medical treatment of cholecystitis is appropriate if the inflammation is based in infectious agents (such as *Salmonella*) or stasis from lack of contraction (such as occurs in the absence of duodenal stimulation in prolonged fasting, nasogastric aspiration and total parenteral nutrition). Antibiotic treatment may be adequate in the former, and choleretic agents and endocrine stimulation, as with cholecystokinin, in the latter.

There is a good case to be made that the presence of gall stones in the gall bladder discovered incidentally in an asymptomatic patient does not necessitate removal. If the patient were at risk greater than average should symptoms evolve (because of age, diabetes, compromised reserve or immune status), cholecystectomy could be advised even without the development of symptoms. In such an indication laparoscopic cholecystectomy might be the treatment of choice.

For the patient with evidence of biliary tract obstruction from stenotic segments of duct, or from likely malignant disease, exploration, resection evaluation, and reconstruction might involve a more extensive procedure than that which should be undertaken by laparoscopy, and laparotomy would be indicated for such patients.

Medical therapy for the dissolution of stones, and ECSWL for the disruption of stones have each been less successful in the biliary tract than minimally invasive surgical excision. In contrast with the utility of ECSWL for renal calculi, the use for biliary calculi has not been as applicable.

PART IV
ANATOMICAL SURGICAL REVIEW ITEMS

DIRECTIONS: Each of the following numbered items or incomplete statements is followed by a list of answers or completions of the statement. Select the **ONE** best response from the lettered options that is the best completion or correct answer to the statement in the stem.

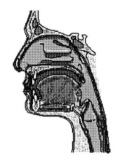

HEAD AND NECK SURGERY

Items 711-720

711. A mass in the midline of the neck just above the tracheal cartilage has been notable for some months in an 8 year-old girl but in the last four days there has been some reddening and discomfort. Which of the following statements is most likely to be correct?

   (A)   it has a high probability of malignancy

   (B)   it would most likely resolve completely with antibiotics

   (C)   it would rise higher in the neck when she protrudes her tongue

   (D)   incision and drainage is adequate treatment

   (E)   it is associated with anomalies of the ear

712. Each of the following factors contributes to the likelihood that a mass in the neck is malignant **EXCEPT**:

   (A)   the patient is alcoholic

   (B)   the patient had another malignancy outside the neck

   (C)   the patient is quite sure it was not present a week ago

   (D)   the patient was a heavy smoker, but quit two years ago

   (E)   the patient had facial irradiation for treatment of acne

713. A 19 year-old man is thrown forward in an automobile accident, striking his face on the dashboard. In the ER, his face was bloody and swollen with edematous tongue and a free floating mandible with multiple fractures of each ramus. There is an unresolved question of posterior cervical pain. Emergency management should include

   (A)   nasotracheal intubation

   (B)   emergency tracheotomy

   (C)   cricothyroidotomy

   (D)   oxygen by nasal catheter

   (E)   splinting the neck in extension

714. Each of the following treatments is appropriate for Stage I carcinoma of the larynx **EXCEPT**:

(A) laryngoscopic laser excision
(B) primary radiotherapy
(C) total laryngectomy
(D) partial surgical excision
(E) larynx-conserving subtotal hemilaryngectomy

715. Which of the following statements concerning parotid tumors is true?

(A) 80% are benign
(B) diagnosis is by incisional biopsy
(C) facial nerve palsy is a definite sign of malignancy
(D) tumors that extend into the deep lobe of the parotid are unresectable
(E) radiation is an appropriate curative treatment

716. Which of the following statements is **NOT** true of vocal nodules?

(A) they are a malignant tumor of the larynx
(B) they are associated with chronic voice abuse as in screaming
(C) they are sometimes called "singer's nodules"
(D) they do regress with speech therapy
(E) they are bilateral and located between anterior middle thirds of both true vocal cords

717. A debilitated patient in the inner city who has a problem with chronic alcoholism presents with weight loss, posterior cervical nodularity with ulceration, and leakage of a watery fluid that persisted in drainage for several months following outpatient incisional biopsy of neck nodes without any evidence of cancer. This clinical picture may represent a form of

(A) bronchogenic cleft fistula
(B) tuberculosis
(C) squamous cell carcinoma
(D) thyroid carcinoma
(E) radiation necrosis

718. A 2 year-old child has been diagnosed with a capillary hemangioma which was noted shortly after birth and got larger along the left nasal margin between eye and lip for several months after it was first detected. It appears now to be regressing as the child grows, but the parents are asking if it can be treated before the child becomes self-conscious about its presence. Appropriate advice would be

(A) to excise it with rotational full thickness skin-flap coverage
(B) irradiation
(C) surgical tattooing
(D) embolization
(E) temporizing

719. Each of the following is an indication for tonsillectomy **EXCEPT**:

    (A)   dysphagia — interference with swallowing

    (B)   dyspnea — interference with breathing from mass effect in the nasopharynx

    (C)   peritonsillar abscess

    (D)   bacterial allergy from focal infection

    (E)   a second acute tonsillitis episode in a 4 year-old whose older brother is also scheduled for tonsillectomy

720. Following commando composite resection (mandibulectomy and anterior glossectomy for floor of the mouth squamous cell carcinoma), combined with bilateral radical neck dissection, a patient is seen in follow-up nine months post-operation. On examination you find three firm nontender nodules vertically aligned and spaced along the posterior cervical triangle, on the right, and — to your surprise — similar nodules on the opposite side in mirror image. The patient has no complaints. The most likely diagnosis is

    (A)   metastatic squamous cell carcinoma

    (B)   reactive lymph node hyperplasia

    (C)   fibrous scar

    (D)   varicosities at ligated tributaries of the excised jugular

    (E)   neuromas

ANSWERS AND TUTORIALS ON ITEMS 711-720

The answers are: **711-C; 712-C; 713-B; 714-C; 715-A; 716-A; 717-B; 718-E; 719-E; 720-E**.

711. This description is that of a thyroglossal duct cyst. These may occasionally become inflamed as it appears to have recently in this instance, and antibiotic therapy will not cause its complete resolution, since the embryologic abnormality remains even when the inflammation subsides. Incision and drainage will not be adequate therapy, and may produce a fistula which will persist so long as the cells remain in the embryologic development track. Simple excision is inadequate, since the extent goes from the base of the tongue through the hyoid bone to the thyroid gland, and incision must be carried out to the base of the tongue and include the midportion of the hyoid if recurrence is to be avoided (Sistrunk procedure).

It is not an uncommon congenital abnormality with no likelihood of malignancy at the time of this girl's presentation, and unlike pharyngeal arch abnormalities, there should be no associated anomalies of the ear. Because of its attachment from the foramen cecum, motion of the tongue such as protrusion or swallowing causes the cyst to move its position in the neck, an observation that can confirm its origin in the thyroglossal duct.

712. The reliability of this finding is somewhat dependent on the observance of the patient, but if that seems trustworthy, it is unlikely to be malignant. The "rule of sevens" is a reference to this, that if a lesion has been present seven days it is inflammatory, seven months it is malignant, seven years it is congenital. Alcoholism and tobacco use are the highest correlations, and radiation at a very young age would be even more suspicious than therapeutic radiation for acne in the teenage years which is less likely to produce thyroid malignancy, but is, nonetheless, a risk factor.

Smoking is probably the most highly correlated risk factor, and that would include a cumulative risk even if recent cessation had followed an earlier history. It is obvious that metastatic spread can occur from a tumor elsewhere, but the presence of a known tumor elsewhere in the body additionally increases the likelihood of a new primary cancer found in the head and neck region.

713. There is no point to cervical splinting in a patient who has lost the strut that tethers the tongue anteriorly, since the tongue will fall back with or without cervical extension in the absence of the mandibular arch. Cricothyroidotomy is a temporizing procedure, and the patient is going to require tracheostomy both immediately and for the foreseeable future because of the multiple injury, anticipated swelling, and loss of bony support as well as soft tissue trauma.

Extension of the neck is also contraindicated until the status of the cervical spine is determined. Nasal catheterization for oxygen delivery will be ineffective if the obstruction is in the pharynx where the swollen tongue has fallen back. Hyperextension of the neck as is required for endotracheal intubation would cause the tongue to fall back during that process, which also puts at risk the

cervical spine which is as yet unevaluated. Tracheostomy is both the first and last indicated procedure for securing this patient's airway.

714. This is over-treatment for the T-1 size laryngeal cancer in the larynx, since the presentation of laryngeal cancer is often early because of changes in the voice marking a sensitive indication for screening. Radiotherapy may be the preferred treatment, but laser laryngoscopy with repeated follow-up to detect the occurrence of any new nodules, benign or malignant, may be a second choice. If that has already occurred, then a partial excision or hemilaryngectomy is the appropriate treatment, but total laryn-gectomy with loss of the larynx for voice purposes is reserved for larger tumor sizes which cannot be treated by these more conservative limited means.

715. In a surprise reversal for head and neck tumors in the adult, the majority of parotid tumors are benign. In fact, in comparison with the other salivary glands, the obverse is true in that 80% of tumors arising in these glands are malignant, a fact probably designed purely for test-taking purposes! The primary parotid tumors can grow to be huge, and although facial nerve palsy suggests malignancy, benign tumors may also give the same feature; neither the nerve palsy nor extension into the deep lobe are contraindications to resection. Surgical therapy is the treatment, although even the benign tumors have a recurrence rate that is high, but radiation therapy is not a successful curative treatment, and is unlikely to be indicated for the vast majority of benign parotid tumors.

716. There is an important distinction to be made between vocal polyps and vocal nodules. Vocal polyps are unilateral. They are not typically associated with voice abuse and do not respond to speech therapy, and require operation, probably in contemporary practice with laser treatment. Vocal nodules are bilateral lesions at the "kissing" contact points at the anterior junction between the front and middle thirds of each vocal chord. The voice lessons can help resolve this by decreasing stress to this area, and surgery is rarely indicated for these "singer's nodules".

717. Malignancy is a very high likelihood given this patient's presentation. However, there are distinctive differences that might lead to consideration of other diagnoses. The presentation is not at all typical for thyroid cancer. The patient is unlikely to have a congenital abnormality that first presents in adult life with this amount of inflammation, even if alcoholism and debilitation may contribute to weakened defenses. Squamous cell carcinoma is a very highly likely possibility, but at least one unsuccessful attempt was made to confirm this. It may have been missed, but it is not typical for epidermoid carcinoma to give draining sinuses. Radiation may contribute to tissue necrosis and ulceration, and devitalized tissue may constitute foreign body nidus with a continuing drainage. There is a strong inflammatory component to this, and in the patient's suppressed state any number of etiologic agents that might not cause disease in someone with good nutrition might become pathogenic.

In this case, the diagnosis turns out to be atypical tuberculosis. In this instance, antimicrobial therapy is not as useful as complete excision of the draining sinus tracks to eliminate the local focus of infection which is serving as a foreign body nidus to the giant cell reaction. Draining cervical lymphadenitis has the term "scrofula" applied to it as well as the delightful historic reference of the "King's Evil" since the touch of the king was supposed to relieve the patient of this problem; it certainly would if that touch is extended to curettage and excision of the involved cervical lymphadenitis!

718. Any of the more radical treatments advised should be applied quickly before the lesion goes away! Particularly in this cosmetically sensitive location, no disfigurement from excision, grafting, radiation (and its associated risks to growth and later carcinogenesis) or permanent cosmetic cover should be attempted. Embolization would not be very easy given the possible feeding vessels, and spontaneous thrombosis is likely without this manipulation. Parents are also to be told that local manipulation (compressing it with taped-on coins, heat, cold, or daily cosmetic application) would perhaps do more to induce the self-consciousness that they are concerned about than the ongoing devolution of what is a transient stage in this lesion. There is a role for tattooing of permanent cosmetic features such as some "portwine stains". But for the cavernous hemangioma the appropriate treatment is the passage of time.

719. Tonsillectomy is not indicated for tonsillitis in children, but it may be for the complications of tonsillitis. Tonsillitis is a primary indication for antibiotic treatment and local management for symptomatic relief. However, there are complications that stem from secondary infectious sequelae, such as peritonsillar abscess or an allergy from resident bacteria or upper air or food passage disruption based on a mass effect from very hypertrophic tonsils.

In times past, six patients with the same last name would be posted sequentially on the OR schedule with a homey note in the hospital news bulletin with a caption under a photograph saying something like "the family Robinson is having its tonsils removed today". This gimmickry is inappropriate, since tonsils do not need removing because they are there. Even primary pathology is not an indication, unless there is a second order phenomenon that would justify this procedure with a benefit that is anticipated to outweigh the risk.

720. Along the posterior border of the field of radical neck dissection, the cervical plexus of cutaneous nerves is encountered in the segmental distribution from auricular nerves inferiorly. These are each sectioned in turn as expendable, with attention directed to the preservation of cranial nerves to the extent possible, a necessity for certain nerves such as the vagus and desirable for the spinal accessory nerve which is not sectioned unless necessary and with the consequent disability of the "winged scapula". This sectioning produces neuromas that are rarely hypersensitive and usually are sensitive only for a short time. They may be confused with lymph nodes (which should mostly have been cleared in the dissection bloc) or metastatic deposits but their anatomic regularity makes them more easily recognized as benign consequences of the radical neck dissection. Ligated vein tributaries shrivel following thrombosis, and postoperative scarring would not be so anatomically regular in this pattern.

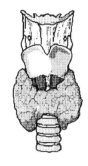

THYROID SURGERY

Items 721-730

721. Each of the following conditions is a primary indication for thyroidectomy **EXCEPT**:

(A) thyroiditis
(B) two cm thyroid nodule with hoarseness
(C) recurrent Graves' disease in second trimester pregnancy
(D) dysphagia with submanubrial goiter
(E) positive fine needle aspirate cytology

722. Which of the following studies is both necessary and sufficient in the absence of other compelling clinical features to indicate thyroidectomy?

(A) technetium scan
(B) iodine scan
(C) ultrasound
(D) arteriogram
(E) fine needle aspiration cytology

723. Each of the following statements is true regarding a two cm differentiated papillary thyroid cancer in a 24 year-old woman **EXCEPT**:

(A) involvement of adjacent cervical lymph nodes with papillary cancer changes the staging of the primary tumor with a worse prognosis

(B) tumor free survival rate following treatment is expected at greater than 90% in ten years

(C) radical neck dissection should not be combined with total thyroidectomy from the side of the lobe with the primary tumor

(D) such a nodule is most often cold on scan

(E) operation is elective and could be postponed four weeks on the basis of patient's request that it not interfere with a personal matter she does not care to divulge

724. Which of the following lesions in the thyroid is typically unifocal with unlikely disease elsewhere in the thyroid gland?

(A) Plummer's syndrome
(B) medullary thyroid cancer in a teenager
(C) follicular carcinoma
(D) papillary carcinoma
(E) *struma lymphomatosa*

725. Each of the following statements concerning medullary thyroid cancer is true **EXCEPT**:

(A) it may occur in families with a genetic predisposition for it

(B) it is nearly always multi-centric when found in young patients

(C) radioiodine treatment is the therapy of choice for control of lymph node metastases

(D) metastatic disease in the liver, lungs or regional spread can be detected in the absence of imaging studies by characteristic secretions from the tumor

(E) the prognosis following surgical treatment is much worse than that for papillary carcinoma of comparable stage

726. Which of the following statements regarding follicular thyroid carcinoma is true?

(A) its incidence is highest in populations where iodine deficiency is widespread

(B) prevalence of follicular carcinoma in the United States has increased remarkably in this century

(C) it is the most common cancer found in patients who report a history of head and neck irradiation

(D) multicentricity is the rule rather than the exception

(E) lymphatic metastases are a principle means of spread

727. Which of the following tumor cell types has the worst prognosis in the thyroid gland?

(A) lymphoma
(B) anaplastic carcinoma
(C) medullary carcinoma
(D) papillary carcinoma
(E) follicular carcinoma

728. A young man with follicular carcinoma of the thyroid treated by total thyroidectomy is asymptomatic, but follow-up scan when he has been off thyroid replacement shows bilateral pulmonary uptake of the isotope. Which of the following statements is true regarding this condition?

(A) this distribution is an artifact, and there is no confirmed evidence of metastasis until lung biopsy is carried out
(B) the patient is doomed to a very short life expectancy from this heavy metastatic tumor burden
(C) wedge resections of lung should be undertaken in bilateral staged thoracotomies to reduce the bulk of the pulmonary metastases
(D) following radioiodine therapy, prolonged tumor-free survival is anticipated
(E) chemotherapy should be initiated with cytotoxic drugs used in combination

729. Which of the following characteristics of a patient with thyroid cancer has the most effect on prognosis?

(A) degree of differentiation
(B) tumor stage
(C) lymph node involvement
(D) tumor size
(E) patient's age

730. Each of the following complications of subtotal thyroidectomy for Graves' disease is unique to operative treatment and does not occur with radioiodine EXCEPT:

(A) hemorrhage
(B) hypoparathyroidism
(C) hypothyroidism
(D) recurrent laryngeal nerve injury
(E) superior laryngeal nerve injury

ANSWERS AND TUTORIALS ON ITEMS 721-730

The answers are: **721-A; 722-E; 723-A; 724-C; 725-C; 726-A; 727-B; 728-D; 729-E; 730-C**.

721. Thyroiditis may cause hyperthyroidism when, early in its course, it stimulates production and release of thyroid hormones (so-called Hashimoto's toxic thyroiditis), but inflammatory processes in the thyroid are usually self-limited, and often result in a "burnout" in the end-stage. The patient may experience some discomfort, but this can be handled with analgesics and anti-inflammatories, and thyroid operation would likely only speed up the onset of hypothyroidism. This problem is more common in women, and is getting increasingly more frequent for reasons that are not known. Treatment is most generally symptomatic if there is some degree of hyperfunction, and long-term thyroid replacement is the treatment in the hypothyroid later stages of fibrosis. The presence of, or high probability of, thyroid malignancy is an indication for operation, and fine needle aspiration cytology has refined that possibility to a probability. Clinical evidence is still useful, however, and hoarseness with a thyroid nodule that has caused either recurrent laryngeal paralysis or laryngeal invasion is indicative of malignancy with or without cytologic confirmation.

Compression of the upper air or food passages is strong indication for relief of the compression, as is most frequently the case with goiters with large expanding intrathoracic components inside enclosure that compromises the airway. The patient with recurrent Graves' disease is an appropriate candidate for surgery, particularly if pregnant. These conditions are "staples" in thyroid surgery, but must be distinguished from the larger number of benign goiters that will not require surgical treatment.

722. Each of the radiographic imaging studies constitute "shadow producing procedures". That the thyroid nodule occupies space is likely known already from the clinical examination since that is the presentation of most thyroid nodules. Further information about this mass is limited in knowing its blood flow (technetium and arteriography) or its iodine concentration ability (iodine scan). The ultrasound can tell us whether it is solid or cystic, information strongly suggested on clinical examination as well, and none of the diagnostic studies just mentioned would give opportunity for treatment simultaneously as would needle aspiration in the event that the lesion turned out to be cystic. Since the information yield has not been critical (i.e., malignant lesions can be hot or cold, relatively more or less vascular, and some have cystic degeneration) the only value added to the information obtained in imaging is a microscopic appreciation of the nature of the mass.

Cutting tissue with a core needle biopsy could give histology which is helpful, but a more rapid assessment can be done with cytology through fine needle aspiration, which is now the method of choice for the assessment of a thyroid nodule based on clinical features that recommend its cytologic identification, generally now in preference to one of the shadow producing procedures, since much more value is added than a confirmation that the mass can be imaged.

723. It comes as a surprise to many who are accustomed to the staging systems for adenocarcinomas elsewhere that cervical lymph node involvement does not change papillary thyroid cancer staging. The prognosis is not impaired by lymph node involvement, and lymph node status does not significantly alter treatment. That the nodes were found to be involved is likely because they were taken with the thyroidectomy specimen, and residual cellular disease not excised is likely to be ablated by radioiodine follow-up in the absence of the "iodine sink" when the thyroid is gone. This treatment does not need to be combined with radical neck dissection, and this therapy would result in excess of 90% disease free survival long-term. These nodules are not invariably cold, although they tend to be, since differentiated thyroid cancer frequently concentrates iodine, and in fact, that is the basis of radioiodine follow-up therapy. This usually requires enhanced TSH, which also occurs naturally after thyroidectomy if thyroid replacement is withheld until radio-iodine adjunctive administration. Operation can be scheduled electively, and there is every reason to honor the patient's request, since there is negligible risk of tumor spread in the interval suggested.

724. Plummer's syndrome is the hyper-functioning of an autonomous nodule in a preexisting multinodular goiter. Since nearly all of the thyroid gland is involved with the multinodular goiter, this disqualifies this benign condition as it does *struma lymphomatosa* which is chronic thyroiditis of the Hashimoto type, affecting all parts of the thyroid in inflammation. Familial medullary thyroid carcinoma originates in both lobes wherever parafollicular C-cells are scattered in their multicentric malignant degeneration. Papillary carcinoma is more often than not multicentric, which is one of the rationales employed in advocating at least lobectomy and probably thyroidectomy to eradicate the other foci of the disease besides the primary presenting nodule. Of the lesions listed, only follicular carcinoma typically stands alone, and it may arise in an otherwise normal thyroid gland.

725. Medullary thyroid cancer originates from C-cells, which are parafollicular and do not iodinate thyronine. Therefore, whether inside or out of the thyroid in lymphatic or other locations, concentration of radioiodine does not occur and

radioiodine therapy for lymphatic metastases would be ineffective. It can occur in families, and when it does so, younger affected patients have nearly always multicentric disease. It can be found by stimulated release of calcitonin in response to calcium or pentagastrin through venous catheters positioned for sampling from potential metastatic sites. Its prognosis is much poorer than papillary carcinoma in even the most advanced stage of the latter in comparison with even earlier stages of the former, since spread is early and aggressive in most instances, and especially so in the hereditary type called MEA-IIB.

726. Because follicular carcinoma is associated with iodine deficiency, the widespread use of iodized salt in the United States has caused a remarkable decrease in the incidence of follicular cancer within this century. Unlike papillary carcinoma, in which multicentricity is the rule, follicular carcinomas are usually unifocal. They spread by capsular and vascular invasion, and lymphatic metas-tases are not a prominent method of metastases. The most common form of cancer discovered in patients who have reported head and neck irradiation is papillary carcinoma although follicular carcinomas may rarely be seen in such patients.

727. Anaplastic carcinoma is essentially an untreatable disease, with nearly uni-formly fatal outcome despite the treatments that have been tried. It spreads quickly and early and is not controlled by radioiodine, radiation or chemotherapy. Extensive surgical efforts have resulted in some relief of obstructive disease while tumor spread usually continues unchecked. In order of

232

malignant behavior, medullary thyroid carcinoma would be next worst, followed by follicular, lymphoma (which may present primarily in the thyroid gland) and papillary with the best prognosis.

728. In very fortunate contrast to other tumors such as sarcoma that might spread by the hematogenous route to fill the lungs with metastases, this form of thyroid cancer has a good prognosis, due largely to the "magic bullet" of iodine concentration in the thyroid tissue that can be further enhanced with the TSH stimulation that occurs naturally in hypothyroidism. This directed "smart weapon" is magnified in the "homing signal" provided by that iodine concentrating capacity that is evident in the uptake of this metastatic disease. It is unlikely to be present in small pulmonary nodules in the pattern of sarcoma spread, so bilateral thoracotomy for the purpose of metastatic wedge resection would be futile, and unnecessary given the superior treatment results with radioiodine. Cytotoxic chemotherapy has not proven effective in thyroid cancer and would not be given.

729. The biologic factors predominate in prognosis of thyroid cancers and many of them are "given" rather than controllable. The single most important is the patient's age, since if all other features were held constant, the younger patient has a better prognosis. Lymph node involvement, as previously noted, is not a principle factor in changing the staging of tumors of the same size, but size is a factor, and staging is principally determined by T-stage with much less contribution from N-staging. Differentiation of the tumor for a given cell type, such as papillary, is a significant prognostic factor for groups of patients, but

is not as significant as age. Since most of the patients have well differentiated tumors, it is also humbling to note that one prognostic factor absent as a principle determinant of how well patients do is treatment, about which each clinician carries such passionate belief that it is difficult to test treatment options to determine a superior method which we honestly do not know.

730. Hypothyroidism is a condition that may follow Graves' disease whether treated or not and by any means. The hypothyroidism that follows operation is usually within the period of postoperative follow-up, and is recognized and treated by replacement hormone. The hypothyroidism that follows radioiodine, if effective, is nearly inevitable but usually occurs much later than the follow-up period, and is often insidious and untreated. In fact, late hypothyroidism is the chief disadvantage of radioiodine therapy that does accomplish the control of hyperthyroidism without recurrence. One of the principle advantages to operation is its low incidence of hypothyroidism after surgical therapy, and operation should be preferred since drug-free follow-up and autoregulation of the pituitary-thyroid axis is possible. The surgical complications of hemorrhage, hypoparathyroidism from disturbance of the parathyroid glands or their blood supply, and dysfunction of either superior or recurrent laryngeal nerves is more likely to happen with surgery than radioiodine. However, it should be noted that recurrent laryngeal nerve palsy has happened following radioiodine treatment, and has been reported, even bilaterally, simply with intubation in a patient undergoing operation outside the neck or chest.

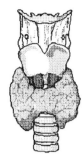

PARATHYROID SURGERY

Items 731-740

731. Which of the following statements is true concerning the parathyroid glands and is useful in identifying them in their embryologically possible ectopic positions?

(A) blood supply of the superior parathyroid usually originates from the superior thyroid artery, and the blood supply of the inferior parathyroid usually arises from the inferior thyroid artery

(B) the inferior parathyroid gland originates in association with a pharyngeal pouch superior to the superior parathyroid gland's origin

(C) neither superior nor inferior parathyroid glands descend into the neck if the thyroid doesn't

(D) the parathyroid is derived from neuroectoderm

(E) the parathyroid glands have no embryologic relationship to the thymus

732. Which of the following lesions is **LEAST** common?

(A) parathyroid cyst
(B) parathyroid hyperplasia
(C) chief cell adenoma
(D) parathyroid carcinoma
(E) oxyphil cell adenoma

733. The most typical presentation of the hypercalcemic patients proven by operation to have primary hyperparathyroidism currently is

(A) asymptomatic
(B) renal stones
(C) bone pain and radiographic evidence of resorption
(D) abdominal pain
(E) disorientation and change in personality

734. One unusual familial syndrome that may be confused with primary hyperparathyroidism which it closely mimics can be distinguished by urinary calcium determination in hypercalcemic patients. This syndrome is

(A) secondary hyperparathyroidism
(B) tertiary hyperparathyroidism
(C) sarcoidosis
(D) hypocalciuric hypercalcemia
(E) renal tubular acidosis

735. After the confident biochemical and endocrine confirmation of primary hyperparathyroidism in the hypercalcemic patient, which of the following studies is required before parathyroid exploration is first attempted?

(A) thallium-technetium scanning
(B) none
(C) ultrasonography
(D) thyrocervical angiography
(E) selective venous sampling for parathormone

736. Total thyroidectomy is an operation frequently carried out, but total parathyroidectomy should be avoided at some considerable effort. The principle reason for this is

(A) total parathyroidectomy has a much higher risk to the recurrent laryngeal nerves
(B) there is no satisfactory replacement for endogenous parathormone
(C) ablation of the parathyroid glands endangers the blood supply to the anterior cervical spinal cord
(D) parathyroidectomy is too technically difficult, and can only be done with an operating microscope
(E) cancer develops in the thyroid gland more frequently than in the parathyroid glands

737. Each of the following surgical procedures is appropriate for secondary hyperparathyroidism EXCEPT:

(A) excision of three and a half parathyroid glands
(B) excision of one large parathyroid gland and biopsy of a second
(C) reduction of all discoverable parathyroid tissue down to approximately 100 mg in residual well vascularized tissue
(D) total parathyroidectomy from all cervical and mediastinal locations and autograft of small portions of one gland in forearm muscle
(E) renal transplantation and observation to see if secondary hyperparathyroidism resolves

738. In all patients in the US who might be demonstrated to have hypercalcemia, the single most prevalent cause is

(A) primary hyperparathyroidism
(B) secondary hyperparathyroidism
(C) malignancy
(D) milk-alkali syndrome
(E) hyperthyroidism

739. The most frequent cause of failure of a primary cervical exploration to correct primary hyperparathyroidism is

(A)   regrowth of subtotally resected parathyroid tissue in secondary hyperparathyroidism
(B)   parathyroidosis
(C)   parathyroid carcinoma
(D)   failure to appreciate multiple gland disease
(E)   familial hypocalciuric hypercalcemia

740. Postoperative hypocalcemia immediately following parathyroid exploration strongly suggests which of the following is true?

(A)   the surgeon has probably excised or devascularized all the parathyroid tissue
(B)   if the patient is asymptomatic, low calcium numbers are not treated, but uncomfortable complaints are managed with calcium replacement
(C)   this condition is an indication for parathyroid allograft
(D)   the patient should receive vitamin D treatment as soon as the serum calcium fall below 10 mg/dl
(E)   unlike hypercalcemia, bone or joint discomfort is *not* a clinical feature in this form of hypocalcemia

ANSWERS AND TUTORIALS ON ITEMS 731-740

The answers are: **731-B; 732-D; 733-A; 734-D; 735-B; 736-B; 737-B; 738-C; 739-D; 740-B.**

731. The parathyroid glands peregrinate around the neck and mediastinum in embryologic development, but they have to carry their blood supply with them, and usually they have a predictable pattern of unpredictability in location. The search for the anatomically possible position, is helped by knowing which gland it is that appears missing. The inferior parathyroid gland has actually descended further from its embryologic origin, and sometimes does not stop in the customary position, but continues on down into the thymic tongue into the mediastinum. When it does so, its blood supply can frequently be identified as a tether dragged behind it, branching from the inferior thyroid artery. The inferior thyroid artery supplies both superior and inferior parathyroid glands, and typically the side on which an enlarged parathyroid gland is located is quickly approximated by the relative size of the inferior thyroid arteries. An enlarged gland also has an enlarged feeding vessel, and it is helpful to follow such an apparent vessel bound into the mediastinum in the event that the inferior parathyroid gland is missing. It is also surgically significant that the chest does not need to be opened, since the arterial control will remain in the neck at the level of the inferior thyroid artery while teasing back the wayward parathyroid gland from its mediastinal hiding place.

732. In the United States, parathyroid carcinoma is remarkably rare, at least as it may present as hyperparathyroidism. It is rarer still when the criterion of diagnosis is metastatic disease that can cause the patient's death. For some reason, there is a much higher incidence in Japan, although some would doubt the clinical significance of this because of the use of different histopathologic criteria. Parathyroid cyst is somewhat more common if the degenerated adenomas with cystic features following involution, often accompanied by hypercalcemic crises, are added. Oxyphil adenoma is rare, and the majority of hyperparathyroidism is based in chief cell hyperplasia. Both hyperplastic oxyphil cell and chief cell tissue cannot be distinguished in a single specimen from a process called adenoma in one gland. In the confusion between the terms two gland hyperplasia or double adenomas becomes futile. The best description for hyperfunctioning parathyroid tissue is that it exists in single or multiple gland disease.

733. Hyperparathyroidism is now nearly uniformly found as an incidental biochemical abnormality on screening blood examination. It is probably the most valuable yield of the multichannel autoanalyzer, since hypercalcemia is always worth investigation for discovery of diseases that are either treatable, significant with respect to prognosis, or when correction would prevent further problems. The old mnemonic "stones, bones, moans, and abdominal groans" defines the past pattern of advance stage disease which brought patients to have these complaints investigated. Retrospectively, there is some insidious loss of capability (forgetfulness, headache, many features attributed to advancing age) that are only recognized by

their absence when hyperparathyroidism is relieved. However, the minority of patients now present with one of the major complications, and asymptomatic population screening with a rapid, relatively inexpensive and reliable method has found the indicators that are proven to be related to the illness. These findings in asymptomatic patients raise the question of whether the disease is being treated in advance of its appearance other than by biochemical markers when it might not ever cause symptomatic disease. This is often resolved in favor of operation for those with an arbitrarily selected higher value of serum calcium concentration than for those with lower levels of elevation, unless any early clinical features appear to be developing.

734. A familial syndrome has been discovered in patients who have had failed parathyroid explorations for persistent hypercalcemia, until it is found that they have lower urinary excretion of calcium based in a higher "setpoint" for renal threshold for circulating calcium. Hyperparathyroidism is appropriate stimulation of the parathyroid glands, usually from chronic renal failure and hyperphosphatemia. If such patients are transplanted and renal failure resolves, persistent hyperparathyroidism is referred to as tertiary when the reactive hyperparathyroidism of secondary form turns autonomous. Sarcoidosis is, in effect, a hypersensitivity to vitamin D, and renal tubular acidosis is part of the differential diagnosis of hypercalcemia, but has none of the other features of hyperparathyroidism.

735. Of the most sensitive tests for identifying the surgical objective — that is normal or suppressed parathyroid glands which may be much smaller than any radiographic imaging threshold — the primary surgical exploration is the only method that is satisfactory in all and successful in most. The reliability of each radiographic method listed is less than that of most experienced surgeons, and considerably less than experienced endocrine surgeons who are frequently called upon to perform re-exploratory surgery. In these instances, imaging and selective sampling can be most helpful in limiting exploration, not only to find the hyperfunctioning parathyroid tissue, but what is more important to the long-term benefit of the patient, to avoid destruction of residual parathyroid tissue that might be restored to normal function. None of the imaging tests are needed before primary cervical exploration, and a selective approach to only those tests needed to guide re-exploration is appropriate for re-operative work.

736. A patient who is aparathyroid is suffering a crippling disorder with continuous requirement of vitamin D and calcium to inadequately maintain a serum calcium always dangerously close to tetany levels. The other technical and biologic reasons listed are trivial for the technical reasons and false in the biologic assertions. It is true that thyroid cancer is more prevalent than parathyroid cancer, but that would not mean total ablation of all parathyroid glands, since it is usually a unifocal disease, and ablation of the other parathyroids does not enhance the uptake of any given treatment directed at the parathyroid. Total parathyroidectomy or its functional equivalent by interrupting its blood supply is altogether too easy, and is sometimes unintentionally performed in total thyroidectomy (which might more

appropriately be called a "parathyroid preservation procedure").

737. Secondary hyperparathyroidism is a disease in which all glands should be appropriately responding to the hyper-phosphortemia by hyperplasia. It is, simply, multiglandular disease, so the search for a single hyperfunctioning gland and confirmation of the presence of another is — as it would be in most instances of primary hyperparathyroidism that are sporadic (except — notably — any familial disease) — inappropriate treatment in secondary hyperparathyroidism. Two of the responses show reduction of the excessive parathyroid tissue down to a level that should give function without hyperfunction — one of those leaving half of one gland, and the other attempting to leave at least two sites on intact vasculature but not to exceed 100 mg in total. In very experienced hands, total para-thyroidectomy with careful preservation and transplantation techniques have been able to eradicate parathyroid tissue from the neck, and place it in a position where it can not only "take", but in many instances, again become hyperplastic and result in hyperfunction, but in this instance can be reduced by re-excision of the implanted fragments under local anesthesia as an outpatient. It is also possible to treat secondary hyperparathyroidism expectantly, if the primary stimulus to its hyperplastic stimulus response is corrected as with transplantation. If the hyperfunction continues after phosphate clearances improve, this situation is referred to as tertiary hyperparathyroidism, and in this instance of autonomy is treated, once again, as primary hyperparathyroidism.

738. Hypercalcemia is a common and vexing complication of some of the most common types of visceral malignancy, and shortens life and increases morbidity in patients who suffer from it. This especially includes breast cancer, but may also include lung cancer, hypernephroma, prostate cancer, each representing tumors with a predilection for bone metastases. It is for this reason that it was stated earlier that hypercalcemia is always a significant pickup on multichannel blood tests, in this instance because of its prognostic significance and management requirement rather that potential for cure. Most patients with secondary hyperparathyroidism would not be suffering from an unknown condition since most of them are on dialysis. Sarcoidosis and milk-alkali syndrome can give hypercalcemia, and hyperthyroidism can also. One group of patients in whom the hypercalcemia may be the first indication of any illness since they are otherwise asymptomatic would be the patients with primary hyperparathyroidism, and this group runs a close second behind malignancy in prevalence in hypercalcemic patients.

739. Multiple gland disease that is treated as though it were primary hyperparathyroidism based in single gland pathology is the source of failure in most primary cervical explorations that do not control hypercalcemia. The patient who is at risk for this undertreatment is the patient with secondary hyperparathyroidism in which there may be supernumerary glands, that is, more than the four identified and three and a half that were excised. This is nearly always the case in familial hyperparathyroidism, since multiple gland disease is the rule. If the first enlarged parathyroid encountered is removed, and another less imposing gland identified as "normal", this patient will have recurrence, if not persistence. Persistence is referred to as hypercalcemia that is present within six months of the operation (usually it is obvious on the same day) and recurrence refers to hypercalcemia that follows operation by more than six months during which hypercalcemia is absent. Parathyroid carcinoma may spread and hyperfunction, but it is rare to begin with, and rarer still that it would be a source of persistent hypercalcemia. FHH might be a source of failure when operation is done on a propositus of a kindred as yet unknown, but testing urinary calcium clearance in this patient should identify hypercalcemic relatives who have the same problem. As yet, this syndrome — although reported in many families — is cumulatively not large enough to account for a clinically significant number of primary parathyroid operation failures.

740. The very hypocalcemia that is expected to result from excision of a large hyperfunctioning parathyroid gland is the signal that would stimulate the hypoplastic parathyroids to recover function normally, so early treatment of hypocalcemia in the absence of patient symptoms is not indicated because it may protract recovery of residual parathyroid secretion. There is a syndrome of postparathyroidectomy arthritis due to pseudogout, so that paradoxically the bone pain that was said to be symptomatic of hypercalcemia may be a complication of its correction early in the hypocalcemic course. It is not likely that all the parathyroid tissue has been destroyed, although that is a remote possibility, and will only be determined when the parathormone secretion doesn't return after a period of hypocalcemic stimulus. Vitamin D therapy would be unnecessary, and would be called for only if a patient required calcium supplementation and that was inadequate alone to relieve hypocalcemic symptoms.

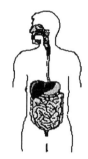

ESOPHAGEAL SURGERY

Items 741-750

741. The one type of hiatal hernia for which operation is indicated based on its demonstrated presence is

   (A) sliding hiatal hernia
   (B) para-esophageal hiatal hernia
   (C) "short esophagus"
   (D) Barrett's esophagitis
   (E) hiatal hernia with reflux esophagitis

742. A sensitive diagnostic test for clinical determination of symptomatic reflux esophagitis is

   (A) barium swallow
   (B) esophageal manometry
   (C) esophagoscopy
   (D) Bernstein's test
   (E) compression of abdomen or tilt test

743. Medical management of symptomatic reflux esophagitis includes each of the following **EXCEPT**:

   (A) bedblocks tilting the bed to elevate the head
   (B) aspirin
   (C) antacids
   (D) metoclopramide
   (E) H_2-receptor antagonists

744. Which of the following operations wraps the lower esophagus with a cuff of stomach in fundoplication?

   (A) Belsey (Mark IV)
   (B) Allison
   (C) Nissen
   (D) Hill
   (E) Collis

745. Which of the following esophageal abnormalities is premalignant?

   (A) reflux esophagitis
   (B) Barrett's esophagitis
   (C) presbyesophagus
   (D) scleroderma
   (E) alkaline stricture

746. Survival following optimum therapy for esophageal carcinoma three years after treatment is reported to be

   (A) greater than 90%
   (B) 75%
   (C) 50%
   (D) 25%
   (E) less than 5%

240

747. Of the anatomic layers of the esophagus, which statement is true for the serosal layer?

(A) it is effective in temporarily halting the spread of carcinoma
(B) it lubricates the esophageal thoracic mobility during swallowing
(C) it is useful in suturing anastomoses to the esophageal stump
(D) it helps seal perforations or leaks that may develop in the esophagus
(E) it does not exist

748. The treatment recommended as primary therapy for bleeding esophageal varices is

(A) endoscopic sclerotherapy
(B) the Tanner operation — esophageal transection
(C) mesocaval shunt
(D) splenorenal shunt
(E) devascularization of varices over the cardia and hiatus

749. Flexible esophagogastroduoden-oscopy (EGD) is a contraindicated primary procedure in which of the following?

(A) bleeding esophageal varices
(B) burns from recent lye ingestion
(C) actively bleeding duodenal ulcer
(D) scleroderma
(E) malignant gastric ulcer

750. A 32 year-old woman complains of difficulty swallowing, foul breath, and regurgitation of undigested food. Her most likely diagnosis is

(A) esophageal cancer
(B) achalasia
(C) Zenker's diverticulum (pulsion)
(D) esophageal stenosis from reflux esophagitis
(E) traction diverticulum

ANSWERS AND TUTORIALS ON ITEMS 741-750

The answers are: **741-B; 742-D; 743-B; 744-C; 745-B; 746-E; 747-E; 748-A; 749-B; 750-C**.

741. Para-esophageal hernia is the presence of a portion of the stomach through the diaphragm in the chest adjacent to the esophagus. The stomach may become incarcerated with considerable discomfort and risk of infarction of the strangulated stomach. This is attended with very high risk of hemorrhage. The presence of a para-esophageal hernia is an indication for its surgical correction; whereas, a sliding esophageal hiatal hernia, even one with some reflux esophagitis, is treated medically. The hernia is not the indication for operation but significant complications of it may be. Short esophagus is a term used for one contracted from prolonged esophagitis. Barrett's esophagitis is ulceration in the esophagus due to an ectopic patch of gastric mucosa that is secreting and causing erosion of adjacent esophageal mucosa. The only condition requiring urgent repair is the demonstrated presence of a para-esophageal hiatal hernia.

742. The Bernstein's test is the placement of a distal esophageal catheter and a dilute solution of hydrochloric acid is instilled through it. If the acid instillation reproduces the patient's clinical symptoms, the patient's complaint is likely related to esophageal reflux of gastric acid. Upper GI series cannot demonstrate symptomatic findings, and are sensitive only to later stages in esophageal mucosal inflammation. Esophagoscopy is more sensitive in determining the degree of esophagitis, but cannot conclusively prove the etiology of the esophagitis. Esophageal manometry is helpful in determining motility disorders, and can demonstrate sphincter incompetence at the lower esophagus. But manometry cannot demonstrate the clinical results of what this acid infusion test may be.

743. Elevation of the head of the bed or avoiding constricting garments or posture that increase intra-abdominal pressure or not lying down until several hours have passed since meals each give hydrostatic advantage to prevent reflux. To decrease acidity of the gastric contents, antacids or H_2-receptor antagonists are helpful. Metoclopramide (Reglan) may stimulate sphincter competence. Alcohol reduces sphincter tone, and would make reflux more likely, particularly when taken in association with meals when pressure in the gastric lumen is higher or between meals when the acid present in the stomach is more concentrated. Aspirin is itself an acid irritant to the mucosa, and would be contraindicated.

744. Each of the operations listed by the name of the promoter for the procedure attempts to fix the stomach in intra-abdominal position: by suturing crura of the diaphragm (Allison), to the median arcuate ligament (Hill), by gastropexy posteriorly (Collis), or pulling the esophagus and its junction with the stomach down into the abdomen (Belsey). In the Nissen fundoplication, a wrap of the gastric fundus is sutured around the lower esophagus (which is stinted with a bougie) to prevent reflux, but over-correcting may make it difficult for the patient to belch, preventing either fluid — air or liquid — return from stomach to esophagus.

745. In the case of Barrett's esophagitis, columnar metaplasia is chronic that may lead to adenocarcinoma. Esophageal stricture whether from acid reflux or from a lye burn is a fibrosing stenosis which is non-malignant but highly symptomatic. Presbyesophagus results in a motility disorder as does scleroderma, but the one most clearly associated with adeno-carcinoma is Barrett's esophagitis.

746. Esophageal carcinoma, even under optimal treatment is a miserable disease with a very poor prognosis. With such dismal results, improvements in therapy are less likely to be expected to yield satisfying patient salvage as much as methods of prevention, since these results reflect that in all honesty there is no treatment for esophageal carcinoma despite best efforts applied to it with what information is available presently.

747. The anatomic feature about the esophagus that is distinct from many other components of the gastrointestinal tract lower down, is that it lacks a serosal layer, which is biologically significant as well as technically a handicap in esophageal operations. Without a serosa, there is no barrier to early spread of malignancy through the mediastinum or at least temporary containment of leakage or a flap that might seal perforations. The absence of the serosa is a very significant anatomic fact with clinical implications for esophageal disorders.

748. Immediate control of bleeding esophageal varices can best be obtained by approaching them directly, and endoscopic identification of them can be followed by some form of hemostatic procedure, either sclerotherapy or laser fulguration. The other means listed attempt to decompress the portal circulation so as to decrease the pressure head on the varices in the esophagus that are bleeding or by disconnecting them from the remainder of the portal system, mesocaval or splenorenal shunting achieving the former, and esophageal transection or devascularization attempting the latter. Mortality of such major operations in patients in such urgent crisis is forbidding, and esophagoscopy is a less morbid procedure.

749. Fiberendoscopy is a very useful procedure that has become widely employed as a primary diagnostic and sometimes therapeutic intervention in many upper GI disorders, since it can retrieve both information and definitive sampling for diagnosis as well as control some forms of bleeding. However, in the acute phase after corrosive lye ingestion, the esophageal injury is a friable mushy mixture of inflammation and necrosis that could be readily perforated with the semirigid endoscope and the introduction of any stiff instrument or foreign body into

the injured esophagus under these circumstances is contraindicated.

750. A pulsion diverticulum develops at the junction of the decussation in pharyngeal musculature with the esophagus in the cervical proximal extension of the esophagus, and this posterior diverticulum often fills with food after swallowing. It may become filled with foul smelling food and not empty while in the act of esophageal contraction which closes the diverticular opening. Because of the difficulty it may give in the clinical symptoms described, it is frequently either excised or tacked up so as to empty appropriately into the esophagus in the act of swallowing. Esophageal carcinoma is much more likely in a patient with severe symptoms and at a more advanced age, and the same would be true with respect to severity of symptoms at a younger age for esophageal stenosis or achalasia. The traction diverticulum is most likely due to an inflammatory event and scarring in the adjacent mediastinum as might be the case with tuberculosis or other focal reaction, and would not give the same complex of symptoms seen in this instance.

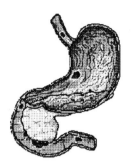

GASTRIC SURGERY

Items 751-760

751. Which is the correct statement regarding the vagus nerves?

   (A) they are sympathetic trunks
   (B) the right vagus nerve is anterior on the stomach
   (C) the left vagus nerve is posterior on the stomach
   (D) both vagal trunks send fibers along the lesser curve to the distal stomach
   (E) vagal stimulation inhibits parietal cell acid secretion

752. Which of these therapeutic maneuvers remarkably increases the likelihood of recurrent ulcer?

   (A) high, subtotal gastrectomy
   (B) retained antrum connected to duodenum
   (C) prolonged treatment with ranitidine
   (D) prolonged treatment with omeprazole
   (E) prolonged antacid administration with alkali

753. Duodenal ulcer is a likely event in patients with

   (A) gastrinoma
   (B) gastric carcinoma
   (C) pernicious anemia
   (D) pancreatic cholera (WDHA)
   (E) truncal vagotomy

754. Each of the following are advantages of superselective (parietal cell) vagotomy **EXCEPT**:

   (A) no gastric drainage procedure is necessary
   (B) incidence of diarrhea is reduced
   (C) vagal innervation of biliary tree is not impaired
   (D) no anastomotic suture lines required with risk of leak
   (E) ulcer recurrence rate is abolished

755. Which of these statements is **NOT** true of dumping syndrome?

   (A) it is unlikely with a functioning intact pylorus
   (B) dizziness, palpitations and flushing are common clinical features
   (C) it would be less likely to occur in the prolonged fasting state
   (D) it usually resolves untreated over a short time
   (E) operation is sometimes required to take down the gastric connections to the lower gut

756. Which is the **LEAST** likely cause for upper gastrointestinal bleeding in the patient with known chronic alcoholism?

(A)   gastrinoma
(B)   duodenal ulcer
(C)   gastric mucosal tears (Mallory-Weiss)
(D)   gastroesophageal varices
(E)   erosive gastritis

757. Which of the following studies is most likely to make the diagnosis of a malignant ulcer in gastric carcinoma?

(A)   barium upper GI contrast
(B)   CT scan
(C)   nonhealing on three weeks of treatment
(D)   gastroscopic biopsy
(E)   random nasogastric aspirate for cytology

758. Which of these findings indicates a resection for curative intent in a gastric tumor?

(A)   lower peritoneal mass palpable by rectal exam
(B)   malignant nodule in umbilicus
(C)   gastroscopic biopsy of lymphoma
(D)   malignant ascites
(E)   positive supraclavicular lymph node

759. Which of the following is **NOT** a risk factor for gastric cancer?

(A)   alcoholism
(B)   Oriental race
(C)   blood group O
(D)   pernicious anemia
(E)   smokers

760. Which of the following post-operative supportive measures is **NOT** indicated following total gastrectomy?

(A)   vitamin B-12 replacement
(B)   chloride repletion
(C)   frequent small high calorie feedings
(D)   monitoring of hemoglobin for anemia
(E)   clinical monitoring for metastatic disease

ANSWERS AND TUTORIALS ON ITEMS 751-760

The answers are: **751-D; 752-B; 753-A; 754-E; 755-D; 756-A; 757-D; 758-C; 759-C; 760-B.**

751. The right vagus nerve runs posteriorly and the left vagus nerve anteriorly on the surface of the stomach, but both contribute fibers called "nerves of Latarjet" along the lesser curvature to the distal stomach. The vagus nerve is parasympathetic, and stimulation causes parietal cells to increase acid secretion.

752. Excision of the major portion of the acid secreting stomach reduces the likelihood of ulcer, as do protracted treatments with antacids of alkali, H_2-receptor antagonists, or proton-pump inhibition. However, if antrum is left in contact with duodenum following stomach resection, the physiologic situation called the "Mann-Williamson preparation" exists in which chronic antral gastrin release gives a near inevitability of peptic ulcer recurrence. It is for that reason that many gastric resections are designed for antral exclusion or resection.

753. Patients with pernicious anemia frequently have associated atrophic gastritis with a failure of gastric acid secretion. This is also true for the syndrome known as pancreatic cholera or "watery diarrhea, hypokalemia, and achlorhydria" with which patients also produce less acid. Truncal vagotomy would interrupt the cephalic phase of gastric acid stimulation and gastrectomy would eliminate the acid producing cells, making duodenal ulcer very unlikely.

Patients with gastrinoma (Zollinger-Ellison syndrome) have a sustained autonomous secretion of gastrin which makes peptic ulceration very likely, since whatever parietal cells are present will be under constant stimulation. It is for that reason that total gastrectomy was suggested as a treatment for Zollinger-Ellison syndrome, since if there is "no acid, no ulcer".

754. Selective vagotomy allows other viscera to have intact vagal innervation so that diarrhea incidence is less, and biliary innervation is preserved, although this latter is of questionable significance. Superselective vagotomy denervates only parietal cells in its intent, and therefore motor nerves to the antrum should be spared and no gastric drainage procedure

would be necessary. In fact, no entry into the gut is required, and no anastomotic suture lines would be subject to risk.

However, parietal cell vagotomy may require a meticulous procedure that could be incomplete, and this may lead to complications from over-zealous interruption of nerve and vascular supply to the lesser curve and may cause a vascular necrosis of the lesser curvature of the stomach, or less than adequate interruption of all the fibers may lead to recurrence of the ulcer from incomplete denervation.

755. Dumping syndrome occurs when there is a rapid entry of hypertonic gastric contents into the duodenum or jejunum, which is, therefore, very unlikely if the pylorus is present and functioning. If it is bypassed, hypotension may occur from the dilution occasioned by the osmotic load in the gut, and flushing and palpitations are common. Because of the anatomic rerouting of the gastric contents, the syndrome typically does not go away, and is not accommodated within a short period of time from the gastric resection.

Medical therapy is generally successful in ameliorating the condition by decreasing carbohydrates and anticholin-ergic treatment as well as careful monitoring of fluid intake so as not to drink during meals to allow greater time for gastric mixing. The syndrome does not occur in the fasting state. Only rarely are symptoms so severe and unmanageable that takedown of the gastric bypass is required or a slower mixing of gastric contents engineered by adding resistance to outflow by a reversed antiperistaltic loop of gut.

756. The patient with chronic alcoholism usually has some degree of cirrhosis and portal hypertension. The latter accounts for the likelihood of varices and their propensity to bleed. However, the cirrhosis also decreases histaminase activity in the liver, and all foodstuffs or the blood itself in the gastrointestinal tract will be absorbed and, with its histamines, be absorbed into the portal circulation where the histamine is deaminated in the liver. If the liver is impaired in this process and there is shunting of the histamine to the systemic circulation, the patient is under chronic histamine stimulation for gastric acid production and duodenal ulcer or gastritis may result.

Vomiting is frequently a problem, and the recurrent retching and vomiting may give rise to Mallory-Weiss tears of the gastric lining. Gastrinoma is rare and would have no higher incidence in the alcoholic than is the population at large.

757. Nonhealing of an ulcer on appropriate therapy may be suggestive of malignancy, but is also a property of persistent or recurrent ulcer diathesis. Random gastric fluid sampling for cytologic examination may get lucky with some identification if food particles, blood and other degenerating debris do not confuse sampling, but gastric brushing gives better cytology and gastric biopsy gives the definitive diagnosis. Both barium radiography and CT would only give suggestions as to characteristic shape, but the definitive procedure for differentiation is gastric biopsy.

758. The implants within the peritoneum or at distant sites have been described as contraindications: the supraclavicular lymph node (Virchow's node), the "Blumer's shelf" palpable by rectal exam, or the "Sister Mary Joseph's node" in the umbilicus or malignant ascites detected by paracentesis are all contraindications for curative exploration. In contrast, a diagnosis of lymphoma by gastroscopy is actually a helpful sign, since gastrectomy for lymphoma rather than adenocarcinoma has a much better prognosis following surgical attempt at cure.

759. The highest incidence of gastric cancer is seen in Japan and the Orient, and it is highest in lower socioeconomic groups with a high intake of alcohol and tobacco. Pernicious anemia patients have low acid secretion and are at higher risk. It is blood group A that is associated with a higher incidence, and other evidence of genetic linkage is two to six times the risk in a positive family history.

760. One of the principle problems following gastrectomy is maintenance of a normal hemoglobin, since vitamin B-12 absorption is made possible by intrinsic factor and can be replaced with vitamin B-12 administration. It is frequently difficult to maintain weight in the absence of the stomach, since the capacitance for food intake is reduced, and dumping or diarrhea may follow as well. Frequent feeding and a check on the caloric intake is important nutritional follow-up, and there should be monitoring to differentiate the weight loss and cachexia of metastatic recurrent disease from that of nutritional crippling from the absence of the stomach. There is no need to replace chloride, since it is not being secreted by the stomach, and in any event when secreted when the stomach is present, it is reabsorbed, so there is no net loss of this abundant anion in the changes following gastrectomy.

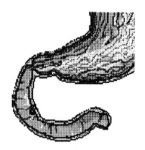

DUODENAL SURGERY

Items 761-770

761. Which is the **LEAST** likely cause of duodenal obstruction that might be expected to be encountered in the patient with gastric outlet obstruction?

   (A)   primary duodenal carcinoma
   (B)   pancreatic carcinoma
   (C)   duodenal stenosis from healed ulcer
   (D)   benign polyp or leiomyoma
   (E)   benign or malignant biliary pathology encroaching on the duodenum

762. Duodenal obstruction in the newborn is **LEAST** likely to be associated with which of the following?

   (A)   pyloric stenosis
   (B)   duodenal web
   (C)   annular pancreas
   (D)   bowel malrotation
   (E)   ulceration and stenosis

763. Which of the following characteristics of an anterior perforating duodenal ulcer is **LEAST** likely?

   (A)   exsanguinating hemorrhage
   (B)   rigid board-like abdomen
   (C)   abrupt onset in a previously well unsuspecting patient
   (D)   normal amylase
   (E)   an acute abdominal emergency

764. A 32 year-old patient with known duodenal ulcer under treatment becomes pale, sweaty and faint. His abdominal X-ray shows no free air, but he has epigastric tenderness and an amylase of 850 mg/dl. The most likely urgent crisis he faces is

   (A)   fulminant pancreatitis
   (B)   peritoneal soilage and peritonitis
   (C)   life-threatening hemorrhage
   (D)   pancreatic pseudocyst
   (E)   gastric outlet obstruction

765. Afferent loop syndrome is **LEAST** likely to result in which of the following complications?

   (A)   recurrent ulcer
   (B)   duodenal stump blowout
   (C)   bacterial overgrowth
   (D)   bloating from distention and necrosis
   (E)   carcinogenesis

766. Which of the following neoplasms is **MOST** frequently sited in the duodenum?

    (A)   primary adenocarcinoma
    (B)   gastrinoma
    (C)   metastatic colonic adenocarcinoma
    (D)   lymphoma
    (E)   leiomyosarcoma

767. Duodenal mucosa does **NOT** secrete which of the following?

    (A)   hydrochloric acid
    (B)   gastrin
    (C)   secretin
    (D)   cholecystokinin
    (E)   enterogastrone

768. In a gastroduodenostomy (Billroth I) complications may result, including all of the following **EXCEPT**:

    (A)   afferent loop syndrome
    (B)   alkaline reflux gastritis
    (C)   duodenal ulcer recurrence
    (D)   dumping
    (E)   gastric stasis

769. Which of the following stimulations to gastric acid secretion is **NOT** mediated by histamine and cannot be blocked by H_2-receptor antagonists?

    (A)   cephalic phase
    (B)   gastric phase
    (C)   duodenal G cells
    (D)   gastrin from pancreatic islet cells
    (E)   intestinal phase

770. Which of the following agents does **NOT** break down the mucosal barrier to back-diffusion of H^+?

    (A)   alcohol
    (B)   prostaglandin
    (C)   salicylates
    (D)   bile salts
    (E)   potassium concentration

ANSWERS AND TUTORIALS ON ITEMS 761-770

The answers are: **761-A; 762-E; 763-A; 764-C; 765-E; 766-B; 767-A; 768-A; 769-E; 770-B**.

761. The malignant potential obstruction in the duodenum is that of surrounding organ primary disease, since malignancy in the duodenum is the lowest in frequency of any primary site along the gastrointestinal tract. Benign strictures of the duodenum may take place from inflammation and recurrent fibrotic healing with stenosis that results, most frequently from duodenal ulcer, but may be from biliary or pancreatic origin as well. The most frequent carcinomas that give rise to gastric outlet obstruction, are those that originate in the pancreas.

762. The congenital causes of duodenal obstruction are anatomic abnormalities that are first noted after birth such as duodenal web, atresia, or annular pancreas, or the anatomic derangement from a failure of fusion fascia that normally situate the abdominal viscera that results in mal-rotation and "Ladd's bands". Pyloric stenosis is acquired later in life of the infant when it is detected a month or more after birth, but duodenal ulceration would be very unlikely, and chronicity of such an ulcer to the point of fibrotic stenosis would be unheard of, making ulcerative stenosis the least likely cause of gastric outlet obstruction of the newborn.

763. Posterior penetrating duodenal ulcers bleed. Anterior duodenal ulcers perforate. The latter give a previously well patient an abrupt catastrophic intra-abdominal emergency with peritonitis as gastric contents flood the peritoneum and a board-like rigid abdomen results. The posterior penetrating ulcer is usually a more chronic phenomenon in which the ulceration is known or suspected previously, and erodes back into the pancreas giving pancreatitis and the erosive enzymatic digestion of very large visceral blood vessels that can cause exsanguination.

764. The posterior penetrating ulcer has reached this patient's pancreas causing the pancreatitis and the elevated amylase. Both fulminant pancreatitis and its much later sequel of pancreatic pseudocyst are manageable in most instances, as would be gastric outlet obstruction. It is unlikely that he will perforate, since the posterior location of the ulcer makes communication with the free peritoneum unlikely with a lesser risk of peritonitis.

The biggest threat to life in this individual is the proximity of the major blood supply in this area, the gastro-duodenal and the pancreaticoduodenal arteries which lie in the inflammatory mass of autodigestive enzymes and gastric acid output. The hemorrhage that results from disruption of these vessels is catastrophic, and requires treatment — even in advance of precise diagnosis — and such a patient

is taken to the operating room, not for radiographic or endoscopic confirmation, since abrupt loss of half or more of the blood volume over a short period of time is not coming from mucosal origin alone. Life-threatening hemorrhage is the risk associated with posterior penetration of duodenal ulcer.

765. The afferent loop in a Billroth-II reconstruction following partial gastrectomy may become obstructed at the gastrojejunal stoma, and the afferent loop may become distended. This distention can give stasis with bacterial overgrowth.

The duodenal stump may blow out if pressure buildup occurs and recurrent ulceration and necrosis are possible. Although each of these significant complications is part of the afferent loop syndrome, none are implicated in malignant degeneration, and the long-term risk of cancer in the afferent loop syndrome is not a problem.

766. The duodenum is a site remarkable in the GI tract for its low incidence of adenocarcinoma. However, there are other secretory cells in the mucosa, and some of these are endocrine. These endocrine cells may become the site of excessive gastrin secretion. As many as 10% or more of patients with Zollinger-Ellison syndrome may have a duodenal gastrinoma. Lymphoma is possible in the duodenum but not at a higher rate than anywhere along the gastrointestinal tract, and adenocarcinoma from the colon is rarely metastatic in this site preferring travel along lymphatics in the mesentery. Leiomyosarcoma is possible wherever smooth muscle is present, but is very rare in general, and exceedingly so in the duodenum.

767. The enteroendocrine cells located within the duodenum can produce many peptides and do so in physiologic response to duodenal filling when secretin, gastrin, and cholecystokinin are released and enterogastrone inhibits rapid emptying of the stomach. The mucosal goblet cells produce exocrine secretions of mucus, but there are no parietal cells that secrete hydrochloric acid. There may be ectopic "rests" along the gastrointestinal tract at embryologic sites such as the Meckel's diverticulum that contain gastric mucosa and can secrete hydrochloric acid, but these are not typically found in the duodenum. The duodenum is sensitive to hydrochloric acid in high concentrations, and for that reason direct anastomosis with gastric acid secreting cells without the pylorus in between or without modification of the parietal cell secretion of hydrochloric acid is injurious to the duodenum and may give rise to recurrent ulceration.

768. The Billroth I gastroduodenostomy directly connects the stump of the stomach to the duodenum, end-to-end in most instances, without an afferent loop as exists with Billroth II gastrojejunostomy. Because the pylorus is destroyed, dumping is possible, and because the anastomosis may be in the area that has been inflamed previously or might become so with recurrent ulcer disease possible, stenosis and gastric stasis may result in some instances. Because the biliary input now has retrograde access into the stomach, alkaline reflux gastritis is possible. Of the complications listed, the only one not possible is the afferent loop syndrome since there is no afferent loop in gastroduodenostomy.

769. The cephalic phase of gastric acid stimulation is by vagal efferents which stimulate parietal cells and the G cells through histamine release. That same effect comes from gastrin whether from gastric, duodenal, or pancreatic islet origin, each of which have a histamine intermediary and therefore are capable of being blocked by an antihistamine that is antagonistic to H_2 receptors. The intestinal phase has another group of enteric endocrine peptides, not all of which are histamine intermediated, and therefore are not uniformly susceptible to interception with an H_2-receptor antagonist.

770. The mucosal barrier is sensitive to the H^+ secreted in highly concentrated form by the gastric parietal cells. That duodenal mucosa is further sensitive to the H^+ in the presence of alcohol, salicylate, and bile salts, and concentrated potassium may cause erosion as well. Prostaglandin has been used experimentally to improve the mucosal barrier and protect it from ulceration, and is a suggested future treatment for the peptic ulcer diathesis.

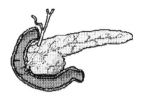

BILIARY TRACT SURGERY

Items 771-780

771. In a young nonjaundiced woman with right upper quadrant pain, nasogastric suction is begun with IV fluids pushed and an oral cholecystogram attempted by administration of telepaque (iodide complex) tablets, but no visualization is seen on radiography eight hours later. The most likely cause for these findings is

   (A) the elevation of the bilirubin
   (B) hepatic parenchymal disease
   (C) pancreatitis
   (D) gastric aspiration of the telepaque
   (E) choledocholithiasis

772. Each of the following treatments is indicated for acute obstructive biliary tract disease with cholangitis **EXCEPT**:

   (A) nasogastric aspiration
   (B) morphine analgesia
   (C) intravenous rehydration
   (D) symptomatic treatment for itching
   (E) intravenous antibiotics

773. Which of the following statements is true of the cystic artery in acute cholecystitis?

   (A) it is frequently congenitally absent
   (B) it is frequently thrombosed
   (C) it arises from the left hepatic artery
   (D) it is most often aberrant
   (E) it can be ignored in dissection of the gall bladder

774. Gallstone ileus is almost always associated with

   (A) hemoglobin pigment gallstones
   (B) a fistula eroded between biliary tree and gut
   (C) ascending infection originating in the ampulla
   (D) a traumatic blow to the right upper quadrant
   (E) megacolon

775. A 19 year-old woman complains of fever, abdominal and pelvic pain, and on physical examination has diffuse tenderness over the right upper quadrant. Her bilirubin is 1.0 mg/dl and her white blood count 23,000 cells/mm³. A likely diagnosis is

   (A) hepatitis
   (B) perihepatitis
   (C) acalculous cholecystitis
   (D) cholecystitis with cholesterol gallstones
   (E) gallstone ileus

776. Each of the following conditions may predispose to acalculous cholecystitis **EXCEPT:**

(A) hereditary spherocytosis
(B) typhoid fever
(C) diabetes mellitus
(D) cystic duct obstruction
(E) reflux from common channel

777. An increased output of bile from the liver and/or gall bladder is inhibited by

(A) the vagus nerves
(B) fasting
(C) secretin
(D) cholecystokinin
(E) bile salts

778. Which of the following treatments would increase the likelihood for cholecystitis?

(A) total parenteral nutrition
(B) overhydration
(C) choluretics
(D) low fat feeding
(E) oral medium chain triglycerides

779. A painless distended gallbladder palpable on physical examination of a jaundiced patient is strongly suggestive of

(A) empyema
(B) gallstone impacted in the cystic duct
(C) gallstone impacted in the ampulla at the sphincter of Oddi
(D) pancreatic carcinoma
(E) hepatitis

780. In a flatplate X-ray (KUB) looking for kidney stones, an incidentally noted calcific right upper quadrant opaque object is interpreted as a 2 cm gallstone in the gallbladder of which this 55 year-old otherwise healthy man is totally unaware. The appropriate treatment is

(A) schedule oral cholecystogram
(B) ^{99m}Tc HIDA scan
(C) laparoscopic cholecystectomy
(D) cholecystectomy by laparotomy and common duct exploration
(E) observation

ANSWERS AND TUTORIALS ON ITEMS 771-780

The answers are: **771-D; 772-B; 773-B; 774-B; 775-B; 776-A; 777-B; 778-A; 779-D; 780-E.**

771. In order for opacification of the gall bladder to take place, the iodinated contrast medium must be absorbed and circulate through the liver, where functioning hepatic parenchymal cells must excrete it, and it must be conducted to the gall bladder for water reabsorption and thus concentration of the contrast medium. It is true that inflammation of the gall bladder would interfere with this water reabsorption and nonvisualization would result, but each of the prior steps must take place for this conclusion to be drawn. The naso-gastric tube inserted for relief of the nausea and vomiting in biliary tract disease would remove any orally administered contrast medium to prevent its absorption even if it could be excreted and concentrated, and this example of nonvisualization is an artifact of treatment.

772. Bedrest and gut relaxation are important to the patient with biliary tract obstruction, so nasogastric evacuation and hospitalization are appropriate. Patients with hyperbilirubinemia frequently complain of itching, and symptomatic treatment is appropriate. Life threatening sepsis may result from cholangitis, and antibiotics are indicated. In contrast to relaxation of the gut, morphine causes increased contraction of the sphincter of Oddi. This analgesic, with its secondary histamine release properties, is contra-indicated in biliary tract obstruction; whereas, other analgesics such as meperidine may be appropriate.

773. In acute cholecystitis, inflammation can involve the blood supply of the gall bladder itself, and the arteritis frequently results in thrombosis of the cystic artery. This is an effect, rather than a cause, of cholecystitis since the gall bladder has collateral blood supply from the liver as well, and simple ligation of the cystic artery would be unlikely to result in necrosis of the gall bladder. However, in severe inflammation of the gall bladder, these collateral arterial supplies may also thrombose, and gall bladder necrosis may result secondarily from the combined process of inflammation and ischemia. The cystic artery generally arises from the right hepatic artery, and although it may be aberrant, it is not more often so in patients with cholecystitis and it should never be ignored during dissection.

774. Gallstone ileus is a rare mani-festation of stones that escape from the biliary tract into the gut, almost always by eroding through the biliary tree and fistulizing to the upper GI tract. Infection is not a necessary component of this, and would not originate at the ampulla which is often not involved in the process, since the size of the gallstone to cause interference in GI motility may be too large to reach the lower biliary tree. The stones involved are typically the most common ones of cholesterol origin, and there is no antecedent or subsequent primary colon pathology common to these cases.

775. Pelvic inflammatory disease, which may be strongly suggested by her pelvic tenderness, is often reflected in right upper quadrant tenderness from perihepatitis (Curtis-Fitzhugh's syndrome). There is less likelihood of her having cholecystitis, particularly of the cholesterol stone variety, and acalculous cholecystitis is infrequent with gallstone ileus being a complication that is far rarer still. Hepatitis would not be likely in a nonjaundiced patient with a normal bilirubin, so her likely diagnosis would be perihepatitis from a primary inflammatory source elsewhere from the pelvis.

776. Diabetes predisposes to acalculous cholecystitis by involving small vessel vasculitis, and bacterial or parasitic infections such as typhoid fever may be responsible for it. Cystic duct obstruction would prevent bile from entering or leaving the gall bladder and pancreatic reflux in a "common channel" might result in chemical irritation and inflammation. The hematologic abnormalities, however, lead to an excess hemoglobin breakdown and pigmented stones. Therefore, acal-

254

culous cholecystitis is rare in patients with pigment breakdown excess load. Ninety percent of the cholecystitis in US patients is associated with stones and the options listed except for hemoglobin abnormalities accounts for the acalculous minority.

777. Food, particularly the hydrochloric acid component from the stomach, entering the duodenum results in secretin release, which is a strong stimulus to bile production. The vagus nerves also stimulate secretion as do bile salts in the gut. Cholecystokinin released from mucosal endocrine cells is triggered by fat entering the duodenum. It causes contraction of the gallbladder. Fasting would remove these neural and endocrine stimuli and inhibit bile secretion.

778. Total parenteral nutrition (TPN) puts the gut at rest for prolonged periods and without stimulation of the duodenum and release of cholecystokinin, stasis in the gallbladder may result. Thus, TPN is implicated in the origin of some acalculous cholecystitis. Choluretics actually improve the flow of bile, as do each of the regimens that involve oral feeding. Presently there are protocols to attempt to reduce the incidence of acalculous cholecystitis during prolonged TPN by periodic administration of cholecystokinin despite lack, through fasting, of stimulation that would otherwise take place through the duodenum.

779. This finding is characteristic of malignant biliary tract obstruction and was first described by Courvoisier and is called "Courvoisier's sign". Almost any cholecystitis associated with stones will have the cardinal manifestations of inflammation, which include pain. Painless jaundice is unlikely to be due to an inflammatory biliary tract disease with or without stones, and would be either associated with parenchymal liver abnormality or a malignant obstruction distal in the biliary tree. Hepatitis would give rise to jaundice, but the inflamed hepatocyte would not be secreting bile. The palpable gallbladder that is nontender in this jaundiced patient strongly suggests distal biliary tract malignancy which is most likely at the head of the pancreas.

780. This patient has what is referred to as a "silent gallstone" picked up incidentally without any symptoms or hazard associated with it. He is to be informed of the finding, and this information will be valuable should any problems be referable to this stone. It is large enough to be highly unlikely to get outside the gallbladder through the cystic duct into the common bile duct which is the very hazardous complication that could lead to obstruction or cholangitis, and cholecystitis would come to his attention. Absent other significant health risks, this stone would not pose a threat to life when he is aware of its presence.

The oral cholecystogram and ^{99m}Tc HIDA scan would both be irrelevant, since normal liver function is assumed in this nonjaundiced patient, and it is highly unlikely that the gallbladder would reabsorb water and become visualized, since some degree of low-grade chronic cholecystitis is assumed on the basis of the presence of the stone. Cholecystectomy is not justified simply on the basis of the presence of the stone either by open or closed technique, and there is no indication for common bile duct exploration.

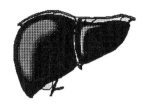

HEPATIC SURGERY

Items 781-790

781. The most common cancer in the liver is

(A) hepatoma
(B) cholangiocarcinoma
(C) hepatocholangioma
(D) fibrolamellar
(E) metastatic

782. The anatomic division of the liver for right lobar hepatectomy may be defined by each of the following **EXCEPT**:

(A) the falciform ligament
(B) the distribution of the right hepatic artery
(C) the distribution of the right portal vein
(D) the drainage area of the right hepatic veins
(E) an imaginary line drawn through the gallbladder fossa to the vena cava

783. Alpha-fetoprotein is **NOT** useful and **NOT** indicated for

(A) primary screening for hepatoma
(B) detection of persistent tumor after resection
(C) detection of recurrence during follow-up after therapy
(D) an indication for adjunctive chemotherapy
(E) help in indicating reoperation or thrombosis of tumor

784. One method of pre-operative therapy that has been helpful in facilitating liver resection for tumor has been

(A) pre-operative external beam radiation
(B) arteriographic vascular occlusion
(C) portal venous thrombosis
(D) intensive cancer chemotherapy with leucovorin rescue
(E) three weeks of total parenteral nutrition

785. If the residual, well-vascularized, hepatic remnant is normal and not involved with cirrhotic fibrosis or inflammation, what is the maximum portion of functioning liver that can be removed with normal survival?

(A) 10%
(B) 25%
(C) 40%
(D) 60%
(E) 80%

786. Of the following transmissible agents that may give rise to focal liver infections, which may cause an anaphylactic response if the contents are spilled in the event of resection or rupture?

   (A)   *Entamoeba histolytica*
   (B)   *Staphylococcus aureus*
   (C)   *Clonorchis sinensis*
   (D)   *Echinococcus granulosus*
   (E)   *Proteus mirabilis*

787. A 24 year-old woman experiences an acute abdomen with hemorrhage and shock following minor trauma when falling over a chair and striking her abdomen. At operation, a ruptured tumor in the liver is encountered. The only medicine she has ever taken has been oral contraceptives for the past seven years. The likely diagnosis is

   (A)   hepatoma
   (B)   arteriovenous malformation
   (C)   fibronodular hyperplasia
   (D)   endometrioma
   (E)   metastatic adenocarcinoma

788. Which of the following statements is **NOT** true concerning pyle-phlebitis?

   (A)   it is caused by bacteria in the urinary collecting system
   (B)   it may lead to portal vein thrombosis
   (C)   it is frequently associated with hepatic abscess
   (D)   patients typically have severe illness in sepsis
   (E)   the bacterial origin is often from the colon

789. Which statement about cancer in the liver is true?

   (A)   primary hepatoma and metastatic liver cancer each exhibit 85% or better 5-year survival
   (B)   primary hepatoma has an 85% 5-year survival but metastatic liver cancer shows less than 10% 5-year survival
   (C)   primary hepatoma shows less than 10% 5-year survival but metastatic liver cancer shows greater than 80% 5-year survival
   (D)   both primary hepatoma and metastatic liver cancer show equivalent survivals with equivalent average duration of survival
   (E)   primary hepatoma and metastatic liver cancer each show less than 10% 5-year survival

790. Each of the following factors are important in determining operability and resectability of a liver tumor **EXCEPT**:

   (A)   the patient's age
   (B)   number of liver segments involved in tumor and resection proposed
   (C)   prothrombin time
   (D)   presence or absence of cirrhosis in the residual liver following proposed resection
   (E)   ongoing active hepatitis

ANSWERS AND TUTORIALS ON ITEMS 781-790

The answers are: **781-E; 782-A; 783-A; 784-B; 785-E; 786-D; 787-C; 788-A; 789-E; 790-C.**

781. In the US, hepatoma is much less common than other primary adeno-carcinomas in the GI tract, particularly of the colon. Any tumor that disseminates by way of the portal circulation from the gut has a propensity for hepatic metastases, which are the vast majority of cancers in the liver that originate elsewhere in the gut.

782. The anatomic division of the liver is very important for the three part blood flow which is an important consideration in hepatic resection. The neat anatomic division of the falciform ligament actually separates the left lateral lobe of the liver from the median superior and median inferior components of the left lobe and it is not the true dividing line for hepatic lobectomy. The right and left lobes are divided through an anatomic line that would pass through the gallbladder fossa to the vena cava, which correlates with the distribution of the right hepatic artery, portal and venous systems.

783. Alpha-fetoprotein is helpful after the diagnosis of hepatoma in following the patient through treatment, but has not been useful or cost-effective for screening for primary diagnosis and is not so indicated. It may be helpful to serve as a proxy for the presence of the tumor when the level had previously fallen after treatment and the elevations in alpha-fetoprotein secondarily may indicate treatment without further collateral proof of recurrence.

784. Hepatoma is not a radiosensitive tumor and no pre-operative utility would be expected from radiotherapy or intensive cytotoxic chemotherapy, since it is also highly unresponsive to drug therapy. Immunotherapy and nutritional therapy might make a marginal difference in the host response to operation, but are inadequate to make any marginal difference that would be worth a delay.

The one technique listed that has been proven effective in selective instances is devascularization of the liver segment anticipated to be resected, which gives a head-start on the regeneration of liver function in adjacent liver to be preserved. It is also suggested to decrease the tumor neovascularity involved in the tumor-bearing segment, but this is difficult to judge prospectively and impossible to control in comparative trials. Radiographic occlusion is nonetheless advocated for some selected pre-operative hepatoma management.

785. The liver has amazing abilities of restoration through hyperplasia that allow regeneration of both anatomic mass and physiologic function back to normal following removal of up to 80% of the liver. Not only is this regenerative capacity amazing, but it also seems to know when to stop! The factors which govern this regenerative capacity have been studied and remain an intriguing puzzle, but messenger RNA is involved.

786. Pyogenic abscesses, such as that with *Staphylococcus* or *Proteus* may cause febrile reactions and can lead to septicemia, but not hypersensitivity reactions. *Clonorchis sinensis* is an Oriental liver fluke that takes up residence in the biliary tree, and is a source of inflammatory response, but not anaphylaxis. Amoeba are protozoans that in some zymogen classes not only give rise to colonic inflammation but invade the portal blood stream and can set up hepatic abscess, which when drained does not give anaphylaxis. This is not the case with hydatid cyst caused by *Echinococcus granulosus*. Not only can rupture of the cyst result in implantation and dissemination of daughter cysts, *Echinococcus* can cause a lethal hypersensitivity reaction as well if spilled into the peritoneum.

787. Hepatic nodular hyperplasia is the so-called "pill tumor" found in young women who have had prolonged exposure to oral contraceptive agents with progestational combinations. A young patient is unlikely to have either primary hepatoma or metastatic carcinoma in the liver at her age with no antecedent history of ill health or medication, and arteriovenous malformations don't often rupture into the abdominal cavity. An endometrioma is a possibility, but unlikely to produce hemorrhage in its superficial implantation of the severity that would give shock. The "pill tumor" often presents with hemorrhage following minimal abdominal trauma and this incidental discovery is often the only way this otherwise benign lesion is recognized — as it became known when first described.

788. Pyelonephritis is not to be confused with pylephlebitis which is an inflammation of the portal vein, most often because of bacterial infection. This bacterial infection frequently originates in the colon, and this blood-borne bacterial infection causes inflammation within the portal system and is often associated with hepatic abscesses with the patient severely ill in sepsis. The urinary tract is not drained by the portal system, and there should be no connection of these anatomic regions despite the confusion in similar sounding names between pylephlebitis and pyelonephritis.

789. There is a mean period of average survival for primary hepatoma that is about three times greater than that for metastatic liver cancer, but neither show a favorable prognosis despite treatment. Few survivors of either diagnosis are alive one year from diagnosis.

790. Each of the factors determine whether sufficient viable liver can be expected to remain to support life in the patient in the event that resection must encompass three segments or greater than 85% of the liver parenchyma, or whether the section of liver remaining is necrotic, cirrhotic or inflamed with hepatitis. There is a greater capacity for regeneration in the younger patient, and advanced age would rule out 80% hepatectomy for the compromised reserves that would need to be called upon. Prothrombin time is a measure of the liver production of a labile clotting factor, that can be reconstituted with vitamin K administration that would correct the prothrombin time even if it were prolonged.

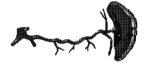 **SPLENIC SURGERY**

Items 791-800

791. Each of the following conditions exhibits splenomegaly **EXCEPT**:

(A) early acute malaria
(B) Gaucher's disease
(C) myelofibrosis
(D) end-stage chronic malaria
(E) hypersplenism

792. Splenic repair rather that splenectomy should be attempted in all of the following conditions **EXCEPT**:

(A) multiple trauma with severe head injury and extremity fractures
(B) stab wound to the spleen
(C) avulsion of splenic capsule from short gastric arteries during vagotomy
(D) splenic vein tear during pancreatic exploration
(E) 8 year-old boy with arm fracture, abdominal bruise following a fall from tree with positive abdominal tap and normal blood pressure

793. Each of the following conditions is an indication for splenectomy **EXCEPT**:

(A) thrombocytopenia
(B) traumatic splenic laceration in a child with minimum blood loss
(C) a splenic artery aneurysm within the splenic pulp
(D) splenic abscess
(E) hereditary spherocytosis

794. Surgical identification and excision of an accessory spleen is important in

(A) splenectomy for hematologic indication
(B) staging laparotomy
(C) splenectomy for trauma
(D) splenosis
(E) factor VIII deficiency

795. Adjunctive methods that may facilitate splenectomy for hematologic disease and benefit the patient include each of the following **EXCEPT**:

(A) polyvalent pneumococcal vaccine
(B) heparinization
(C) platelet transfusion
(D) corticosteroids
(E) immediate splenic artery ligation

796. Each of the following results after splenectomy would be considered complications because they are not part of the normal expected post-splenectomy course EXCEPT:

(A) pancreatitis
(B) thrombocytosis
(C) subphrenic abscess
(D) hemorrhage requiring reoperation
(E) anemia

797. Which of the following conditions is expected to co-exist with hyper-splenism in a patient with hereditary spherocytosis?

(A) thrombophlebitis
(B) gallstones
(C) bone pain
(D) repeated crises of general abdominal pain
(E) extramedullary myelopoiesis

798. Each of the organisms listed may be associated with severe septi-cemia eight years following splenectomy in a 4 year-old child EXCEPT:

(A) *Pneumococcus*
(B) *Pseudomonas*
(C) *Hemophilus*
(D) *Neisseria*
(E) *Meningococcus*

799. One factor weighing AGAINST splenectomy in a patient with splenomegaly from myelofibrosis is

(A) a potential for painful splenic infarction
(B) the threat of intra-abdominal hemorrhage
(C) the majority of blood forming cells may be in the spleen
(D) displacement of abdominal viscera by the massive splenic enlargement
(E) the operative risk of the splenectomy for massive splenomegaly

800. Splenectomy for hereditary spherocytosis is curative for which of the following abnormalities?

(A) anemia
(B) osmotic red cell fragility
(C) cholecystitis
(D) iron absorption
(E) spherocytosis

ANSWERS AND TUTORIALS ON ITEMS 791-800

The answers are: **791-D; 792-A; 793-B; 794-A; 795-B; 796-B; 797-B; 798-B; 799-C; 800-A.**

791. The early stages of malaria have splenomegaly as a prominent feature, particularly in children. In fact, an epidemiologic survey method for determining the prevalence of malaria is the splenomegaly rate in the pediatric population. Over repeated attacks, the spleen suffers multiple sequential infarcts and eventually fibroses down to the small fibrotic organ that is not only clinically not palpable, but in some instances not discoverable on surgical exploration following this "autosplenectomy".

Gaucher's disease is a glucocerebroside accumulation disorder due to deficiency in lysosomal glucocerebrosidase which produces some of the largest spleens recorded. Myelofibrosis, from its extramedullary myeloproliferative disorders, also produces massive splenomegaly in nearly all cases, and hypersplenism is the product of a spleen that is much enlarged as a rule. Of the options listed, only end-stage malaria exhibits a spleen that is not only not palpable clinically, but most likely shriveled below normal size which approximates about 150 grams in the average adult.

792. Splenic conservation should be attempted whenever it is safe and appropriate, particularly in the young. That would include both trauma as described for the boy who fell from a tree or a knife stab wound as well. It particularly applies to intra-operative incidental injuries such as that encountered during vagotomy or pancreatic exploration. However, it has no place in the patient with severe multiple injuries, when the time and attention devoted to splenic repair would pose excessive risk in view of multiple systems which require operative attention.

793. Thrombocytopenia from idiopathic or other acquired origins may respond to splenectomy if steroid therapy no longer induces a response in raising platelets. Spherocytosis is a frequent hemolytic indication for splenectomy as one of the only treatments and with excellent success

rate. Splenic abscess and splenic artery aneurysm both are treated by splenectomy if simple drainage is inadequate or an exterior splenic artery aneurysmectomy is not possible. In children, however, splenectomy is to be avoided for trauma unless there is hemodynamic instability and no other way to control the intra-abdominal hemorrhage. With minimal blood loss and stable vital signs, minimal splenic disruption can be managed by observation in order that the splenic filtration and immunologic function be preserved. If surgical exploration is undertaken, attempts at repair of minor traumatic splenic injuries are recommended, particularly in children, and splenectomy reserved for unsalvageable disruption or patients with multiple other injuries requiring urgent attention.

794. To control consumption of blood cells and platelets, all accessible splenic tissue should be excised, including that in ectopic or accessory locations. Such exploration and excision is not indicated in staging laparotomy, and no disturbance of any splenic tissue not actively bleeding or irreparable should be attempted for trauma. Splenosis is the implantation of viable splenic fragments, and would be irrelevant except if there were hematologic abnormalities secondary to these fragments. At one time, factor VIII deficiency was thought to be improved with splenic implant, and although disproved, there would be no indication for removal of splenic tissue.

795. In dealing with splenomegaly, particularly of the hyperactive spleen which is engorged with blood and consuming platelets and other blood cells, early splenic artery ligation as soon as exposure permits is important, while venous "autotransfusion" from the enlarged spleen continues as the spleen is mobilized. At this point, the patient would be able to retain transfused platelets, which would help in hemostasis for the operative dissection. Prior vaccination of pneumococcal vaccine would protect to some degree from at least some strains of encapsulated gram-positive organisms for which splenectomized patients are at risk.

Heparin anticoagulation would be contraindicated, and would make hemostasis more difficult in the patient already likely to bleed, particularly in the large potential space left behind following excision of an enlarged spleen.

796. The potential space left behind may fill with some minimal bleeding, but reoperation for hemorrhage control is a complication. Subphrenic abscess is not unheard of, but should be brought to a near-zero level by meticulous attention to technique and represents a significant complication when it occurs. The same attention to technique will avoid injury to the tail of the pancreas which lies in close proximity to the splenic hilum, since distal pancreatic injury may give rise to some degree of pancreatitis which is dangerous considering the ligated vessels and the enzymatic sequelae of pancreatic injury, particularly with a patient with impaired clotting abilities. Anemia signifies inadequate blood replacement or a continuing blood loss, and the post-operative red cell indices should be normal.

Thrombocytosis is a normal and expected result of complete splenic ablation. The platelet count should rise to levels that are expected to be approximately two to five times normal for a period of up to a year, but would require no treatment unless the platelet count of more than $10^6/mm^3$ persists.

797. The breakdown products of splenic filtration of spherocytes include the heavy pigment load to the liver for excretion, with pigmented gallstones being so likely as to recommend cholecystectomy for patients undergoing splenectomy for this indication. Sequential repeated abdominal pain crises and bone pain are characteristic of sickle cell anemia from ischemic attacks and infarcts when hypoxic. Thrombophlebitis is no more common in patients with red cell disorders than in the general population, and in a patient with hypersplenism the thrombosis would be less likely. Although the production of replacements for the red cells removed from circulation would be speeded up, in this condition the bone marrow has sufficient reserves that extramedullary sources are not likely to be involved.

798. Gram-positive encapsulated organisms are most typically associated with severe sepsis following splenectomy, and *Pneumococcus* is the principle species. *Hemophilus*, *Meningococcus* and *Neisseria* share the capsular characteristics of the organisms responsible for post-splenectomy sepsis syndrome, but *Pseudomonas* does not.

799. An operative risk is always a consideration, but splenectomy is not a very technically demanding operation even when the spleen is massively enlarged. In fact, mobilization of the massive spleen is sometimes easier, since it becomes a midline abdominal organ with very large and quite easily identifiable and relatively constant vascular attachments. Splenic infarction and the pain and risk of hemorrhage associated with it is a serious consideration indicating splenectomy as is the discomfort from the enlarged spleen moving around the abdomen and displacing other abdominal viscera or causing early satiety following meals.

A very real risk of splenectomy in a patient with myelofibrosis is that the majority of hematopoietic cells are in the enlarged spleen, and the patient may have an impaired ability to produce blood cells requiring transfusion for an extended period if there exists a "packed marrow" that no longer has capacity to produce blood.

800. Splenectomy should reduce hemolysis and therefore correct anemia long-term. The operation would have no effect on iron absorption, nor the continued production of red cells that exhibit osmotic fragility and spherocytic morphology. The excessive pigment breakdown load delivered to the liver for excretion even early in life had most likely produced pigmented gallstones; and, this occurrence, which is present even in children, is not reversed by splenectomy.

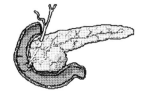

EXOCRINE PANCREATIC SURGERY

Items 801-810

801. Which of the following statements describes the anatomy of the pancreas?

(A) the normal adult human pancreas averages 250 grams
(B) 1/10th of 1% of pancreatic tissue is endocrine
(C) the pancreatic vein is the principle conduit of venous effluent from the pancreas
(D) endocrine and exocrine tissue in the pancreas are approximately evenly distributed through the pancreas in 50/50 equivalents by weight
(E) the adult pancreas averages 80 grams, one gram of which is endocrine

802. Acute traumatic hemorrhagic pancreatitis may result in each of the following **EXCEPT**:

(A) hypoparathyroidism
(B) hypocalcemia
(C) respiratory insufficiency
(D) diabetes
(E) steatorrhea

803. Which are the reasons the total excision of the pancreas also removes the duodenum in pancreaticoduodenectomy (Whipple operation)?

(A) it is technically impossible to separate the pancreas from the duodenum by careful dissection

(B) pancreatectomy involves division of the portal vein

(C) total excision of the pancreas interrupts the arterial supply of the duodenum

(D) the pancreas grows into the duodenum and duodenectomy is necessary for complete pancreatic excision

(E) it is much easier to dissect "*en bloc*" the duodenum and pancreas as a unit

804. Which of the following statements is generally **NOT** true of pancreatic operations?

(A) they are undertaken with intent for curative resection

(B) they evaluate for and attempt to relieve gastric outflow obstruction

(C) they evaluate and attempt biliary obstruction relief

(D) they are rarely effective in accomplishing satisfactory relief of pain

(E) they do not lengthen the patient's life expectancy

805. A pancreatic pseudocyst

(A) should be drained externally

(B) requires operation as soon as confirmed

(C) is lined with an epithelium

(D) should have elective internal decompression only when mature

(E) carries a negligible risk of hemorrhage

806. An elevated serum amylase

(A) is diagnostic of pancreatitis

(B) is only associated with inflammation of the pancreas

(C) must be present or pancreatitis is ruled out

(D) is not always present in late-stage chronic pancreatitis

(E) is more reliable that urine amylase in evaluating pancreatitis

807. A solid, solitary, asymptomatic 4 cm mass in the pancreas in a 48 year-old man discovered incidentally on CT examination for evaluation of "slipped disc" is most likely

(A) cystadenoma

(B) insulinoma

(C) nonfunctioning islet cell adenoma

(D) pancreatic carcinoma

(E) metastatic carcinoma originating elsewhere

808. Surgery is usually indicated for

(A) acute pancreatitis
(B) chronic pancreatitis
(C) multiple small pseudocysts
(D) only some complications of pancreatitis
(E) salvage of endocrine pancreatic function

809. Which of the following statements is true for population screening for pancreatic carcinoma?

(A) the population at risk is easily identified
(B) the diagnostic testing is sensitive, specific and reliable
(C) treatment of early stage disease is simple and widely available
(D) treatment yields satisfactory outcome results
(E) none of the above

810. Which of the following is **NOT** a contraindication for operation for pancreatic carcinoma?

(A) peri-ampullary location
(B) tumor invades portal vein
(C) malignant ascites
(D) invasion of duodenal wall and adjacent vessels
(E) liver metastases

ANSWERS AND TUTORIALS ON ITEMS 801-810

The answers are: **801-E; 802-A; 803-C; 804-A; 805-D; 806-D; 807-D; 808-D; 809-E; 810-A**.

801. The human pancreas is a predominantly exocrine organ with approximately one gram of endocrine tissue scattered rather uniformly through the exocrine gland in 1- 2 million microscopic islets. An enlarged or heavier pancreas (> 100 grams) is likely to represent inflammatory, fibrotic or neoplastic change. Because of this intimate connection and distribution of endocrine tissue throughout the exocrine gland, both functions are affected by any generalized parenchymal disease, although there is far more reserve in the endocrine components which are under separate control mechanisms.

802. Fulminant pancreatitis destroys both exocrine and endocrine tissue, the former earlier than the latter. This means that the inability to digest fat leads to steatorrhea and islet cell destruction leads to glucose intolerance. Saponification of calcium may lead to hypocalcemia. The parathyroid glands would not hypofunction under these circumstances but should react with increased parathormone secretion. The increase in circulating enzymes has a lytic effect both in the retroperitoneum and in distant target organs such the lungs, and respiratory insufficiency may result from both subphrenic irritation and pleural effusion as well as alveolar-capillary permeability.

803. The "Whipple operation" is a treatment with curative intent in operable patients for resectable pancreatic carcinoma — most often in the head of the pancreas where presentation occurs earlier by biliary obstruction. Pancreaticoduodenectomy is an extensive operation, and would not be undertaken for ease of *"en bloc"* dissection or because separation would not be possible, since difficult and involved hookups for any distal pancreatic remnant and biliary conduits are made necessary by the Whipple procedure. The portal vein is not divided in Whipple procedure, although the splenic vein contribution to it is ligated, and it is the splenic vein that is the principle effluent for pancreatic endocrine secretion into the venous drainage from the pancreas. Duodenectomy is a part of the Whipple operation because interruption of the feeding arterial supply of the pancreas would devascularize the arterial connection to the duodenum and necrosis or stenosis might result with interference in enteric and biliary flow.

804. Most operations on patients who have a postoperative diagnosis of pancreatic carcinoma do not encounter resectable tumor. Most of those that undergo resection are not cured. Therefore, most of the results of operation beyond confirming the diagnosis would be in palliation, and that is principally of biliary or gastrointestinal obstruction and much less effectively pain control. Almost all pancreatic operations for cancer do not change the patient's life expectancy.

805. A pseudocyst, when suspected and confirmed should not undergo immediate operation, since external drainage is undesirable, creating a pancreatic fistula with fluid and electrolyte loss. Early operation would take place before the pseudocyst capsule is mature enough to hold sutures for internal diversion. The cyst is "pseudo" because it is not lined with an epithelium, and essentially represents an inflammatory front of autodigestion into an area with many major blood vessels. The threat of massive hemorrhage in an evolving pseudocyst is very significant. When the thickened "rind" is sufficient to create a reliable anastomosis in enterostomy or gastrostomy, and when the mature pseudocyst is obviously large enough that it is unlikely to spontaneously resolve, elective internal drainage into the gut is the preferred management.

806. Serum amylase is nearly always elevated in acute pancreatitis at some time, but not all times when the blood is drawn. Other sources of increased amylase can include salivary glands, biliary tract, or inflammatory disease of the gut. Urinary amylase determination is a method of averaging the fluctuating serum amylase level and is more reliable. In late-stage chronic pancreatitis, fibrosis and exocrine pancreatic loss make it less likely that serum amylase elevations can be sustained.

807. The most common neoplasm in the pancreas is pancreatic carcinoma. Unfortunately, most of the time it is not early in its presentation. Islet cell neoplasms are rare, and the patient would be symptomatic with an insulinoma that has grown to this size. Cystadenoma would not be solid, and is a very uncommon lesion. The pancreas is not a frequent site of metastasis from cancers elsewhere as much as it is unfortunately a primary site of malignancy with unfavorable outlook, even if presenting, as in this case, before it has become symptomatic by its spread.

808. Acute pancreatitis is actually a contraindication to operation unless the patient is *in extremis*. Salvage is attempted by suctioning out the necrotic and septic focus of devitalized tissue. It is not pancreatitis that is operated on but certain complications of it, and they are selected on the basis of a greater benefit than harm in which timing is critical. The endocrine function of the pancreas has considerable reserve, and salvage of endocrine function is an inappropriate indication for operation but a consideration if operation is performed for indications otherwise present. Multiple small pseudocysts generally resolve spontaneously or coalesce into a larger and maturing pseudocyst which might lead to a later operative indication. Neither acute nor chronic pancreatitis is an indication for operation, but often extenuating circumstances such as pain add up against other risks to bring operative treatment to consideration.

809. Pancreatic carcinoma is unfortunately a miserable disease with difficulty in diagnosis. Treatment is expensive and unsatisfactory with a dismal outcome even if early cases could be identified by some screening methods not yet developed. For all these reasons, perhaps the greatest yield will come from investigations in etiology and prevention rather than any anticipated breakthrough in diagnosis and treatment.

810. A peri-ampullary location of pancreatic adenocarcinoma is the most hopeful anatomic site, largely because tumor growth there gives the earliest evidence of its presence, sometimes before nodal, hepatic, duodenal, portal, or superior mesenteric arterial invasion or malignant ascites occur, each of which are contra-

indications for operation with curative intent.

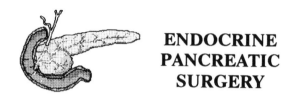

ENDOCRINE PANCREATIC SURGERY

Items 811-820

811. Pancreatic islet cells are

   (A) innervated by the vagus
   (B) concentrated in the head of the pancreas
   (C) found nowhere but inside the anatomic confines of the pancreas
   (D) secreting peptide hormones into the portal venous circulation
   (E) secreting catecholamines

812. Which of the following statements concerning gastrin is **NOT** true?

   (A) secreted by antral G-cells
   (B) secreted by some cells in the duodenal mucosa
   (C) secreted by some pancreatic islet cells
   (D) inhibited by a rising blood glucose
   (E) inhibited by somatostatin

813. Which product is **NOT** secreted from pancreatic islet cells?

(A) serotonin
(B) glucagon
(C) aldosterone
(D) somatostatin
(E) vasoactive intestinal peptide

814. The most common islet cell adenoma and syndrome originating from the endocrine pancreas is

(A) gastrinoma
(B) pancreatic cholera (WDHA)
(C) glucagonoma
(D) somatostatinoma
(E) insulinoma

815. Which of the following is **NOT** a component of Whipple's triad?

(A) inappropriate glucose/insulin ratio
(B) hypoglycemic symptoms with fasting
(C) hypoglycemia following exertion
(D) fasting blood sugar less than 50 mg/dl
(E) symptoms relieved by glucose administration

816. Treatment of Zollinger-Ellison syndrome includes each of the following **EXCEPT**:

(A) H$_2$-receptor antagonist therapy
(B) omeprazole
(C) pancreaticoduodenectomy (Whipple)
(D) total gastrectomy
(E) somatostatin analog

817. Which of the following is **NOT** characteristic of gastrinoma (Zollinger-Ellison syndrome) patients?

(A) secretory diarrhea exhibits low pH
(B) jejunal ulceration is pathognomonic
(C) basal acid output equals maximum acid output
(D) nasogastric suction has no effect on diarrhea output
(E) serum gastrin is always elevated

818. Which of the following is true for Zollinger-Ellison syndrome?

(A) almost never occurs in familial form
(B) most gastrinomas are small and solitary
(C) rarely is the gastrinoma malignant
(D) the tumor is slow growing and the syndrome is very long-lasting
(E) gastrinomas show up readily on angiography in most cases

819. Successful methods of palliation for islet cell carcinoma include all of the following **EXCEPT**:

(A) streptozotocin
(B) somatostatin
(C) diazoxide
(D) subtotal tumor reduction by surgery
(E) radiation therapy

820. Which of the following statements about insulinoma is **NOT** true?

(A) insulinoma is usually solitary and small

(B) insulinoma is almost always malignant

(C) angiography is effective in localizing the majority of insulinomas

(D) blood sugar can be sustained with diazoxide therapy in persistent insulinoma

(E) somatostatin is often effective in inhibiting insulin secretion

ANSWERS AND TUTORIALS ON ITEMS 811-820

The answers are: **811-D; 812-D; 813-C; 814-E; 815-A; 816-C; 817-D; 818-D; 819-E; 820-B**.

811. The pancreatic islets are a collection of neuroendocrine cells that are under the control of peptides and are neither innervated by the vagus nor secrete catecholamines. However, they secrete peptide messengers into the portal circulation in response to changes in blood glucose and other stimuli that are reacted to immediately. They are distributed rather uniformly through the pancreas, but are not confined to the anatomic limits of the pancreas, and may be present in adjacent areas or even in the duodenal mucosa.

812. Gastrin is produced by similar cells in a variety of locations along the upper gastrointestinal tract and pancreas. It is responsive to several stimuli, one of which

is not a rising blood glucose; it is inhibited by somatostatin, and the somatostatin analog is effective in reducing its hypersecretion.

813. The pancreatic islet cells are genetically programmed for polypeptide synthesis but are not specialized for steroid biosynthesis. Therefore, aldosterone cannot be produced by islet cells; whereas, all of the peptides listed above and several candidate hormones for which no function is yet identified can be identified both in secretion from islets or by immunohisto-chemistry in islet cells.

814. The β-islet cell adenoma producing excess insulin is the most common pancreatic islet cell tumor and one of the earliest pancreatic endocrine syndromes known. Allen O. Whipple popularized the symptomatic triad, and several thousand cases have been registered so that it is not uncommon and is a part of most general hospital's experience. Gastrinoma has been known for the past forty years and is also a very recognizable syndrome with several thousand patients registered with the diagnosis. Both glucagonoma and pancreatic cholera have been reported in only a few hundred patients, and less than a hundred for somatostatinoma. It is instructive, therefore, to learn about these syndromes only to fill in the physiology of pancreatic islet abnormalities; whereas, insulinoma and gastrinoma are clinically useful syndromes to learn.

815. Whipple's triad involved hypo-glycemia following fasting or exertion with a low fasting blood sugar. During the time of Whipple's description of insulinoma and its characteristic clinical triad, the only measurements available were those of

blood glucose, and the measurement of hypoglycemia under the circumstances listed with its symptomatic resolution with sugar administration. Since no immuno-assays or other means of detecting insulin in circulation were available, no glucose to insulin ratios were possible at that time. Now the diagnostic standard for the diagnosis of insulinoma, is the glucose:insulin ratio determinations made if suggested by any part of Whipple's triad.

816. Because gastrinoma tumors are multicentric and often malignant with metastases frequent, radical surgical excision such as a Whipple operation would be contraindicated, particularly since the patients do not die rapidly of the oncologic spread of this disease but suffer morbidity of symptomatic endocrine abnormality which may be controlled. That control includes H_2-receptor antagonist therapy, and omeprazole when the former is less effective. Still further treatment is available in somatostatin analog inhibition of gastrin release. If there is no acid there is no ulcer, and no acid is produced in the absence of the stomach, so total gastrec-tomy still has a role in the management of hypersecretion from this syndrome in the event of failing medical management of the mucosal barrier. For the disseminated forms of gastrinoma, eradication is less the objective than secretion reduction and symptomatic control.

817. Hypersecretion of gastric acid is characteristic of Zollinger-Ellison syndrome in which the patient's basal acid output is the same as maximum acid output since they are under chronic gastrin stimulation to maximum secretion. This may produce diarrhea in some patients and the diarrhea has low pH.

One way of distinguishing Zollinger-Ellison syndrome from pancreatic cholera is that the nasogastric tube aspiration of the stomach contents quickly and immediately reduces to zero the irritation that is ulcerogenic as well as the secretory diarrhea. The original description of the syndrome made reference to an atypical location for peptic ulceration in the jejunum, and that remains diagnostic of the syndrome.

818. Most gastrinomas are multiple, malignant, and metastatic when first encountered. Very rarely is any pancreatic gastrinoma found that is solitary, benign, and resectable. It is frequently found in familial multiple endocrine adenopathy, and in such circumstances it is nearly uniformly multicentric. However, the tumor is very indolent in its growth, and patients can live with the syndrome for four or five decades if their endocrine symptoms are controlled.

819. External beam radiation therapy has no benefit in a very slow growing tumor whose predictable morbidity is that from hypersecretion. Management of hyper-secretion can take place successfully by reduction in the number of secreting cells, and subtotal resection of tumor generally yields benefits to patients with these hypersecretory islet cell tumors. The same control method can be managed with reduced activity of the hyperfunctioning cells, and that can take the form of diazoxide which reduces insulin secretion in insulinoma patients, supporting blood sugar; somatostatin which is even more effective in controlling excess of both insulin and gastrin production without causing the normal peptide secretions to go below normal; and streptozotocin which is a less effective endocrinologic control, but adds a chemotherapeutic method for slowing cell growth. Since these are already very slow growing tumors, limited benefit can be expected from conventional chemotherapy.

820. Nearly all insulinomas are solitary, benign and resectable. They are often highly symptomatic from the excess insulin secretion, and both somatostatin which inhibits insulin release and diazoxide which supports the blood sugar can be useful in following a patient who has a persistent *in situ* insulinoma while these medical treatments control the potentially dangerous hypoglycemia. The majority of insulinomas can be localized by arteriography, since they are not generally multicentric, or widely spread out in metastatic locations.

"Regimen is superior to medicine."
Voltaire (1674-1778)

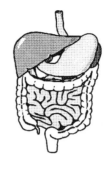

SMALL INTESTINAL SURGERY

Items 821-830

821. The first system to be affected by hydrostatic dysfunction as the intraluminal pressure in the gut rises early in bowel obstruction is

(A) visceral afferent nerves
(B) mesenteric arterial
(C) lymphatic
(D) somatic epicritic innervation
(E) portal venous

822. Which of the following diseases is **LEAST** likely to affect the jejunum?

(A) carcinoid
(B) giardiasis
(C) sprue
(D) Crohn's disease
(E) adenocarcinoma

823. Which of the following rare neoplasms in the small bowel would require a Meckel's diverticulum for its presence?

(A) lymphoma
(B) gastric adenocarcinoma
(C) leiomyosarcoma
(D) carcinoid
(E) metastatic melanoma

272

824. Which of the following statements about small bowel carcinoid tumor is **NOT** true?

    (A)   it is the most frequent primary tumor in the small bowel

    (B)   it is usually clinically evident since it usually causes the carcinoid syndrome

    (C)   it is multicentric in origin

    (D)   metastases exponentially outgrow the primary tumor

    (E)   in late stages it gives rise to liver metastases

825. The strongest layer of the small bowel — that from which the suture called "gut" was originally derived — is the

    (A)   serosa
    (B)   outer longitudinal muscle
    (C)   inner circular muscle
    (D)   submucosa
    (E)   mucosa

826. Which of these conditions is **NOT** a component of small bowel intussusception?

    (A)   dense fibrotic peri-intestinal adhesions
    (B)   age less than two
    (C)   intestinal polyp
    (D)   lead point
    (E)   submucosal edematous congestion

827. Which of the following conditions is **NOT** often seen with mesenteric vascular occlusion?

    (A)   acidosis
    (B)   ileus
    (C)   normal cardiac function
    (D)   elevated LDH
    (E)   multisystem vascular disease

828. Which of the following findings is **NOT** typically a component of a small bowel ileus?

    (A)   abdominal distention
    (B)   vomiting
    (C)   small bowel gas visible on X-ray
    (D)   high pitched bowel sounds
    (E)   obstipation

829. Which of the following conditions would be **LEAST** likely to explain the small bowel obstruction present in a male patient who has an acute abdomen, and at age thirty has never had any previous abdominal operation?

    (A)   internal hernia
    (B)   volvulus
    (C)   adhesions
    (D)   tumor
    (E)   Crohn's disease

830. Which procedure is the most likely to find evidence of other pathology in a patient found incidentally at exploration for appendicitis to have multiple carcinoid tumors confined to the terminal ileum?

(A) a chest X-ray
(B) EKG
(C) CT of the liver
(D) colonoscopy
(E) urinary 5 HIAA

ANSWERS AND TUTORIALS ON ITEMS 821-830

The answers are: **821-C; 822-E; 823-B; 824-B; 825-D; 826-A; 827-C; 828-D; 829-C; 830-D.**

821. As luminal pressure rises, it is translated into the lower pressure vascular systems which are affected in the rising order of pressures determining their flows. First is lymphatic and the consequence is edema; second is portal venous, and stasis and congestion with bluish discoloration from red cell diapedesis is the result. When venous pressure rises to the level of arterial pressure, blood flow stops and infarction follows, all that remains is for the luminal pressure to burst the weakened necrotic bowel to complete the natural history of unresolved bowel obstruction. Visceral afferent nerves are stimulated principally by distention in the bowel wall, which is reflected in clinical symptoms of malaise and nausea and vague discomfort referred to the umbilicus, the route through which the midgut had retreated into the peritoneal cavity during development. When the primary bowel irritation inflames the parietal peritoneum, then the much more discriminating epicritic somatic nerves are stimulated and the sensation of localized pain is appreciated.

822. The upper intestinal tract is rarely the site of primary adenocarcinoma. It is postulated that the rapid motility of any external carcinogens ingested may limit the exposure in the upper gastrointestinal tract unlike their protracted residence in stomach or colon. The upper gastrointestinal tract is also free of microflora that may convert some ingested substances into carcinogens. The rarity of adenocarcinoma of mucosa in the upper intestine is not true of endocrine neoplasms, and carcinoid is the most frequent primary tumor of the small bowel. *Giardia lamblia* is a parasite that can give rise to inflammation with pain and malabsorption from its taking up residence in the upper small bowel where it is most frequently found. Both sprue and Crohn's disease are inflammatory enteropathies, the former giving rise to malabsorption and acquired from some factors in tropical external environments, and the latter is a primary endogenous inflammatory bowel pathology presumably autoimmune in origin. Of these processes, the most infrequently encountered in the jejunum is adenocarcinoma.

823. Meckel's diverticulum contains ectopic gastric mucosa and secretes hydrochloric acid in the unusual milieu of the mid-small bowel mucosa. As a consequence, peptic ulceration can occur in the ileum adjacent to the Meckel's diverticulum where this mucosa is unprotected from the ulceration. In very rare instances, a neoplasm can develop within the Meckel's diverticulum. Gastric adenocarcinoma anywhere else in the gastrointestinal tract apart from the stomach, Meckel's diverticulum, or Barrett's esophagitis would be metastatic from a primary source likely in the stomach. Lymphoma may occur throughout the area of the submucosa, with a greater frequency wherever the Peyer's patches are highest in incidence. Carcinoid is an endocrine neoplasm that usually arises spontaneously in multicentric foci of K-cells scattered through small bowel mucosa, and leiomyosarcoma may arise wherever small bowel smooth muscle can give rise to it. Melanoma is frequently metastatic to the submucosa in gut and lymphatics where it may constitute a lead point for intussusception.

824. Carcinoid tumor is the most frequent primary neoplasm of small bowel. However, it only rarely gives rise to the carcinoid syndrome, and that is not a property of the primary tumor in the small bowel site, nor even in its mesenteric metastases which exponentially outgrow the primary tumor size, but is a property of the hepatic metastases in carcinoid which occur in its later stages. Only some of these hepatic metastases may give rise to the carcinoid syndrome, which requires the hepatic metastases rather than the primary tumor alone for its presence. Therefore, only the minority of carcinoid tumors ever result in the carcinoid syndrome, and the usual carcinoid tumor is not clinically evident and is discovered incidentally, often in multicentric locations where it arises primarily from multifocal origin.

825. The strongest layer of the bowel for holding suture — and that from which suture itself was made — is the submucosa. "Catgut" was originally made of sheep intestine's submucosa — and this nearly

pure collagen layer was processed as the gut itself ("plain") or tanned with chromate salts ("chromic catgut") for longer life *in situ*. The bowel layer that is important in holding sutures remains this submucosal "gut" layer, and no integrity to sutures placed only through muscle — circular or longitudinal, (here or elsewhere in the body) — can be expected. Mucosa is sometimes closed, not for strength but for hemostasis from submucosal vessels, and serosal approximation helps to "seal" a two-layer bowel anastomotic suture line, nearly all the strength of which resides in the submucosal approximation sutures.

826. Small bowel intussusception almost always has a lead point. A lead point is a mass in part of the bowel that invaginates and is pulled downstream, pulling its bowel wall along with it. This is particularly true at ages older than infancy, since primary intussusception is most common in children less than two. Beyond that age, either a polyp or some form of tumor lead point such as a lipoma, adenoma, lymphoma or cancer intruding into the lumen is propelled by bowel motility. When this happens, a partial obstruction results with edema and congestion rapidly engorging the intussuscepted bowel, particularly the mucosa and submucosa, which then act as a further lead point until swollen to complete bowel obstruction. If dense fibrotic adhesions form an external bowel fixation, intussusception is precluded, and bowel propulsive motility would be unlikely to be strong enough to overcome the tethering of these adhesive bands even if a lead point were present.

827. A surgical axiom that reflects this correct response is "in bowel ischemia, treat the heart and not the gut". Mesenteric vascular disease is very rarely isolated from generalized multisystem vascular disease, with the one organ most likely the source of mesenteric occlusion being the heart. Ileus is the rule, since ischemic or infarcted bowel loses motility, becoming a functionally obstructed bowel that may be proximal to the segment affected. Acidosis and elevated LDH may be some of the few laboratory signs suggestive of bowel infarction in these patients who are often seriously ill from low flow dysfunction of other organ systems that allowed the vascular thrombosis in the gut.

828. Ileus is a reflexive small bowel atony, and so bowel sounds, associated with bowel propulsion, would be absent or diminished. Not only would high-pitched tinkling bowel sounds not be likely in ileus, but they would suggest an alternate diagnosis of small bowel obstruction. Abdominal distention and obstipation are seen in both conditions, and vomiting may take place with either, since the stomach is not often affected in small bowel ileus. Gas is visible in the small bowel in ileus, but there is a distinctive pattern to the distribution of that gas in multiple levels called "stepladder" in bowel obstruction since the two fluids quickly equilibrate to the same level unless there is an area of resistance obstructing flow between them.

829. The primary bowel obstruction in a patient without prior operation is unlikely to be from peritoneal adhesions unless there is some antecedent history of some primary inflammatory process in the peritoneum which is unlikely, especially in the male patient. A cause, therefore, must be postulated, and the alternate options are more likely. Volvulus can take place if an embryologic point of fixation is formed, or if a foreign body is present such as a bezoar which itself can be a cause of obstruction. A primary tumor, more likely benign than malignant in a younger age group, may serve as a lead point for intussusception, or primary bowel inflammatory disease such as Crohn's may present as obstruction in this age group. Physical and radiographic findings may suggest the level of obstruction which can be helpful in a differential diagnosis, but it is likely that the patient with the first presentation of primary bowel obstruction without prior inflammatory process in the abdomen should undergo urgent operation to correct both the bowel obstruction and confirm its cause.

830. Patients with the finding of multiple small carcinoid tumors are unlikely to have carcinoid syndrome, since it is very unlikely that the disease will have metastasized, and probably not to the dimensions of creating secreting hepatic metastatic deposits capable of giving rise to the carcinoid syndrome. Therefore, the CT scan of the liver and the 5-HIAA urinary studies are unlikely to be positive. Most likely the chest X-ray and EKG will also be normal, or at least not reflect anything related to the incidental finding of the multicentric carcinoid.

However, patients with primary small bowel carcinoid have up to two-thirds chance of having other benign or malignant tumors in the gut, most of them being other carcinoids. Up to one-fifth of the patients also have primary adeno-carcinoma, an aggressively malignant disease that does not share the indolent behavior of the carcinoid tumor. Because the additional tumors are most likely to be in the colon, and because the most sensitive study for their discovery is colonoscopy, incidental carcinoid discovery would be strong indication for colonoscopic examination.

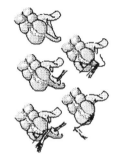

APPENDICEAL SURGERY

Items 831-840

831. Each of the following is a known cause of appendicitis **EXCEPT**:

(A) intraluminal worms
(B) hypertrophy of Peyer's patches
(C) stenosis from hypertrophic circular muscle wall
(D) inspissated barium
(E) benign tumor at cecal junction

832. Each of the following causes peritonitis that can be confused with appendicitis **EXCEPT**:

(A) ruptured ovarian cyst
(B) regional enteritis
(C) tubo-ovarian abscess
(D) renal cortical infarct
(E) sigmoid diverticulitis

833. Which of the following statements regarding appendicitis is true?

(A) 6% of the US population is affected by this disease at some point in their lives
(B) perforation is the most common presenting feature of appendicitis diagnosed in the teenage years
(C) incidence of appendicitis in black patients is evenly distributed worldwide
(D) teenage girls have almost twice the incidence of appendicitis over teenage males
(E) appendicitis does not occur in the elderly

834. Which of the following techniques is proven to prevent appendicitis?

(A) high fiber diet
(B) systemic antibiotics
(C) nonabsorbable antibiotics taken by mouth
(D) corticosteroids
(E) appendectomy

835. All of the following radiographic findings are likely with ruptured retrocecal appendicitis **EXCEPT**:

(A) a "sentinel loop"
(B) free air under the diaphragm
(C) an air fluid level in the right lower quadrant
(D) ileus
(E) a fecolith

836. A 23 year-old man is seen in your office for complaint of right lower quadrant pain. It has been occurring sporadically for over three months, with increasing intensity in the last three days. On your examination you find a temperature and white blood count elevation and he has a tender mass in the right lower quadrant. The most likely diagnosis is

(A) appendiceal abscess
(B) chronic appendicitis
(C) carcinoid tumor
(D) regional enteritis
(E) diverticulitis

837. The biggest advantage of the right lower quadrant transverse (Rockey-Davis) incision for appendectomy is

(A) it permits evaluation of the ovaries in females
(B) it is easily extended for evaluation of sigmoid colon
(C) it is muscle-splitting, with secure closure and low wound complication rate
(D) it can be used to expose the gall bladder for evaluation and excision
(E) it is optimal position for exit of abdominal drainage lines

838. A patient with a large recurrent right inguinal hernia undergoes groin exploration for repair with prosthetic mesh. As the hernial sac that was missed in previous exploration is opened, the cecum and dangling appendix are exposed in the wound. All of the following procedures are appropriate **EXCEPT**:

(A) reduction of the visceral content and high ligation of the sack
(B) inversion of the intact appendix with purse string suture
(C) incidental appendectomy in the course of hernia repair
(D) closure of the hernia incision and removal of the appendix through separate abdominal incision
(E) soaking the prosthetic mesh in antibiotics

839. Which is the preferred method of irrigation following appendectomy for ruptured appendicitis?

(A) copious volume irrigation of as much of the abdomen as can be irrigated
(B) kanamycin added to the irrigant
(C) tetracycline added to the irrigant
(D) local right lower quadrant irrigation with a limited amount of saline
(E) sharp debridement of all visibly inflamed peritoneal surface and triple antibiotic solution irrigation

840. A 30 year-old man undergoes appendectomy for symptoms of appendicitis. At operation the appendix is minimally injected without evidence of gangrene or perforation, and the postoperative diagnosis is acute appendicitis. The patient is eating and ready for discharge 48 hours later when the pathologist calls to add to the histologic confirmation of acute appendicitis the presence of a one and a half centimeter carcinoid tumor one centimeter from the margin of the appendectomy stump. No lymph nodes are found in the specimen. The most appropriate management at this point is

(A) discharge for later admission and second-look operation

(B) scheduled right hemicolectomy electively after bowel preparation in six weeks

(C) cancel discharge, and return patient to operating room for re-operation and local re-excision including adjacent mesentery

(D) discharge patient for routine appendicitis follow-up

(E) order urinary 5-hydroxy-indolacetic acid (5-HIAA) determination

ANSWERS AND TUTORIALS ON ITEMS 831-840

The answers are: **831-C; 832-D; 833-A; 834-E; 835-B; 836-D; 837-C; 838-C; 839-D; 840-D**.

831. There is no known phenomenon of physiologic obstruction of the appendiceal outlet by stenosis of the kind that might be considered an analog of pyloric stenosis. Obstruction of the lumen can take place with intestinal worms, solidifying barium, or benign tumors, including carcinoid, lipomas, or even swollen submucosal lymphoid tissue. When carcinoid is found in the appendix, it is not often found to be obstructing the neck but is coincidently present.

832. A follicular cyst or an enlarged ovarian cyst can rupture physiologically (Mittelschmerz) or pathologically in the event that cystic teratoma is present. Ileitis and tubo-ovarian abscess both give rise to inflammatory changes in the peritoneum, and may mimic appendicitis as with diverticulitis. Peritoneal inflammation is common to each of these, but it is unlikely that a renal cortical infarct would cause similar symptoms of peritonitis as it is retroperitoneal. Only in a very late stage in which a secondary inflammation of the peritoneum occurs (and that would only be a feature of those infarcts in the anterior kidney with peritoneal proximity) could this event be likely to cause confusion. Retrocecal appendicitis can give retro-peritoneal findings that might be com-parable. The distinction is on the basis of the peritonitis common to each of the other options which is usually associated with appendicitis in its usual anatomic position.

833. Appendicitis has a wide geographic variability and a skewed age distribution. It is nearly unknown in some areas of the world among the same racial groups with highest incidence elsewhere. In Africans living in rural central Africa, it is unheard of, but the same population may migrate to

certain western environments and achieve an incidence of appendicitis higher than that seen in the population that has lived for generations in this same environment to which the formerly low incidence group has migrated. It is slightly more common in males than females, particularly in teenage years. Perforation is an uncommon presentation, but may be a complication of late diagnosis or atypical findings. The unusually high prevalence of this source of an acute abdominal emergency in the US makes it a public health problem of major consideration. It happens less frequently in the elderly, but for that reason and that it exhibits atypical presentation when it does, the complication rate is higher in such patients, in part due to late diagnosis.

834.   Although it might seem obvious, without an appendix there is no appendicitis. Incidental appendectomy to remove a normal appendix is advocated in some surgical operations, undertaken for other indications. Although appendicitis may not occur following elective appendectomy, diverticulitis (a subspecies of which *is* appendicitis) can occur, and control of the factors leading to conditions whereby inflammation may take place in any of these "bayous off the flora-chocked colon" have been attempted. The most successful of these appears to be a high fiber diet.

Appendicitis is definitely not treated by systemic antibiotics nor is there any evidence that such treatment prevents it. Similarly, bowel preparation with nonabsorbable oral antibiotics yields a very temporary reduction in flora which repopulate rapidly, especially with re-feeding of the patient. Corticosteroids have a role in suppressing inflammation, but they have a prominent role in suppressing

immunoresponse to the infectious factors that may trigger inflammation and thereby they suppress resistance to their further spread. At present, adequate fiber in the diet is the best known preventive measure for reducing inflammatory processes in the lower gut, and incidental appendectomy may be indicated in some operations to which it may be added as accessory. Weighed against the advisability of interval appendectomy is the 94% likelihood that an American (the one population with the highest incidence of this disease) will never develop appendicitis even without the application of any known, expected, or yet-to-be-developed preventive measures.

835.   A fecolith in the appendix, known as an appendicolith, may often be seen on radiography and strongly suggests appendicitis. The local collection of an air-water interface suggests appendiceal abscess with perforation with localization in the right lower quadrant. This is a retro-peritoneal appendix, so free air in the abdomen would not be anticipated, and if present would be likely accompanied by much more vigorous peritoneal reaction and abdominal peritoneal signs. Ileus is a common response to bowel inflammation, and a peculiar local form of ileus is a segment of atonic small bowel adjacent to the inflammatory site of the abscess which does not propel air forward in the gut. Bowel motility usually precludes any air being seen in small bowel on flat plate abdominal X-ray because of its rapid transit. The arrest of this air distending an atonic bowel loop is the radiographic pattern referred to as a "sentinel loop" suggesting an adjacent inflammatory focus.

836.   Chronic appendicitis is not a recognized entity, although not all instances of appendicitis go on to gangrenous infarction and perforation. This patient has peritoneal signs and a mass which suggest a segment of inflammation, and both appendiceal abscess and diverticulitis are possible. The latter is less likely in this age group, and the former is rarely indolent developing over months, particularly in a patient at this age and in this setting. Carcinoid tumor is also a possibility, but the most probable diagnosis given the duration and physical finding described is regional enteritis. A mass is characteristically present from the edematous and inflamed bowel, and the course is often more protracted than the abrupt intra-abdominal crisis seen with appendiceal rupture and abscess formation.

837. The right lower quadrant Rockey-Davis incision is ideal for appendectomy when the diagnosis is correct, the appendicitis is limited, the appendix is in the right position, and no major surprises are encountered. However, many surgeons have cursed the inventor for profound lack of imagination when appendicitis is not encountered as the explanation for the abdominal pain and in some instances when the appendix itself is not encountered through this limited approach. It is nearly impossible to evaluate other parts of the abdomen which are at risk of significant pathology through this minimal incision designed for essentially one purpose. Extension is possible, but not satisfactory in exposure of the pelvic organs such as ovaries and sigmoid colon, and not at all for the epigastrium and biliary tree. Often, if the appendix is not found or the problem causing the peritonitis is not appendicitis, the Rockey-Davis incision is closed or abandoned for the moment, and a new incision is made to give better exposure of other organs involved or for atypical positions of appendiceal complications. For that reason, the abdomen should be prepared and draped for sterile extension. In these instances, the Rockey-Davis incision is not even optimum for drainage, since the valve-like tension of the muscles closes off the layers almost without suturing.

Drainage sites are selected for dependant drainage rather than for exposure. It is for this very reason that makes for disadvantage in drainage that the Rockey-Davis is nearly ideal for the more usual encounter with acute appendicitis. The muscle-splitting approach means that the direction of the fibers assist in secure layers with tension at right angles in successive planes, and a secure abdominal wall in which incisional herniation is extremely rare.

838. When appendectomy is carried out, the classification of the operation changes on the operating room nurse's categories from clean to contaminated. Particularly in a recurrent hernia repair, one would not wish to introduce the risk of contamination, and this is nearly an absolute contraindication in the repair of a recurrent hernia with a prosthesis implanted. One does not rescue this bad judgment through a misapplication of antibiotics, and if antibiotics are used to soak the prosthesis, it is for other indications than for neutralization of the risk of an ill-advised incidental appendectomy. The most appropriate surgical judgment might be to return the visceral contents with the appendix and perform the high ligation of the sack originally missed and then attempt repair without employing the prosthesis. Much the second best method — and only if there is some extraordinary reason for the compulsion to ablate the innocent appendix — would be to invert the appendix without opening it like pushing the toe of the sock through the anklet into the cecum where this intussusception is closed with a purse-string suture. It might there slough into the gut, but the inversion of this stump might cause a filling defect in the cecum for later confusion in barium enema interpretation!

839. Debridement of peritonitis has not been proven to benefit or even to accelerate resolution of peritonitis and has increased complication rates attending it. The use of antibiotic solutions in irrigation appears intuitively helpful; however, questions would have to be asked as to what effective action the antibiotic can be expected to have and what complications might attend its use from other properties it may possess. Kanamycin is active against the spectrum of flora expected; however, it has the property of potentiating muscle paralysis caused by anesthesia. Prolonged apnea, oto- and nephrotoxicity may attend its use in abdominal instillation. Tetracycline also has the right antibiotic spectrum, but is a sclerosing agent that would give a greater chemical peritonitis than that bacterial component which it was expected to relieve.

Almost all irrigation referenced in operative notes is modified with the term "copious" a seemingly inseparable prefix to the term "saline". However, the use of high volumes and pressures in irrigating as much of the abdominal cavity as can be reached might actually spread the flora from the local right lower quadrant contamination that the local defense factors mustered by the peritoneum (including the omentum) have been at such pains to wall off. Copious saline would further dilute the

macrophages and other defensive elements within the peritoneum and probably raise the possibility of intra-abdominal sepsis and scatter it in multiple locations.

For these reasons, simple local irrigation confined to the principle contamination site will remove much of the debris and devitalized tissue without disrupting the containment of abdominal defensive protection. The most effective way to deliver antibiotic to this inoculum site is that which is injected in the vein, since a number of antibiotics are carried by white blood cells in response to chemotaxic factors originating in the inflammatory response at the site of the inoculum.

840. A carcinoid tumor found in this appendix incidentally represents a finding and not a disease. The patient has been treated and, presumably cured, of his presenting illness, and follow-up should be for the standard practice of routine appendicitis postoperative care. Immediate re-operation would be to no purpose without indication of presence of residual disease and its location, and interval re-admission with bowel preparation for an extensive resection of innocent tissue is not indicated on any information that suggests a higher risk for either residual or multiple primary carcinoid or other tumors related to appendiceal carcinoids.

Urinary 5-HIAA determination would be a way of evaluating indole metabolites which are highly unlikely in a patient with this small primary carcinoid tumor, since they would be a reflection of carcinoid syndrome from hepatic metastases which is nearly unheard of even following a long period of potential growth and spread whether or not this incidental appendiceal carcinoid had been removed.

The patient should be informed of the incidental finding, followed by post-appendectomy routine, and advised to have colorectal screening and comparable advice given to anyone with risk factors that now additionally include the incidental finding of the small appendiceal carcinoid.

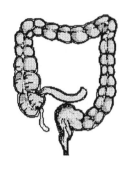

COLONIC SURGERY

Items 841-850

841. Adenocarcinoma of the colon is

    (A)   more common than skin cancer
    (B)   significantly higher in men than women in the US
    (C)   geographically distributed across the globe
    (D)   the most frequent visceral cancer in the US
    (E)   often cured by chemotherapy

842. Which of the following conditions is **NOT** a risk factor in predilection for the development of colon cancer?

    (A)   gender
    (B)   genetics
    (C)   diet
    (D)   age
    (E)   environment

843. Which of these antecedent conditions predisposes to the higher risk of the development of colon cancer?

    (A)   Crohn's disease
    (B)   ulcerative colitis
    (C)   diverticulosis
    (D)   urinary bladder cancer
    (E)   melanoma

844. The principle population screening method for detecting colo-rectal abnormalities is

    (A)   barium enema
    (B)   sigmoidoscopy
    (C)   digital rectal exam
    (D)   occult fecal blood
    (E)   colonoscopy

845. The most likely cause of occult blood loss in a 68 year-old who undergoes routine physical examination after retirement is

    (A)   hemorrhoids
    (B)   *fissure-in-ano*
    (C)   diverticulosis
    (D)   carcinoma
    (E)   adenomatous polyp

846. An annular "napkin ring" appearance on barium enema is most characteristic of

    (A)   carcinoma of the cecum
    (B)   squamous epidermoid cancer of the anus
    (C)   cancer of the sigmoid colon
    (D)   cancer of the rectal ampulla
    (E)   villous adenoma

847. The highest percentage of colon cancers are first found in the

(A) liver
(B) cecum
(C) ascending colon
(D) descending colon
(E) rectosigmoid

848. The design of curative operations for colon cancer resections are patterned according to

(A) the ease of operative excision
(B) the instruments available for surgical utilization
(C) the anatomic distribution of adjacent lymphatics
(D) the minimum colon required for fluid reabsorption
(E) siting of colostomy

849. Indications for colon resection in a patient with a large sigmoid carcinoma and hepatic metastases include each of the following **EXCEPT**:

(A) relief of bowel obstruction
(B) the best chance for a cure
(C) control of hemorrhage
(D) prevention of necrosis
(E) disobstruction of the ureter

850. Which of the following studies is contraindicated in defining the extent of a partial obstruction?

(A) colonoscopy
(B) gastrograffin swallow
(C) barium enema
(D) barium UGI
(E) gastrograffin enema

ANSWERS AND TUTORIALS ON ITEMS 841-850

The answers are: **841-D; 842-A; 843-B; 844-D; 845-D; 846-C; 847-E; 848-C; 849-B; 850-D**.

841. The incidence of colon cancer is second only to skin cancers, in the US, but a majority of the skin cancers are trivial with respect to threat to life. Adenocarcinoma of the colon is the most frequent visceral cancer in the US constituting 14% of all nonskin cancers in both males and females which it affects equally. There is a remarkable asymmetry in geographic distribution, since it is nearly unknown in less developed parts of the world and is a component part of Western life style and diseases of development. It is very much a surgical disease, since chemotherapy offers very little palliation and no curative control.

842. Colon cancer constitutes 14% of visceral cancers in males and an identical percentage in females. That there may be a greater number of females at advanced age than males means that the prevalence of colon cancer is higher in females only because of this longevity and not because of a predilection based in biology or behavior difference between the sexes.

An increasing incidence of colon cancer is correlated strongly with an increase in age, and genetic predisposition appears evident from two to three times greater incidence in family members of those affected. However, this is difficult to separate from the environmental factors which are overwhelmingly obvious, since people from areas of the world where colon cancer is nearly unheard of can immigrate to Western urban centers and adopt the life style of modernization and within a generation develop an incidence of colon cancer that sometimes surpasses that of the indigenous Westerners. Some part of this environment is provably associated with low fiber, high fat and refined carbohydrate.

843. There appears to be a random association of colon cancer with other coincident tumors such as melanoma or urinary bladder cancer, but there is a correlation with breast carcinoma and a strong association with carcinoid. Inflammatory disease of the bowel is sharply distinguished between Crohn's disease, which does not appear to be a predisposing risk factor, and ulcerative colitis which has a very high correlation with later development of adenocarcinoma of the colon increasing with duration of the colitis. The anatomic finding of diverticulosis may be associated with same proximate causes — for example, low fiber diet and Western life style, but there is no correlation of the diverticulosis and colon cancer risk primarily.

844. Since the principle easily detected physical finding associated with colon carcinoma is occult blood loss in the stool, this method is a sensitive way of case finding. However, it is very non-specific. For that reason, the much more specific studies of radiographic barium, or physical examination by rectal exam, sigmoid-oscopy, or colonoscopy are indicated for those of the general population who screen positive on the more sensitive examination which will uncover a large number of patients who are false positives or who have benign problems discovered by true positive occult blood detection.

845. Hemorrhoids are common, but bleeding from them less so, which is more common with *fissure-in-ano*. However, both of these do not produce occult blood loss but streaking that is visible to the patient. Diverticulosis can cause blood loss, but it is typically not occult when it happens, as it does infrequently, when it may cause massive bleeding. An adeno-matous polyp rarely bleeds unless it is large enough to be ischemic, and then often blood loss is part of its passage. The important point to be carried from this question to the clinic is that colon cancer is the single most common cause of occult blood loss in the older patient.

846. Adenocarcinoma of the colon grows into the bowel wall and spreads along the submucosal lymphatics, which are arranged in a circumferential pattern in an area where the structure and function of the colon is principally for propulsion. In the right side of the colon the principle functions are capacitance and water absorption, and tumors tend toward endophytic polypoid growth — although there is frequent overlap between these patterns. Villous adenoma is a frond-like extension that may be sessile when seen on barium enema, but is characteristically polypoid rather than annular wherever it occurs.

Although not principally annular in configuration, both rectal ampulla and perineal lesions would not be described as napkin rings on barium enema, since barium enema does not define the pattern in the lower reaches of the rectum and anus since the barium does not opacify them and there is a rectal ballooned catheter present that interferes with definition on radiographs of this lower extreme end of the colon.

847. The rule of thumb — if not of index finger — is that one-third of colon carcinomas are found within range of digital rectal exam and two-thirds within the range of the sigmoidoscope, or 25 cm. Less frequent are the cancers on the right side of the colon, but they often — but not always — are associated with characteristic clinical syndromes. The majority of colon cancers still offer presentation from symptoms relating to the colon, rather than to metastatic sites such as the liver.

848. Curative resection of colon cancers encompasses not only the area of the primary tumor and adjacent bowel, but also the mesenteric fan or lymphatic distribution in encompassing not only the primary tumor but the most likely sites of potential metastatic spread *en bloc*. These lymphatics closely follow the pattern of portal venous effluent, so the extension is often carried back to the root of the major venous drainage of this region of the bowel. Ease of operation, the instrumentation available, and siting of the stoma are technical considerations as well as the residual colon and its storage and reabsorption capacity for the patient, but each is secondary to the primary concern that the patient undergo a curative resection procedure.

849. Palliative operations for sigmoid cancer are limited in indication if the patient does not have morbidity directly related to the presence of the tumor. These factors would include continuing blood loss or necrosing tumor with the threat of bowel disruption. Bowel obstruction should certainly be relieved, but it is not generally a good idea to perform this much in advance of imminent obstruction, since the patient's survival may be a shorter time than the obstruction requires to develop, and this interval would best be served for the patient's own uses rather than hospitalization and recovery. Ureteral obstruction is rare, and typically does not impair renal function if the opposite kidney is uninvolved, but may cause pain and may be relieved incidentally during operation for other indication. A patient is not curable with hepatic metastases already present, and therefore the operation should be limited in scope, without effort to encompass all secondary metastatic areas of spread, since tertiary levels are already involved. The design of the operation will be tailored for the strategy of the indication, namely symptomatic palliation.

850. High grade obstruction in the GI tract, particularly in such an area as the left colon where it may frequently occur, may be studied safely from below with barium or gastrograffin contrast and colonoscopy, since such introduced materials are retrievable. Barium introduced by mouth must be able to pass through the gastrointestinal tract, however, and in the event of a partial high grade bowel obstruction, the oral barium contrast can complete the obstruction making it difficult to retrieve not only the barium, but to pass anything else through the gut and require emergency operation. Judicious use of gastrograffin contrast, conscious of its osmotic activity, can be employed in these instances, but the proximal part of the bowel is already likely to be distended upstream from a site of obstruction, and such bowel distention can decompensate with additional osmotic intraluminal pressure increase. A general rule for partial bowel obstruction is that such obstructions should be studied from the downstream side, that is, distal from the point of obstruction.

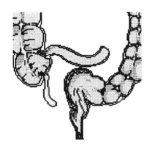

ANORECTAL SURGERY

Items 851-860

851. Treatment for uncomplicated external hemorrhoids observed on physical examination should include each of the following **EXCEPT**:

  (A) anoscopy
  (B) digital rectal exam
  (C) diet high in soluble fiber
  (D) frequent Sitz baths
  (E) elective hemorrhoidectomy

852. An important clinical difference between internal and external hemorrhoids is

  (A) one thromboses, the other does not
  (B) one may bleed, the other does not
  (C) one has somatic innervation, the other does not
  (D) one is associated with portal hypertension, the other is not
  (E) one should be excised, the other incised

853. To perform adequate hemorrhoidectomy, each of the following procedures is indicated **EXCEPT**:

  (A) circumferential excision of the hemorrhoidal skin
  (B) sigmoidoscopy
  (C) high ligation of the hemorrhoidal vein
  (D) suture closure of the mucosa
  (E) avoidance of disruption of muscular sphincter

854. *Fistula-in-ano* is likely to be associated with each of the following conditions **EXCEPT**:

  (A) radiation proctitis
  (B) abdomino-perineal resection
  (C) tuberculosis
  (D) Crohn's disease
  (E) foreign body reaction

855. Which of the following is **LEAST** likely to be a clinical feature of *fissure-in-ano*?

  (A) asymptomatic
  (B) usually posterior midline associated with trauma
  (C) bleeding is prominent
  (D) streaking on outside of stool
  (E) "sentinel pile"

856. Which of the following conditions is **LEAST** likely to be associated with villous adenoma of the rectum?

  (A) prolapse
  (B) diarrhea
  (C) electrolyte loss
  (D) malignant degeneration
  (E) asymptomatic finding

857. A proctocolectomy is an operation contraindicated for

(A) ulcerative colitis
(B) familial polyposis
(C) granulomatous colitis
(D) Stage IV sigmoid carcinoma
(E) rectal stump recurrent cancer at low lying suture line

858. Rubber band ligation is recommended for

(A) a single uncomplicated internal hemorrhoid
(B) all three large clusters of internal hemorrhoids during initial procedure
(C) skin tag
(D) "sentinel pile"
(E) bleeding external hemorrhoid

859. Each of the following features is an advantage for the technique of suture closed external hemorrhoidectomy EXCEPT:

(A) decreased bleeding
(B) decreased discomfort
(C) increased peri-anal hygiene
(D) decreased abscess rate
(E) more comfortable Sitz bathing

860. "Pull through" operations in which the muscular layers of the rectum and sphincters are preserved while more proximal gut is brought down following mucosal excision would be indicated for each of the following EXCEPT:

(A) Duke's C Stage I rectal carcinoma
(B) high level imperforate anus
(C) aganglionic segment of distal colon (Hirschsprung's disease)
(D) familial polyposis
(E) early stage ulcerative colitis

ANSWERS AND TUTORIALS ON ITEMS 851-860

The answers are: **851-E; 852-C; 853-A; 854-B; 855-A; 856-E; 857-D; 858-A; 859-D; 860-A**.

851. Most hemorrhoids resolve spontaneously without operation. The indication for hemorrhoidectomy is not the presence of hemorrhoids, but complications of their presence or failure of other management methods to resolve them over a protracted trial with good compliance. The presence of external hemorrhoids is not a contraindication for the appropriate rectal examination and anoscopy. The best dietary advice includes the essential requirement of soluble fiber in regular dietary components such as fresh fruits and vegetables, bran and cereals or in supplement form.

852. An important distinction for both patient and clinician is the sensation based in somatic innervation in groups of internal and external hemorrhoids. Since there are no somatic nerve fibers in the mucosa of internal hemorrhoids, successful out-patient ablative procedures can be carried out without anesthesia, such as rubber band ligation. Both types of hemorrhoid may reflect portal hypertension, both may thrombose, and each may be a source of blood loss.

853. Adequate hemorrhoidectomy includes proximal ligation of the vein draining the hemorrhoid excised, and the mucosal re-approximation with suture, whereas the skin of the external hemorrhoidectomy excision site may be left open or closed depending on the patient's condition and the surgeon's preference. However, under no circumstances should circumferential anal skin excision take place, since the resultant fibrosis and scarring may result in very troublesome anal stenosis. The site of the skin excision is often resurfaced by advance of the more rapidly proliferating mucosa so that secreting surface epithelium is present in the exposed perineum creating a "wet anus". These defects are a complication called the "Whitehead deformity" and are resulting from the formerly proposed "Whitehead radical hemorrhoidectomy", an obsolete operation abandoned because of this very morbid complication.

Avoidance of injury to the muscular sphincter is desirable in any anal surgical procedure, but if necessary, the sphincter may be cut in one position only, so as to allow a fistula to heal in. This may be done over time such as with a "seton". The scarring will allow competence of the muscular sphincter if gradually divided at one position, but if it is cut in two

positions, the sphincter becomes incompetent and incontinence results. The Whitehead deformity and sphincter incompetence are far more troublesome sequelae than the much more likely recurrence of hemorrhoids.

854. *Fistula-in-ano* is frequently associated with continuing inflammatory disease as occurs in Crohn's disease (in which *fistula-in-ano* may be a sentinel lesion) or radiation proctitis. A foreign body reaction is also a continuing inflammatory stimulus. *Mycobacterium* infection can give rise to *fistula-in-ano*. Following excision of the anus there can be no *fistula-in-ano*, and that is a component part of the abdomino-perineal procedure referred to as the Mile's operation.

855. *Fissure-in-ano* is highly unlikely to be asymptomatic. It causes very painful defecation, visible bleeding usually streaking on the outside of stool and may even result in such extremely painful circumstance as continuing spasm of the voluntary muscle contraction in the external sphincter called "tenesmus". There is often a fibrotic area at the anal verge adjacent to the fissure from the scarring following inflammation, and this may result in obstruction to hemorrhoidal venous return creating what is referred to as a "sentinel pile". This is a clue on the physical examination as to the location of the fissure, which is most frequently in the posterior midline.

856. A villous adenoma, particularly positioned low in the rectal ampulla, often grows very large, may prolapse and secretes actively, giving both fluid and electrolyte loss, particularly potassium deficiency. It is associated with malignant potential, particularly when persistent over a long time and increasing with size. Because of these features and the characteristically bulky endophytic growth, the least likely clinical event is that the villous adenoma would be a silent physical finding in a patient who is asymptomatic.

857. Familial polyposis requires proctocolectomy for removal of all genetically predisposed colonic mucosa with malignant potential. Ulcerative colitis frequently affects the entire colon down to and including the lower rectum, and it also has pre-malignant potential throughout the length of the involved colon. The granulo-matous colitis may have skip areas involved, but it also has a tendency toward recurrent colitis, even if much less malignant degenerative potential than end-stage ulcerative colitis. Carcinoma that is recurrent at the anastomotic suture line in a low lying anastomosis might frequently require completion of proctocolectomy for a chance at cure. Since there is no chance for a cure in a patient who has Stage IV carcinoma of the sigmoid, such a very large and debilitating operation should not be performed in a patient with so limited a prognosis, and it is not an appropriate palliative procedure.

858. If you have chosen C, D, or E, you are either forgetting some sensory information or else have a lack of imagination or empathy! Somatic innervation contraindicates the use of rubberband ligation on external hemorrhoids. Even if local anesthesia were administered at the time of the banding, later discomfort at these cutaneous sites would limit patient's return or compliance with physician follow-up! The correct answer is that a single internal hemorrhoid if uncomplicated is appropriate for band ligation. If there are complications to the internal hemorrhoids or if there are large multiple internal hemorrhoids, each of them should not be banded at the same initial procedure, since the engorgement and swollen circumferential presence of these banded hemorrhoids would constitute obstruction in the anal canal, since they would infarct and slough only after a further period of time and not likely all at once. A considerable amount of anal bleeding could be expected as well. Internal hemorrhoidal band ligation is appropriate sequentially, but the second procedure should follow the sloughing and resolution of the first.

859. The reason that open external hemorrhoidectomy was advocated to begin with is that this area of the body has very high microbial colonization rates and is impossible to decontaminate with repeated soilage. When the wound is left open, there is no potential for abscess, and primary closure of external hemorrhoidectomy makes the possibility of abscess formation present, although acceptably low considering the other advantageous features listed which are true.

860. The Stage I signifies that the patient has a chance at curative excision with the Mile's operation — abdomino-perineal resection — yet the lesion is not confined to the mucosa but has invaded transmurally through muscular walls of the lower rectum and therefore disease would be left persistent for later progression that may cause the patient's death if this chance for curative resection is foregone. The other lesions are those effecting the mucosa throughout the affected length, but limited to the mucosa as in the instance of polyposis and early ulcerative colitis. There are two options of either functional (Hirschsprung's) or anatomic (imperforate anus) atresia, and pulling the bowel through this segment of missing or non-propelling and unresponsive neuromuscular component of the rectum is appropriate treatment indicated for successful management of the primary problem.

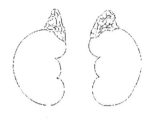

ADRENAL SURGERY

Items 861-870

861. In the Cushing's syndrome that may be a paraneoplastic feature of small cell lung cancer, the pathology expected is

(A) adrenal cortical carcinoma
(B) adrenal cortical adenoma
(C) pituitary basophilism
(D) bilateral adrenal cortical hyperplasia
(E) anterior pituitary tumor

862. Each of these conditions can be expected to produce secondary aldosteronism **EXCEPT**:

(A) nephrotic syndrome
(B) congestive heart failure
(C) renal artery stenosis
(D) cirrhosis with ascites
(E) cortical adrenal adenoma

863. Surgical correction is recommended for each of the following conditions **EXCEPT**:

(A) aldosterone secreting cortical adenoma
(B) renal artery stenosis
(C) coarctation of the aorta
(D) bilateral micronodular hyperplasia of the zona glomerulosa
(E) Cushing's adrenal adenoma

864. Which of the following statements is true regarding adult onset virilizing adrenal tumors?

(A) they are highly malignant in their behavior
(B) they are recognized earlier in males than females
(C) long-term survival is likely with adrenalectomy
(D) cortisol replacement is necessary since all steroid production is shunted into androgens
(E) the patient is usually asymptomatic from the endocrine excess

865. The sources of Cushing's syndrome from APUD tumors include each of the following **EXCEPT**:

(A)   pituitary adenoma
(B)   oat cell carcinoma of the lung
(C)   adrenal cortical tumor
(D)   pancreatic islet cell carcinoma
(E)   hypothalamic neoplasm

866. Metanephrine is excreted in the urine in a patient with an adrenal medullary pheochromocytoma because

(A)   metanephrine is the final breakdown product of all catecholamine metabolism
(B)   the adrenal medulla is the only anatomic location of catechol-O-methyltransferase
(C)   metanephrine is secreted by the kidney in response to the stimulation of other messengers from the adrenal pheochromocytoma
(D)   normetanephrine is too volatile with too short a half-life
(E)   norephenephrine does not break down but is continuously taken back up and resecreted

867. The pheochromocytoma syndrome can result in a tumor in each of the following locations **EXCEPT**:

(A)   adrenal medulla
(B)   carotid body
(C)   adrenal cortex
(D)   para-aortic bodies (Zuckercandl bodies)
(E)   aortic arch

868. Cushing's syndrome is characterized by each of the clinical features listed **EXCEPT**:

(A)   diabetes
(B)   hypokalemia
(C)   hirsutism
(D)   arrhythmia crises
(E)   hypertension

869. Which of the following statements about adrenal cortical carcinoma is **NOT** true?

(A)   most present early when the tumor is small and resection is curative
(B)   there is a recommended successful chemotherapy for maintenance of remission after surgical excision
(C)   intravenous tumor extension is a prominent pathologic feature
(D)   operation with curative intent frequently takes the form of *en bloc* nephro-adrenalectomy
(E)   the tumors are generally radio insensitive

870. Each of the following conditions is required in invasive localization procedures such as arteriography in the patient with pheochromocytoma **EXCEPT**:

(A) the patient must be attended
(B) continuous blood pressure monitoring
(C) cardiographic monitoring of heart rate and rhythm changes
(D) pharmacologic preparation should precede study, and blocking agents must be available for immediate infusion
(E) glucagon infusion should be employed as enhancement for contrast imaging

ANSWERS AND TUTORIALS ON ITEMS 861-870

The answers are: **861-D; 862-E; 863-D; 864-A; 865-C; 866-B; 867-C; 868-D; 869-A; 870-E.**

861. The paraneoplastic syndrome results from a production of an ACTH-like peptide, and this would mean the secondary hypercortisolism of a normally responsive adrenal cortex. There would be no likelihood of autonomous hyperfunction from either cortical adenoma or carcinoma. The pituitary is not involved in the production of the ACTH, and in fact would probably be suppressed by the excess cortisol circulating. Therefore, either the hypothalamic stimulus to ACTH release (pituitary basophilism) or the hyperfunction of the anterior pituitary cells that make the ACTH (pituitary adenoma) would be unlikely, and in fact would be expected to be suppressed rather than stimulated.

862. In each of the options listed except for the last, there is a high renin driving the production of angiotensin which stimulates the adrenal cortex. As a consequence, the source of the aldosterone would be bilateral hyperplasia. In the adrenal cortical adenoma, the aldosterone is elevated primarily from an autonomous secretion. This fact would suppress renin below normal levels. That is what makes this form of aldosteronism primary. Each of the other conditions listed are secondary for appropriately renin-driven forms of aldosteronism, and therefore, are examples of secondary aldosteronism.

863. Aldosteronism that results from bilateral micronodular hyperplasia is not very responsive to surgical therapy. If operation were performed, bilateral adrenalectomy would be necessary, and that requires the patient to be dependent upon corticosteroid replacement, which is too high a price to pay for a condition that does not involve malignant hypertension and can be managed with medication. The lesions that produce hypertension because of high renin output (renal artery stenosis), high aldosterone output (aldosterone secreting adenoma), high cortisol output (Cushing's adrenal adenoma), or hemodynamic and unknown factors (coarctation of the aorta) are each surgically curable conditions and should have the benefit of operation.

864. Virilizing tumors of the adrenal gland are nearly always lethal because of their oncologic spread. Patients are symptomatic with respect to the androgen production, and females note these androgenizing features earlier than males, since male secondary sexual features mask androgens or estrogens in same-sex affected patients. Long-term survival is nearly unheard of, both because of late treatment and early aggressive spread of tumor. Unlike adreno-genital syndrome, this is not an enzymatic defect in which all steroid production is shunted into one form of cortical steroids rather than another, and the normal mechanisms of control of the zona glomerulosa should regulate aldosterone and of the zona fasciculata should control cortisol output without replacement being necessary for either if the adrenal gland is intact on at least one side.

865. APUD tissue has the enolase and other enzymes that result in the production of amine or peptide hormones, and ACTH is a characteristic APUD peptide. It is produced by ectodermally derived tissue, such as the hypothalamus, the anterior pituitary, pancreatic islets and the K-cells in the bronchus, and each of these tissues may produce peptide messengers such as ACTH, or corticotrophin releasing factor or ACTH-like peptides in paraneoplastic syndromes. Distinctly unlike these cells, the adrenal cortex is from mesoderm, and cannot make these messenger peptides: it has instead the enzyme chemistry to secrete a lipid-derived hormone, the steroid. Therefore, tumors in the APUD system make peptides which can only be reflected in Cushing's syndrome by secondarily stimulating the adrenal cortex in the zona fasciculata to produce the cortisol. In the absence of the adrenal cortex, these peptide messengers would not be able to express the characteristic Cushinoid features of the syndrome. Both

the adrenal cortex and the gonads are not derived from ectoderm and do not characteristically have the APUD features of peptide production, and their characteristic endocrine products, the steroids, are likewise not APUD hormones but under the control of trophic hormones that regulate their production.

866. The nature of the excretion products of the catecholamines found in the urine can help localize the chromaffin neoplasm. Nerve endings produce norepinephrine, that is, (in German — "Nulline Ohne Radical", or "catecholamine without the methyl group", which we use in acronym in calling it "norepinephrine"). Unlike the nerve endings, the adrenal medulla has an enzyme called "catechol-O-methyl-transferase". Because of this enzyme, the catecholamine produced has a methyl group, and is the one we call epinephrine. The catecholamine breakdown products are excreted as normetanephrine for the product that comes from nerve endings outside the adrenal medulla or as metanephrine, the breakdown product that comes from the catecholamine process that adds the methyl group within the adrenal medulla. Metanephrine, therefore, reflects in the urine its origin in the adrenal medulla, localizing the tumor. It is true that norepinephrine is taken back up and recycled, but so is epinephrine, and each are broken down by monamine oxidase and excreted as their respective catabolites normetanephrine and metanephrine respectively.

867. The chromaffin cells present in the adrenal medulla have their postganglionic counterparts in the carotid body, aortic arch and at the lumbar retroperitoneum near the bladder adjacent to the inferior mesenteric artery (Zuckerkandl's bodies or organs). These chromaffin cells can secrete catecholamines, but they would typically be norepinephrine secreting, as just described, since the adrenal medulla has the enzyme that can make epinephrine of the same precursors by adding the methyl group. Each of these locations have the ectodermally derived APUD cells that can become neoplastic and produce an autonomous syndrome. The adrenal cortex, by contrast, cannot take up, modify and secrete catecholamines, and therefore does not mimic the pheochromocytoma syndrome.

868. Cushing's syndrome is based in a glucocorticoid, cortisol, therefore gluconeogenesis may be reflected as diabetes. Hypertension is a feature, but it is not episodic crises of hypertension, and distinctly absent are any crises of arrhythmia which are a feature of catecholamine secretions. Cushing's syndrome differs then, from the hypertension and hyperglycemia seen with pheochromocytoma in that cardiac arrhythmias are not prominent, and episodic crises are not characteristic since there is no immediate acute responsiveness in the steroid receptor activation comparable to that which happens at catecholamine receptors. The other features of metabolic hypokalemia and hirsutism are true of Cushing's syndrome, and are not shared by pheochromocytoma.

869. Malignant adrenal cortical tumors are nearly always large, and many massive, at the time of presentation. Size alone is used as a criterion of malignancy in their pathologic evaluation. Because the adrenal is in such an anatomically silent area of the body in terms of mass disruption of adjacent organ function, the tumor can grow to football size before it is appreciated, sometimes by minimal endocrine manifestations. By the time the tumor has reached massive size, it is also likely to have spread, and one of the common forms of spread is intravenous extension. Surgical therapy should take the form of a radical nephrectomy including the adrenal and Gerota's fascia *en bloc* with care to avoid embolization of intravenous tumor. Following this excision, mitotane (OpPDDT) has been successful in maintenance therapy with proven reduction of recurrence potential. However, most of these tumors would recur and cause the patient's death if not treated by radical excision at the time of discovery with adjunctive follow-up chemotherapy extended, and in all probability, for the life of a long-term survivor.

870. The patient undergoing invasive testing with a known or suspected pheochromocytoma must be attended, monitored, pharmacologically prepared, and emergency control of hypertensive or arrhythmia crises be ready at hand if the invasive manipulation is physically or psychologically provocative enough to trigger a crisis. Glucagon which is often given to dilate the gut in which contrast may be better distributed is absolutely contraindicated in the pheochromocytoma patient. Glucagon is among the most powerful catecholamine releasing agents known, and its use in the patient with suspected pheochromocytoma can cause a lethal outcome.

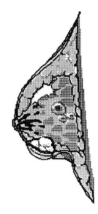

BREAST SURGERY

Items 871-880

871. Each of the following constitutes a risk factor for breast cancer **EXCEPT**:

   (A) heredity
   (B) fibrocystic disease
   (C) nulliparity
   (D) prolonged breast feeding
   (E) prior breast cancer

872. Signs of breast cancer include each of the following **EXCEPT**:

   (A) bloody nipple discharge
   (B) skin dimpling
   (C) Paget's disease of the nipple
   (D) breast discomfort
   (E) unilateral nipple retraction

873. Which of the following cancers of bone is **LEAST** common?

   (A) primary osteosarcoma
   (B) breast carcinoma
   (C) lung carcinoma
   (D) prostate cancer
   (E) thyroid carcinoma

874. In a 36 year-old woman with a painless hard dominant breast lump, the next step should be

   (A) mammography of the lump
   (B) fine needle aspiration cytology
   (C) radiation therapy
   (D) radical mastectomy
   (E) bone scan

875. Which of the following breast lesions is typically benign?

   (A) cystosarcoma phylloides
   (B) comedocarcinoma
   (C) lobular carcinoma
   (D) medullary carcinoma
   (E) intraductal carcinoma

876. Mammography should be employed

   (A) annually for asymptomatic women over age 30
   (B) to screen other areas of the breast in an 18 year-old found to have a fibro-adenoma
   (C) every 6 months in 30 year-old women identified as high risk
   (D) to definitively characterize a dominant mass discovered on physical examination
   (E) no more frequently than annually in asymptomatic women 50 years of age or older

877. Stage I carcinoma of the breast is characterized by each of the following **EXCEPT**:

(A) tumor size smaller than 2 cm
(B) two or more axillary lymph nodes are positive
(C) no distant metastases are present
(D) five year survival is 85% or more
(E) estrogen receptors may be positive or negative

878. Each of the following represents premalignant disease or a risk factor for breast cancer association **EXCEPT**:

(A) proliferative fibrocystic disease
(B) fibroadenoma
(C) Paget's disease
(D) lobular carcinoma *in situ*
(E) atypical ductal hyperplasia

879. Estrogen receptor activity can be characterized by which of the following statements?

(A) positive only in breast cancer
(B) will react only in binding estrogen
(C) is associated with a poor prognosis
(D) is positive only in pre-menopausal patients
(E) is an indication for adjunctive endocrine therapy

880. Current adjunctive therapy for a premenopausal 40 year-old woman following radical mastectomy with a 2.5 cm ductal carcinoma with 2 of 15 lymph nodes involved and an estrogen receptor negative tumor includes

(A) tamoxifen
(B) cytotoxic chemotherapy
(C) androgens
(D) oophorectomy
(E) pituitary irradiation

ANSWERS AND TUTORIALS ON ITEMS 871-880

The answers are: **871-D; 872-D; 873-A; 874-B; 875-A; 876-B; 877-B; 878-E; 879-E; 880-B**.

871. Earlier prior breast cancer in the patient or first order female relatives increases the risk of breast cancer as does prolonged estrogen stimulation as is seen with nulliparity. Dysplastic changes in fibrocystic disease may be precursors of neoplasia. Prolonged breast feeding interrupts estrogen stimulation and is actually protective against the development of breast cancer.

872. Pain is often associated with inflammatory conditions, and if the neoplastic change causes a secondary inflammatory component, breast discomfort may be associated with breast cancer, but it is not typically due to it. Retraction or a specific scaly rash of the nipple (Paget's disease) or a bloody nipple discharge along with a dimpling or depression of the skin are serious signs of breast cancer, often associated with a painless lump.

873. Primary bone cancer is the least likely of those cancers listed. Metastatic disease to the bone is much more frequent, and breast and lung cancers are very frequent carcinomas metastatic to bone. Both thyroid carcinoma and prostatic carcinoma have a high predilection for bony metastasis.

874. Mammography is not indicated for a mass that requires cytologic or histologic identification, so mammography of a suspicious lump will not change the indication for its biopsy. Neither radio-therapy nor mastectomy are appropriate until diagnostic confirmation of carcinoma is confirmed either by cytology or sub-sequent biopsy at which point therapeutic options can be discussed, and bone scan would only be appropriate as a prediction of metastatic disease which still would require primary breast cancer diagnosis and treatment.

875. Despite the misleading name, cystosarcoma phylloides is an atypical rapidly growing variant of fibroadenoma. It is almost always benign, with lymphatic metastases very uncommon and malignancy occurring in less that 10%.

876. Positive axillary lymph nodes represent breast cancer at Stage II disease which decreases survival at five years from 85% to 66%. Stage I disease has no distant metastases, and a small primary tumor size, in which estrogen receptors may or may not be positive.

877. Despite its name, many authors regard lobular carcinoma *in situ* as a pre-

malignant finding rather than true carcinoma, and Paget's disease is often a harbinger of breast cancer. Atypical hyperplasia and florid fibrocystic disease are both associated with excess breast cancer risk, but fibroadenoma is not associated with such risks.

878. Estrogen receptors are found in breast tissue, and other tissues such as colon cancers or colon tissue in either gender. They react with ligand-binders in addition to estrogen, such as antestrogens, e.g., tamoxifen. They are not only associated with premenopausal patients, and confer a better prognosis in those patients largely because they do constitute an additional indication for an adjunctive therapy with endocrine treatment.

879. A clinically discovered mass requires invasive cytologic or histologic diagnosis and not mammography. Other parts of the breast might be examined to determine therapy, but not for an 18 year-old with a suspected fibroadenoma. Even for patients with high risk, repeated mammography at short intervals, particularly at younger ages, should be avoided. The current recommendation is for asymptomatic women to be screened annually after age 50.

880. The patient described has Stage II carcinoma which requires adjunctive therapy in current clinical opinion. The alternative treatments represent endocrine therapy that would be recommended if estrogen receptors were positive, but negative estrogen receptors in this younger woman suggest a poorer prognosis that would be best treated by adjunctive chemotherapy.

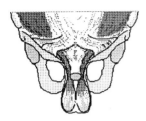

HERNIA SURGERY

Items 881-890

881. The surgical feature common to repair of adult and infant indirect inguinal hernia is

   (A) transplantation of the cord
   (B) Hougouet maneuver
   (C) high ligation of the sac
   (D) fixation of the testis in the scrotum
   (E) closure of the internal inguinal ring

882. The **LEAST** common reason for hernia recurrence is

   (A) failure to identify and ligate indirect inguinal sac
   (B) failure to appreciate associated hernia
   (C) suture breakdown
   (D) excessive tension on approximated structures
   (E) collagen disorder producing wound healing defect

883. The most likely reason for irreducibility of an apparently incarcerated but viable large right inguinal hernia is

   (A) a sliding component
   (B) ingrowth of new vascular attachments from the scrotum
   (C) incompetence of the inguinal canal
   (D) increased intra-abdominal pressure
   (E) loss of domain

884. All of the following statements about Richter's hernia is are true **EXCEPT**:

   (A) is an incarceration
   (B) may be found in sites other than the groin
   (C) perforation is a high risk
   (D) only a partial circumference of the bowel is involved
   (E) operation is not indicated

885. Which of the following hernias is the single most common hernia in young females?

   (A) femoral hernia
   (B) indirect inguinal hernia
   (C) direct inguinal hernia
   (D) Richter's hernia
   (E) para-esophageal hiatus hernia

886. In which of the following hernias should nonoperative reduction be given consideration?

(A) sliding hernia
(B) femoral hernia
(C) indirect hernia incarcerated for the past two hours
(D) indirect inguinal hernia incarcerated for the past 24 hours
(E) Richter's hernia

887. Which of the following statements is true of umbilical hernia?

(A) there is a high risk of bowel obstruction
(B) Richter's hernia is frequent at the umbilicus
(C) most childhood hernias resolve spontaneously
(D) taping some form of support such as a coin helps resolution
(E) they are rarely symptomatic

888. Each of the following statements is true regarding large incisional hernias in the abdominal wall in adults EXCEPT:

(A) they rarely incarcerate
(B) they may require prosthesis in their repair
(C) a corset helps in symptomatic management
(D) they are often the result of wound infection with necrotizing fasciitis
(E) they frequently burst through the skin with minimal trauma

889. Massive scrotal hernias and hydrocoeles are encountered with frequency in some Third World environments, and an epidemiologic factor suggested to be associated with these abnormalities is

(A) hypoalbuminemia
(B) sickle cell anemia
(C) filariasis
(D) malnutrition
(E) ignorance of careful lifting practices

890. Laparoscopic hernia repair is a clinical experiment which may have which of the following advantages over open surgical repair?

(A) decreased operating time
(B) quicker rehabilitation
(C) local anesthesia
(D) outpatient procedure
(E) lower recurrence rate

ANSWERS AND TUTORIALS ON ITEMS 881-890

The answers are: **881-C; 882-E; 883-A; 884-E; 885-B; 886-C; 887-C; 888-E; 889-C; 890-B**.

881. For an operation as frequently performed as inguinal hernia repair, there are a very large variety of methods for carrying it out, with the inference drawn that not one of them is clearly superior. However, despite the variety of defect repairs in securing or replacing transversalis fascia attachments, the one antecedent feature common to each repair in infants and adults is dissection of and high ligation of the hernial sac. There is no further surgical repair indicated in children, whereas, in adults, further steps are taken to decrease recurrence by tightening up fascial defects. Moving the cord to a different layer is a feature of only a few adult operations, and in neither adult nor children is the internal ring strictly closed unless the spermatic cord has been cut as it may sometimes be in very elderly men or in females in which there is no structure to be salvaged at the internal ring. In most adults, the internal ring is tightened , but not obliterated, and even this step is unnecessary in children.

882. Many hernia recurrences are actually persistence of an associated hernia not appreciated at the time of original exploration, such as a concomitant femoral or direct inguinal hernia while an indirect hernia was repaired. Excessive tension is the most common technical failure, and occurs far more frequently than failures of the suture, since attenuated structures approximated under tension without appropriate relaxation incisions or prosthetic substitution would cut through tissue before breaking the suture material. Wound healing deficits are an extremely uncommon patient factor in hernia recurrence, and most of them are due to infection or drug therapy such as corticosteroids rather than an intrinsic collagen disorder in scar formation. Nearly all hernia recurrences are related to physician factors rather patient factors, making improper scar formation the least likely in this list.

883. Some apparently incarcerated hernias cannot be reduced, not because the abdomen is full, or because the inguinal valve cannot retain it, but because only

part of the hernia is represented by sac and there is a retroperitoneal component. This is particularly common on the right side in large hernias. The herniated bowel does not parasitize scrotal blood supply, but has carried it down with the retroperitoneal component in the anatomic features of a sliding hernia. To return this component to the abdomen requires recognition of the sliding feature of the hernia and wrapping of the peritoneum around the blood supply from the groin approach or doing an intra-abdominal operation to pull up the viscera intra-abdominally (the Laroque maneuver). In true incarceration, the bowel would likely become strangulated, and bowel that is apparently viable but not reducible from this ectopic location has likely got some component of the hernia outside the extrusion of the peritoneal sac.

884. A Richter's hernia is the incarceration of a portion of the bowel circumference that still allows passage of luminal contents so it does not cause more than a partial bowel obstruction or none at all. The incarcerated portion of the bowel is at high risk of perforation, and this constitutes an urgent indication for operation. It may occur at points other than the groin, such as the linea semilunaris. If the entire circumference of the bowel insinuated into the linea semilunaris, this would be termed a Spigelian hernia which enters at one site into the abdominal wall and protrudes down the sheath to exit at another site lower down. Richter's hernia would be more common and have a wider variety of sites than the single entry point into the abdominal wall of the Spigelian hernia.

885. It is true that femoral hernias are more frequently seen in females than in males; however, the more frequent hernia in females is the indirect inguinal hernia, the same as is true in males. Both genders should be checked for both potential sites and the other two of the three areas on the physical examination of the groin, since more than one type of hernia may be present in any individual.

886. The indication for nonoperative reduction is for a hernia that can be reduced and will retain viability if reduced. Sliding hernias cannot be reduced. Richter's hernia and femoral hernia reductions should not be attempted because of a higher risk of strangulation and perforation, and an indirect inguinal hernia that has been incarcerated for 24 hours has a very high risk of strangulation and infarction even if it could be reduced. The manipulation in its reduction may make the likelihood of perforation of devitalized bowel much greater.

887. Umbilical hernias are a frequent finding in childhood but rare in adults, and not all of those have had surgical repair, so spontaneous resolution must be the general rule. In adults, they may be acquired at a later age by intra-abdominal pressure increase such as pregnancy or ascites, and they are then quite often symptomatic. Richter's incarceration is rare, and serious complication of umbilical hernia in childhood such as bowel obstruction is rare. In the adult, however, they are frequently symptomatic, particularly with a considerable increase in intra-abdominal pressure, and there is a more likely recommendation for elective operation in the adult than in children.

888. Very large incisional hernias rarely cause trouble through incarceration of the bowel, and may be managed by symptomatic external support. When repaired, they frequently require prosthesis implantation, since many times they are the result of infection which has destroyed the fascia through which they herniate. The skin is a very tough and flexible barrier for their containment, and a ruptured abdomen is very unlikely after healing has taken place.

889. In some African nations the presence of scrotal enlargement from hernia and hydrocele is taken as a proxy of filariasis endemia. The correlation may not be exact, but enlarged lymphatics in the inguinal area may facilitate hernia protrusion. The hernias are not acquired by inattention to diet or any other pattern, since they are not present to excess outside the area where the endemia pattern includes filariasis but where the same diet and activity pattern obtains.

890. Laparoscopic herniorrhaphy cannot be called an advance if it converts a fifteen minute operation under local anesthesia in an outpatient into a four hour procedure under general anesthesia in an inpatient with attendant excess costs and an as yet unproven but suspected inferior recurrence rate. The one advantage suggested is that it may have a decreased recovery time and more rapid patient rehabilitation, but it as yet has not demonstrated a proven acceptability for the standard of care in hernia repair.

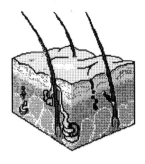

SKIN AND SOFT TISSUE SURGERY

Items 891-900

891. Which of the following treatments is **CONTRAINDICATED** for condylomata acuminata?

    (A)   surgical excision
    (B)   cryotherapy
    (C)   electrofulguration
    (D)   laser ablation
    (E)   podophyllin resin application

892. Which of the following procedures is **CONTRAINDICATED** in the management of a suspicious mole?

    (A)   high frequency electro-coagulation destruction of the mole
    (B)   excisional biopsy
    (C)   punch biopsy
    (D)   extensive palpation of regional lymph nodes
    (E)   chest X-ray

893. A 24 year-old male has a black pigmented nevus on his forearm. It has a central raised tumor with necrosis and ulceration and blood clot, and two satellite spots are noted 3 mm from the periphery. The punch biopsy should be performed

    (A)   in the center of the tumor
    (B)   through the ulceration bed
    (C)   tangentially through the tumor to obtain as much tissue as possible
    (D)   at the margin of the primary tumor to include normal skin
    (E)   encompassing one of the satellite spots

894. Which of the following factors is **LEAST** important in determining outcome following the diagnosis of melanoma?

    (A)   gender
    (B)   age
    (C)   tumor thickness
    (D)   lymph node involvement
    (E)   chemotherapy

895. Characteristic anatomic features of melanoma that are recognized with associated prognosis implications include all of the following **EXCEPT**:

    (A)   Hutchinson's lentigo
    (B)   superficial spreading
    (C)   nodular
    (D)   mucosal melanoma
    (E)   neuromelanoma

896. For which of the following lesions is there an identified gene association?

(A) cutaneous melanoma
(B) retinoblastoma
(C) keratoacanthoma
(D) fibrosarcoma
(E) choriocarcinoma

897. Which of the following cutaneous lesions carries the best prognosis?

(A) basal cell carcinoma
(B) squamous cell carcinoma
(C) melanoma
(D) mast cell tumor
(E) mycosis fungoides

898. Which of the following skin lesions does **NOT** have malignant potential?

(A) junctional nevus
(B) intradermal nevus
(C) keratoacanthoma
(D) actinic keratosis
(E) cutaneous horn

899. Which of the following lesions has the greatest likelihood of degenerating into soft tissue malignancy?

(A) lipoma
(B) neurofibroma
(C) sebaceous cysts
(D) ganglion
(E) hemangioma

900. Which of the following cancers is most likely to spread by means of lymphatic metastases?

(A) basal cell carcinoma
(B) squamous cell carcinoma
(C) leiomyosarcoma
(D) chondrosarcoma
(E) rhabdomyosarcoma

ANSWERS AND TUTORIALS ON ITEMS 891-900

The answers are: **891-A; 892-A; 893-D; 894-E; 895-E; 896-B; 897-A; 898-B; 899-B; 900-B**.

891. Condylomata acuminata are perianal or genital papillomas called venereal warts. They frequently respond to one or more applications of podophyllin, and if they have not been completely resolved, some form of destructive energy might be applied to the wart itself. Excision of the warts and suture closure would result in probable viral implantation and recurrence. Surgical excision is unnecessary as a first treatment with other ablation techniques listed being preferable over excision, reserved for second order treatment.

892. Electrofulguration with a high frequency coagulation destruction of the mole (hyfrecation) destroys the mole without pathologic identification of it. The diagnosis is therefore left uncertain as well as the depth of its invasion should it turn out to be malignant. The primary lesion and the regional nodes and sites of potential spread (such as chest X-ray) should be evaluated should it prove to be malignant. Punch biopsy with margins of normal skin is a preferable diagnostic approach, with punch biopsy being a diagnostic procedure for a later prescription of definitive management.

893. Biopsy of the pigmented skin lesion should be done perpendicular to the plane of the skin. This allows determination of the thickness of the lesion and an estimation of its depth of invasion. This should be done in the margin of the lesion so as to include normal skin, at the presumably laterally growing edge. If the ulcer bed is biopsied, there will be much inflammatory artifact, including blood clot, and necrosis will eliminate some unknown part of the thickness of the primary tumor. Tangential drilling may yield a greater sample of tumor, but it will be worthless for the determination of tumor thickness which is the best measurement to determine further therapy. The satellite spot may or may not be the same as the primary nodule, and that would leave the matter of the primary nodule's diagnosis indeterminate.

894. Melanoma is not very responsive to chemotherapy. In addition to surgical treatment, the one method that has shown promise is immunotherapy. Lymph node involvement is a principle component of clinical staging of the disease and positive nodes worsen prognosis remarkably. Tumor thickness (Breslow's method) is a measurement indicating the likelihood of invasive potential. Age is an important factor, since both the young patients with what is called juvenile melanoma (Spitz tumor) and elderly individuals with spreading melanotic freckle (Hutchinson's lentigo) have very much better prognoses than those in the mid-range of life with nodular melanoma. Across all tumor types and

stages, females seem to have a better prognosis by about 10% comparing stage for stage.

895. Although the pigmented melanocyte is a neural crest derivative, the term neuromelanoma and this association are not recognized as a clinical entity. Of the other options listed, the prognosis ranks in descending order with clinical patterns to each syndrome. Mucosal melanoma often presents in advanced stage and that may considerably limit the prognosis since the melanocytes are incorrectly thought only to be cutaneous in anatomic distribution.

896. Retinoblastoma arises from malignant transformation of pigmented retinal epithelial cells. For this lesion, there is an identified gene responsible for at least some instances of this and other malignancies, none of which are listed in the other options.

897. Basal cell carcinoma may be locally invasive and persistent with frequent recurrence, but it rarely metastasizes. Each of the other tumors listed either have the potential for metastatic spread (squamous cell carcinoma and melanoma) or are systemic from the onset with manifestations in the skin (mast cell tumor and mycosis fungoides).

898. Two of these lesions are composed of melanocytes, and three are squamous cell in character. Each of the epidermoid lesions is malignant or has pre-malignant potential, and are often found in sites exposed to sunlight or radiation. Both intradermal and junctional nevi have melanocytes, but the junctional nevus has melanocytes at the junction or contiguous interface of dermis and epidermis and may be prone to become melanoma if degenerating. The intradermal nevus has no such threat; these melanocytes are in the dermal layer deeper to the more worrisome junctional nevus.

899. Lipomas are benign encapsulated collections of lipocytes and are found with very high frequency in the general population. Their malignant potential is near zero, and they are excised only if they cause discomfort at critical annoying anatomic locations, such as belt lines or under brassiere straps. The ganglion is inappropriately named, since it is a collection of gelatinous mucoid material in the tendon sheath usually across joint surfaces such as at the wrist. Hemangioma is a cavernous collection of endothelium filled with blood without notable malignant potential. Neurofibroma alone is recognized as a pre-malignant lesion, since it may occur in multiple sites in the subcutaneous tissue in patients in a familial pattern with malignant degeneration potential in approximately 10% of these patients (von Recklinghausen's syndrome). When this degeneration occurs, the neurofibrosarcoma may spread as do other sarcomas, typically by hematogenous metastasis to the lungs.

900. Most sarcomas do not spread by lymphatic metastases. Although they may involve lymphatics in areas adjacent to the path of their invasion, they most typically spread by hematogenous dissemination, and therefore the usual first manifestation of their spread is a chest X-ray which suggests pulmonary metastases. Basal cell carcinoma typically does not spread by any means except local recurrent invasion and does not disseminate systemically as a rule. Squamous cell carcinoma, however, is an epidermoid cancer that typically does invade lymphatics and may be found and treated through regional node excision.

"Knowledge does not keep any better than fish."

Alfred North Whitehead (1861-1947)

PART V
GENERAL SURGICAL PRINCIPLES

DIRECTIONS: Each of the following numbered items or incomplete statements is followed by a list of answers or completions of the statement. Select the **ONE** best response from the lettered options that is the best completion or correct answer to the statement in the stem.

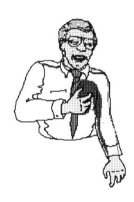

CLINICAL EMERGENCIES

Items 901-910

901.   A 28 year-old man enters the emergency room with sudden onset of severe abdominal pain radiating from left groin to the back and down to the scrotum. He has nausea and urinary frequency and is very restless, without ability to get comfortable in any position, although on physical examination he has no remarkable findings except for his agitation. He has had no previous illness. These findings are suggestive of

(A)   sigmoid diverticulitis
(B)   porphyria attack
(C)   acute cholecystitis
(D)   left ureteral calculus
(E)   acute appendicitis

902.   A 19 year-old woman is brought to the emergency room pale and listless with thready pulse. She has abdominal tenderness and cervical tenderness on pelvic examination which suggests a right pelvic mass. These findings are characteristic of

(A)   ruptured appendicitis with abscess
(B)   torsion of an ovarian cyst
(C)   ruptured ectopic pregnancy
(D)   strangulated internal hernia
(E)   acute tubo-ovarian abscess

903.   A 6 year-old boy is riding his bicycle when he develops a right scrotal pain that brings him crying to his mother. On examination the left side of the scrotum appears normal, but the right testicle appears retracted, tender, dusky, and does not transluminate with a flashlight. These findings are characteristic of

(A)   torsion of the appendix testis
(B)   torsion of the right testicle
(C)   appendicitis
(D)   strangulated right inguinal hernia
(E)   expanding right hydrocele

904. A 29 year-old man is playing tennis and experiences an audible "snap" and pain just below the popliteal space where there is some discoloration in the area and tenderness. The patient is able to walk with some discomfort, and a small "knot" is palpable in the tender area of the upper calf. This is characteristic of

(A)   ruptured popliteal aneurysm
(B)   acute Baker's cyst
(C)   ruptured plantaris muscle
(D)   ruptured Achilles tendon
(E)   ruptured superficial varicose vein

905. A 40 year-old obese woman enters the emergency room with acute onset of upper abdominal pain 30 minutes after a lunch of fried foods. She denies alcohol intake, and any prior history of dyspepsia. The pain radiates through to her back and the abdominal tenderness is located just to the right side of the epigastric midline. The likely clinical scenario suggests

(A)   acute duodenal ulcer
(B)   acute cholecystitis
(C)   acute pancreatitis
(D)   myocardial infarction
(E)   reflux esophagitis

906. A 68 year-old smoker complains of acute onset of right leg pain and numbness with inability to walk since the event began suddenly two hours before. He had two previous myocardial infarctions and is on digitalis, which recently regularized atrial fibrillation for which he had been most recently treated. On examination the left leg is cold below mid-thigh, pale, and pulseless. This clinical pattern is compatible with

(A)   deep venous thrombosis
(B)   superficial thrombophlebitis
(C)   aortic-iliac atherosclerotic disease
(D)   femoral arterial embolism
(E)   angiosclerosis obliterans

907. A 16 year-old boy reports to the emergency room with abdominal pain of 12 hours duration that began in the periumbilical area and migrated to the right lower quadrant. Which of the following physical findings most strongly suggests acute appendicitis?

(A)   direct abdominal tenderness at McBurney's point
(B)   rebound tenderness referred to the umbilicus
(C)   a positive psoas sign
(D)   rectal examination tenderness
(E)   high-pitched tinkling bowel sounds

908. A 72 year-old man is brought to the emergency room after complaining of sudden onset of backache and abdominal pain with one episode of a loose bloody bowel movement. On physical examination, a poorly defined midline abdominal mass is palpable, and his blood pressure is low, although he has been under treatment for hypertension. A likely cause for these findings is

(A) obstructing carcinoma of the colon
(B) sigmoid volvulus
(C) expanding aortic aneurysm
(D) ischemic colitis
(E) mesenteric infarction

909. A 68 year-old woman is brought by her daughter who has found her mumbling incoherently three days after a similar episode in which she was unable to see clearly all of any object placed before her. A transient period of forgetfulness resolved but now similar impairments appear to have returned. The likely diagnosis is

(A) amaurosis fujax
(B) toxic amblyopia
(C) retinal arteritis
(D) expanding intracranial aneurysm
(E) occlusive carotid artery stenosis

910. A 40 year-old woman is rushed to the emergency room following an automobile accident in which the she was slammed into the steering wheel and post. The patient has a large bruise across the anterior chest and has a bluish coloration of the face with distended neck veins. Stethoscope reveals barely audible heart sounds. The likely diagnosis is

(A) tension pneumothorax
(B) traumatic thoracic aortic aneurysm
(C) acute mediastinitis
(D) flail chest
(E) acute pericardial tamponade

ANSWERS AND TUTORIALS ON ITEMS 901-910

The answers are: **901-D; 902-C; 903-B; 904-C; 905-B; 906-D; 907-A; 908-C; 909-A; 910-E**.

901. The passage of a kidney stone in a previously healthy young man is typically characterized by acute flank and groin pain radiating to the scrotum. The other intra-abdominal crises should be manifest by peritoneal signs, and the patient would be typically protecting inflamed peritoneum by trying to minimize motion. Although always a possibility, appendicitis is less likely to give the kind and distribution of acute pain of sudden onset as described, and would likely show further physical findings.

902. The combination of abdominal pain, mass, and shock would suggest hemorrhage from some intra-abdominal catastrophe. Appendicitis and tubo-ovarian abscess are both possible in this age group, but would typically give inflammatory peritoneal symptoms before the abrupt onset of shock. A cyst or internal hernia is possible, but less probable than a tubal pregnancy, the rupture of which results in far more blood loss more quickly. Pregnancy is assumed for any woman of reproductive age, until it is ruled out, and in this instance is the most likely cause of the acute abdominal catastrophe described.

903. Torsion of the appendix testis may give pain and does cause an elevation and tenderness in the testis in the early stages, but it transluminates as a black dot in the scrotum. Hernia and hydrocele would give more presentation in the groin and less evidence of scrotal discomfort; whereas, appendicitis would give abdominal peritoneal findings. Torsion of the testis often presents following some evidence of physical exertion as in the setting described.

904. The patient would be unable to stand let alone walk if it had been the Achilles tendon that ruptured, and the other acute events in the popliteal space are not common in this setting. Although varicose veins may occasionally leak subcutaneously, the acute setting here and the context of the event suggest rupture of the plantaris muscle. It is annoying, but not disabling.

905. The relationship of the onset of pain to meals is frequently helpful for the upper gastrointestinal tract, since peptic ulcer is most significant at times of unopposed acid secretion, therefore is often relieved by eating. Fatty food intolerance is

associated with biliary tract disease, and it in turn may lead to pancreatitis. However, the pain of pancreatitis is often more severe, and is not as localized to the right of the epigastrium. Both myocardial and esophageal symptoms do not typically localize to the abdomen radiating to the back, and usually have some prior signals of antecedent disease.

906. Myocardial infarction can give rise to mural thrombus which may remain in the heart during fibrillation, but with improved contractility and regularization of the ventricular output, thromboembolism may result. The most likely point for impact is in the narrowing of the femoral artery at the adductor canal, giving rise to a threatened limb from distal arterial occlusion. Atherosclerosis and other gradually progressive vascular disorders may also result in ischemia, but are less likely to be as abrupt in onset. Both superficial and deep venous thrombosis can compromise circulation, but on the venous side of the circulation there would be an additional threat of pulmonary thromboembolism from the deep venous system, not made more likely by regularized myocardial rhythm.

907. Direct abdominal tenderness at the site of the appendix is the most suggestive physical finding for the diagnosis of appendicitis at the early stage when the appendix alone is inflamed. Rebound tenderness may detect peritoneal signs when the parietal peritoneum is involved, and psoas and rectal lateralizaton may be helpful for retroperitoneal findings but less frequently. Point tenderness remains a *sine qua non* as an operative indication for acute appendicitis.

908. Abdominal aneurysm is a likelihood in a patient who presents with a midline mass, particularly if pulsating laterally, and the symptoms and evidence of acute bowel ischemia suggest that it is rupturing and occluding visceral branches, as does hypotension. This constitutes a vascular emergency and is life threatening. Colon carcinoma and sigmoid volvulus might give blood loss, but not typically abdominal pain that begins as back pain but progresses rapidly.

909. Transient focal ischemic attacks, particularly involving visual field abnormalities that come and go, are often associated with thromboembolic cerebral circulation impairment. A frequent cause of this is an ulcerated arterial sclerotic plaque which gives rise to platelet aggregates and microthrombi that break loose from the atherosclerotic endothelial ulcerated surface. This finding is an indication for carotid artery flow and imaging studies and correction as indicated.

910. Deceleration injury can result in hemopericardium, either from bleeding into the pericardial space from vessels around the heart or from rupture of one of the heart's chambers. If this blood accumulates under systolic arterial pressure, decompensation is rapid, since outflow will cease, although it takes a longer time for compromise if the pressure is that of the right ventricle or diastolic or systemic venous pressure. Tension pneumothorax can also cause distended neck veins, but would not change heart sounds. A thoracic aneurysm could rupture into the pericardium, but then the acute effect of it would be the same as pericardial tamponade. Acute mediastinitis would not develop this rapidly following injury

whether from esophageal perforation or other origin.

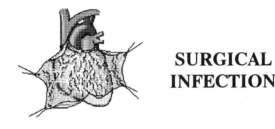

SURGICAL INFECTION

Items 911-920

911. Mechanical bowel preparation can be accomplished through all of the following means **EXCEPT**:

(A) oral administration of an osmotic solution

(B) instillation of saline solution through a nasogastric tube

(C) oral neomycin and erythromycin-base antibiotic administration

(D) intramuscular broad-spectrum cephalosporin administration

(E) oil retention enema

912. Surface decontamination in pre-operative preparation of the surgical field has demonstrated which of the following methods of hair removal is microbiologically superior with a lower risk of surgical wound infection?

(A) no hair removal
(B) electric clipper
(C) dry shaving with razor
(D) lather scrub and razor shave
(E) depilatory cream

913. Which of the following statements is true regarding a comparison of antibiotic monotherapy using imipenem in comparison with combination therapy with clindamycin and tobramycin in septic surgical patients?

(A) imipenem monotherapy is superior to combination therapy in all septic patients studied
(B) combination therapy is superior to imipenem monotherapy in all patients studied
(C) combination therapy is superior to imipenem monotherapy in only the sickest group of patients under study
(D) imipenem monotherapy is superior to combination therapy only in the sickest patients under study
(E) combination antibiotic therapy is the equivalent of imipenem monotherapy in all patients studied

914. Antibiotic prophylaxis is **NOT** indicated in which of the following patient settings?

(A) elective colon resection for carcinoma
(B) implantation of hip prosthesis
(C) aortic valve replacement
(D) thyroidectomy for invasive thyroid cancer
(E) hemorrhoidectomy in patient with rheumatic heart disease

915. The most frequent organisms in highest density that can be isolated from contamination following colon perforation are

(A) gram-positive aerobes
(B) gram-negative aerobes
(C) gram-positive anaerobes
(D) gram-negative anaerobes
(E) protozoan organisms

916. Which of the following groups of microflora are associated with endotoxemia?

(A) gram-positive aerobes
(B) gram-negative aerobes
(C) gram-positive anaerobes
(D) gram-negative anaerobes
(E) protozoan organisms

917. Pseudomembranous colitis is associated with which group of microorganisms?

(A) *Staphylococcus*
(B) *Streptococcus*
(C) coliforms
(D) *Pseudomonas*
(E) *Clostridium*

918. The preferred treatment of an infected foreign body implanted in musculoskeletal tissue is

(A) removal of the foreign body
(B) antibiotic therapy with gram-positive aerobic coverage
(C) implantation of impregnated beads that release antibiotic effective against gram-negative aerobes
(D) irrigation through adjacent catheters with oxidizing solutions
(E) unroofing and exposure of the infected site for granulation

919. Monoclonal anti-endotoxin therapy has been used in patients with results best characterized by which of the following?

(A) only patients with positive blood cultures benefitted
(B) only patients with higher severity of illness scores benefitted
(C) patients were benefitted only if the agents were administered before shock set in
(D) no benefit was seen if the patient had a negative assay for endotoxemia
(E) patient benefits could not be discriminated based on measurable parameters of sepsis or their mediators

920. An organism frequently cultured from indwelling hyperalimentation subclavian catheters in immuno-suppressed patients on broad spectrum antibiotics is

(A) *Pneumocystis carinii*
(B) *Mycobacterium tuberculosis*
(C) *Bacteroides fragilis*
(D) *Pseudomonas aeruginosa*
(E) *Candida albicans*

ANSWERS AND TUTORIALS ON ITEMS 911-920

The answers are: **911-D; 912-A; 913-D; 914-D; 915-D; 916-B; 917-E; 918-A; 919-E; 920-E**.

911. Bowel preparation involves the "pipe cleaners" of nonabsorbable antibiotics which cause brisk catharsis, as does oral administration of osmotic solutions or a saline load or enema use. Systemic administration of cephalosporins may give antibiotic effect where the circulation carries them, but that does not include the resident flora within the gut.

912. If an experimental model were designed to enhance the probability of wound infection, it would be hard to surpass the "standard of care" written into nursing procedure manuals for operating room routines. First, a patient impaired by a disease process and often nutritionally deficient is administered immunosuppressive drugs, then the stratum corneum is scraped off with a razor, denuding the first line of defense. With the excoriations and superficial burns lowering cutaneous resistance, this injured barrier is then recolonized with hospital flora — a group of pathogens selected for its resistance to most commonly used treatment regimens.

With this microflora now established in the injured barrier, further insult comes from scrubbing the burn with a brush, mechanical shearing forces and toxic chemical solutions. An incision is then made through this previously intact resistant barrier to infection.

The best microbiologic protection comes from no hair removal at all at operative incisions. This is particularly critical at such sites as eyebrows, which, once shaved, do not often grow back. If hair must be removed for exposure for the incision or for adherent draping or dressing, the method that least injures skin should be favored — clipping being the next best — which nonetheless leaves a supracuticular stubble.

913. In the most inclusive and carefully controlled antibiotic trial ever conducted for collaborative evaluation of surgical sepsis regimens, imipenem monotherapy was shown to be the equivalent of combination aminoglycoside (tobramycin, in this study) and anti-anaerobic drug (clindamycin in this study) for patients at lesser severity of illness ratings. But, for patients who were significantly more ill, particularly with multiple organ failure onset, monotherapy was significantly superior to combination therapy.

The important feature of this study that set a standard for future clinical trials of antibiotic regimens in surgical sepsis, is that patients must be stratified according to severity of illness for any meaningful outcome results in comparing treatments.

914. Clean elective surgical procedures do not require antibiotic prophylaxis unless there is a high inoculum that cannot be removed by preparation (as is often the case in colon resections), or there is prosthetic material with a local site of reduced resistance (as is true for orthopedic or cardiac prostheses), or there is impaired resistance from an area with natural immunity defect (such as rheumatic valve disease). Thyroid cancer does not constitute a considerable immunologic deficiency, and the inoculum should be negligible following skin preparation in the elective thyroidectomy.

915. Gram-negative anaerobes are the most numerous species in the lower GI tract and can make up to 80% of the dry weight of fecal contents. Other flora are present in the mixed inoculum but with much lower frequency.

916. Endotoxins are products of the coliform class of microorganisms of which *E. coli* is the prototype. Some of the gram-positive organisms and a few of the gram-negative anaerobes may be associated with exotoxins, but endotoxemia is a characteristic associated with gram-negative aerobic sepsis.

917. *Clostridium* is a gram-negative anaerobe, and one species, *Clostridium difficile*, is associated with the production of an exotoxin responsible for the development of pseudomembranous colitis.

918. The treatment of an infected foreign body is its removal. If the foreign body is a prosthesis that is necessary for function, that function must be either bypassed extraanatomically or replaced after eradication of the infection. Antibiotic therapy alone will not clear the source of sepsis if the foreign body remains.

919.   Monoclonal antibody therapy had potential promise in patients suffering endotoxemic shock; however, clinical trials of these agents could not discriminate benefit based on positive or negative blood cultures, endotoxin assays, or severity of illness, and without these indications for rational administration, this class of agents has not yet been approved by the FDA for general use.

920.   Immunosuppressed patients may be susceptible to *Pneumocystis* or tuberculosis, but they do not get it typically as catheter sepsis. Although both *Bacteroides* and *Pseudomonas* are possible, they would not be likely in the setting described. *Candida albicans* is the fungus which is most likely in the setting of the immunosuppressed patient given prolonged antibiotics and hyperosmotic total parenteral nutrition fluid and is a recognized source of catheter sepsis.

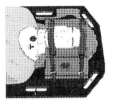

SHOCK/TRAUMA

Items 921-930

921.   Post-traumatic pulmonary insufficiency ("shock lung") with onset suggested in the 24 hours following injury is likely **NOT** to involve incrimination of which of the following insults?

(A)   oxygen toxicity
(B)   pulmonary fat embolism
(C)   toxic gas inhalation
(D)   perfusion with enzymes from pancreatic injury
(E)   microaggregated debris from bank blood

922.   Which of the following perfusion beds in shock has the greatest ability to regulate its blood flow and the greatest adaptation to decreased perfusion pressure?

(A)   liver
(B)   brain
(C)   lung
(D)   heart
(E)   kidney

923. Each of the following treatments has been used in the management of fat embolism, until our information on the syndrome has been improved, so that which is now contraindicated?

(A) controlled increased oxygen tension ventilation
(B) positive end expiratory pressure
(C) heparin therapy
(D) stabilization of long bone fractures
(E) high frequency "jet" ventilation

924. The most clinically significant early physiologic abnormality in post-traumatic pulmonary insufficiency is

(A) increased physiologic shunt
(B) increased dead space
(C) ventilator barotrauma
(D) cardiogenic pulmonary edema
(E) pulmonary fibrosis

925. Which of the following statements is true concerning transfusion with banked whole blood?

(A) it has a hematocrit equal to that of the donor at the time of the blood donation
(B) it contains sufficient numbers of active platelets for hemostasis purposes
(C) it is the treatment of choice for anemic patients with respiratory complications
(D) it is hyperkalemic
(E) it is alkaline

926. Advantages of crystalloid solution over colloid in fluid resuscitation include all of the following **EXCEPT**:

(A) cost
(B) availability
(C) retrievability
(D) low pyrogenicity
(E) edema

927. Military Anti-Shock Trousers (MAST trousers) should be removed from the patient

(A) on arrival in the emergency room
(B) in order to allow the patient to empty the bladder
(C) in the operating room following fluid resuscitation
(D) only after lower extremity and pelvic fractures are stabilized
(E) as soon as possible to facilitate extremity neurologic and vascular examination

928. Which of these patients is **LEAST** likely to be in shock? A patient

(A) making a normal quantity of normal quality urine
(B) with a normal blood pressure
(C) with a cardiac output three times normal
(D) whose extremities are warm and pink
(E) with hypotension and severe bradycardia

929. Caloric energy requirements in patients with a high metabolic demand, such as a major body surface thermal burn or comparable internal surface chemical burn as from peritonitis from perforated ulcer, may require daily caloric intake for the average size adult of

(A) 500 kcal
(B) 1000 kcal
(C) 2000 kcal
(D) 2500 kcal
(E) 3000 kcal

930. Which of the following vital signs most closely represents a patient with closed head trauma that results in loss of consciousness?

(A) increased pulse, increased blood pressure
(B) decreased pulse, increased blood pressure
(C) increased pulse, decreased blood pressure
(D) decreased pulse, decreased blood pressure
(E) normal pulse, normal blood pressure

ANSWERS AND TUTORIALS ON ITEMS 921-930

The answers are: **921-A; 922-E; 923-C; 924-A; 925-D; 926-E; 927-C; 928-A; 929-E; 930-B**.

921. Oxygen toxicity and barotrauma from ventilator therapy are possible complications leading to pulmonary injury following trauma, but not within the first 24 hours. In this event, more direct injury from the inhalation route from toxic gas or from the perfusion side, such as with lytic enzymes or microaggregated debris from bank blood or long bone fracture giving rise to fat embolism, are more likely culprits.

922. Over a wide range of perfusion pressures, the kidney has amazing adaptive responses to adjust its perfusion. First, it autoregulates its resistance vessels so that they relax with decreased perfusion pressure which tends to maintain constant flow. However, when mean arterial pressure is below 80 mm Hg, the kidneys release renin, which results in the pressor activity of angiotensin II, thereby increasing perfusion pressure through peripheral vasoconstriction. A third step is taken by the same angiotensin II in stimulating the outer layer of the adrenal cortex to release the mineralocorticoid aldosterone which ultimately results in sodium retention and volume expansion. These built-in adaptations allow the kidney resiliency in hypoperfusion not shared by such organs with a marginal arterial supply such as the liver with few adaptive responses. The internal vascular resistance of the brain is largely regulated by partial gas tensions (particularly P_{CO_2}), but are quickly used up in adaptive response. Each of the other visceral organs listed does not have the reserves and protective mechanisms of the kidney, and suffer dysfunction earlier in shock.

923. Careful support of respiration by enriched, but not toxic, levels of oxygen and increased end expiratory pressures but short of barotrauma to the lung, (for which jet ventilation may be useful), are measures that support the patient with respiratory distress. Decreasing further fat embolization may take place with early fixation of fractures, by open reduction if necessary. Heparin has lipolytic activity. It was formerly given for this effect, but thereby converted free fat globules to the more toxic free fatty acids, which actually exacerbated pulmonary injury, so that heparin is now contraindicated.

924. Shock lung has increased fluid content, much of it interstitial. This increased fluid volume and decreased gas space has lead to a greater fraction of the lung perfused but not ventilated which is by definition the physiologic shunt. Pulmonary fibrosis occurs at a very late stage and can inhibit gas exchange and impair compliance. This same alveolar capillary blockade can occur from lung injury by high pressures or oxygen tensions administered to the lung. However, the physiologic basis for the inability of the lung to oxygenate blood adequately is the greater fraction of lung perfused without effective ventilation, that is, physiologic shunt.

925. Dr. F.D. Moore described the "ancient and honorable whole blood transfusion" as: "cold, acidotic (sic), hyperkalemic, thrombocytopenic" and without any functioning white cells with only respiratory function in the decaying residual erythrocyte mass. It is not the treatment of choice for anemia. In fact, there are very rare indications for whole blood transfusion and not many of those would involve prolonged storage. For most other purposes of expanding oxygen transport capacity, red blood cells would be more appropriate and for volume expansion crystalloid or colloid would be preferable to whole blood. Donated blood is diluted in the anticoagulant to wind up with a hematocrit lower than that of the donor, and the preservatives are acidic solutions, while potassium increases in concentration as it leeches from devitalized cells.

926. Crystalloid solution is readily available at 1/20th of the cost of albumin, and has fewer associated pyrogenic reactions. It is also possible to retrieve infused crystalloid through diuresis in patients with functioning kidneys. It does cross permeable membranes to accumulate in "third space" components of extracellular fluid; whereas, albumin has a longer circulating half life in patients tending toward congestive edema.

927. Whenever "autotransfusion" results from application of MAST trousers and increased peripheral resistance to prevent pooling in the lower extremities, this same accomplished reinfusion could work against the patient if the MAST trousers were removed prematurely before fluid resuscitation. This should not be carried out in the emergency room to facilitate examination, to return the trousers to the ambulance crew or before adequate resuscitation. MAST trousers are not appropriate as stabilization of fractures. The compressive effect on the urinary bladder from intra-abdominal increase in pressure occurs as soon as the trousers are put on, and voiding or catheterization should occur while they are in place. Hypotension and a reversal of the fluid sequestration from the circulation occurs in premature removal until definitive surgical control can be achieved with adequate volume resuscitation.

928. The kidney is a vital perfusion bed that reflects its blood flow by autoregulating its resistance and endocrine actions that result in pressor activity and volume expansion. Only after these protective mechanisms are exhausted and hypoperfusion occurs does the quality and quantity of urine decrease, so a patient making normal urine is not in shock. In contrast, a patient with a normal blood pressure may have elevated this pressure from hypotensive levels by endogenous or administered catecholamines or other increased resistance. A patient with a higher cardiac output or warm and suffused extremities may be in endotoxic shock. The patient who has intra-abdominal hemorrhage as well as a closed head injury may have hypotension and the Cushing reflex leading to bradycardia from elevated intracranial pressure. Blood pressure and evidence of extremity blood flow are less reliable than the function of one vital visceral perfusion bed that has an output to reflect its perfusion, and the other examples listed would have impaired urine output or concentration.

929. Burn patients experience very high calorie requirements that may be 25 kcal/kg body weight plus 40 kcal per percent of body surface burned.

930. Closed head injury may result in the Cushing reflex which is a reflection of increased intracranial pressure. This gives rise to a strong vagal discharge, and that is reflected in a bradycardia which slows pulse and increased resistance which raises the blood pressure. If a patient has hypotension with a closed head injury, the source of the hypotension must be found in probable blood loss somewhere other than

in the head, with the rare exception being in newborns or infants.

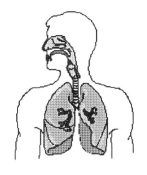

RESPIRATORY INTENSIVE CARE

Items 931-940

931. In setting oxygen tension, ventilatory rate, and tidal volume for ventilator therapy, the best clinical setting would be one that achieves

    (A)   a tidal volume of 700 ml
    (B)   a positive end expiratory pressure of 25 cm of water
    (C)   an arterial partial pressure of oxygen of 450 mm Hg
    (D)   a pH of 7.62
    (E)   arterial oxygen saturation of 90%

932. A negative and undesirable effect of positive end expiratory pressure (PEEP) would be

    (A)   decrease physiologic shunting
    (B)   improve compliance
    (C)   decrease venous return
    (D)   improve arterial partial pressure of oxygen
    (E)   decrease inspired oxygen

933. Candidates for transient extra-pulmonary assistance in oxygenation are those patients with severe but reversible pulmonary insufficiency which would include

(A) *Pneumocystis carinii* pneumonia
(B) bronchiectasis
(C) emphysema
(D) pulmonary fibrosis
(E) pneumoconiosis

934. Oxygen inhalation therapy by nasal prongs is contraindicated in which of the following conditions?

(A) chronic emphysema
(B) acute pulmonary edema
(C) diplococcal pneumonia
(D) myocardial infarction
(E) *Pneumocystis carinii* pneumonia

935. A Stage I epidermoid lung carcinoma in the right upper lobe of a patient with chronic emphysema and a 60 mm Hg oxygen tension on 40% assisted oxygen ventilation in a patient dependant on the ventilator represents a situation in which there is a/an

(A) resectable tumor in an operable patient
(B) nonresectable tumor in an operable patient
(C) resectable tumor in an inoperable patient
(D) nonresectable tumor in an inoperable patient
(E) indication for expeditious thoracotomy and lobectomy

936. Pulmonary emphysema occurring at an early age of onset is associated with

(A) mucoviscidosis
(B) congenital atresia of the opposite lung
(C) alpha-1 antitrypsin deficiency
(D) acetylcysteine therapy
(E) tracheoesophageal fistula

937. Pneumonia secondary to aspiration of gastric contents is a complication frequently seen in all of the following patient conditions EXCEPT:

(A) laryngectomy
(B) chronic alcoholism
(C) closed head injury
(D) heroin addiction
(E) infant asthma

938. Thromboembolism is LEAST likely in which clinical setting?

(A) hip fracture
(B) paraplegia
(C) prolonged abdominal pelvic operation
(D) polycythemia
(E) thrombocytopenia

939. Bronchospasm is treated by each of the following maneuvers EXCEPT:

(A) rigorous endotracheal suctioning
(B) β-adrenergic drugs
(C) somatostatin analog
(D) short-acting muscle paralysis
(E) long-acting muscle relaxation

940. Tube thoracostomy is employed in each of the following procedures **EXCEPT**:

(A) total right pneumonectomy
(B) spontaneous pneumothorax
(C) chylothorax
(D) right upper lobectomy
(E) hemothorax from multiple rib fractures

ANSWERS AND TUTORIALS ON ITEMS 931-940

The answers are: **931-E; 932-C; 933-A; 934-A; 935-C; 936-C; 937-A; 938-E; 939-A; 940-A.**

931. Hemoglobin is the most efficient oxygen carrier known, and once 90% saturation is achieved, the greater oxygen tensions result in very little additional oxygen carriage at much higher toxicity. Alkalosis inhibits oxygen release from oxyhemoglobin. Tidal volume depends on patient size and dead space that is subtracted from it, and end expiratory pressures would be appropriate depending on the positive benefit in reduction of physiologic shunt with minimal impact on venous return and cardiac output. Oxygen saturation of hemoglobin would be the appropriate indicator of clinical ventilator support.

932. PEEP improves the oxygen tension in any given quantity of blood flowing through the pulmonary veins by decreasing pulmonary shunting and improving compliance. However, the positive pressure that affects a greater amount of air in the lungs also affects the low pressure systemic venous blood return and thereby may reduce cardiac output. A greater concentration of oxygen is therefore carried, but in a lesser output of arterialized blood. Early stages of PEEP maximize the beneficial effects, but much higher levels impair delivery of this improved oxygen concentration in a smaller output from the heart.

933. *Pneumocystis carinii* pneumonia is an acute pneumonitis with severe respiratory insufficiency and inability to oxygenate blood with the affected lungs; however, there is an antimicrobial therapy which is effective over a short period of time, and no structural damage is residual in the lung, so such patients could be weaned from extracorporeal oxygenation and back to pulmonary respiration. Pulmonary fibrosis, pneumoconiosis, bronchiectasis and emphysema are all architectural changes with nonreversible pulmonary obstruction which would make the patient unlikely to return to support by pulmonary ventilation.

934. Over a protracted period of chronic lung disease, hypoxia becomes the respiratory drive when the patient accommodates a new higher setpoint of CO_2 tension. If the hypoxia drive is suppressed, ventilatory drive is reduced, and further hypercarbia may result, giving CO_2 tension levels that are anesthetic, dropping respiratory drive altogether. In the acute conditions listed, such as protozoan or bacterial pneumonia or congestive failure, oxygen therapy is a primary indication.

935. Resectability defines the tumor whereas operability is a property of the patient. In this instance we have a tumor that can be resected for surgical excision that is presumably curative in intent for lung cancer, but would further compromise a pulmonary cripple so that life cannot be sustained without — and probably even with — ventilator therapy and oxygen enrichment. This situation represents a tumor that can be resected in a patient that ought not be operated on.

936. An enzyme deficiency is identified with pulmonary emphysema of early onset. Cystic fibrosis or mucoviscidosis is more characteristically associated with bronchiectasis and acetylcysteine is helpful in its treatment. Both tracheoesophageal fistulae and pulmonary agenesis are not conditions associated with pulmonary emphysema of early onset.

937. Any condition that decreases sensitivity toward aspiration response such as suppression of cough reflex with narcotics, obtundation and coma from injury or toxicity predisposes toward gastric contents aspiration, particularly if nausea and vomiting are simultaneously stimulated. A number of infant asthma attacks, particularly those that happen when the patient is supine following eating, are found to be secondary to aspiration. Laryngectomy creates a permanent laryngostomy, and although aspiration of environmental contaminants is possible, gastric aspiration is precluded by this diversion.

938. Prolonged stasis from immobilization with orthopedic or neurologic impairment sets up the conditions whereby lower extremity deep venous thrombosis and embolism may result. Hypercoagulability as with some cancers or viscous blood flow such as

polycythemia may allow blood to clot in vessels more readily. Thrombocytopenia makes blood clotting and embolism less likely.

939. Bronchospasm is a condition of smooth muscle contraction constricting the airways, sometimes stimulated by and often made worse by the mechanical action by endotracheal suctioning. To overcome the smooth muscle tonic contraction, bronchodilators may be used that either employ the β-adrenergic effect of catecholamines, or relax smooth musculature directly in muscular blockade paralysis. A specific bronchodilator operating independent of either muscular blockade or catecholamine effect (and useful in instances of bradykinin bronchoconstriction in which catecholamines are contraindicated, such as carcinoid syndrome) is the use of somatostatin analog octreotide.

940. A chest tube is used to evacuate fluid from the pleural space in order to reexpand the residual lung. These fluids could be lymph, blood, or air; however, if the lung on that side of the mediastinum is completely removed, fluid accumulates to form a later fibrothorax, so no tube is used with pneumonectomy.

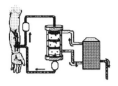

FLUID, ELECTROLYTES, AND BLOOD RESUSCITATION

Items 941-950

941. Infusion of which fluid would be **INAPPROPRIATE** therapy for a patient four hours post 40% full thickness body surface burn?

   (A) Ringer's lactate
   (B) 25% albumin
   (C) packed red blood cells
   (D) plasma
   (E) hetastarch

942. What does the blood type "O+" signify?

   (A) the patient is positive for type "O" antigens on the red cells
   (B) the patient is a universal donor
   (C) the patient is negative for antigens "A" and "B" but positive for rhesus antigen
   (D) a unit of this blood should not be given to a 50 year-old man who is type "AB-" with a negative cross-match
   (E) a unit of this blood should be given to a 5 five year-old girl who is "O-" if the cross-match is negative

943. What percent body surface is burned if a patient is scalded by a spray that strikes the right side of the body circumferentially burning right leg and arm and the torso to the front and back midline, sparing the head and genitalia?

   (A) 18%
   (B) 36%
   (C) 45%
   (D) 63%
   (E) 72%

944. What would be the anticipated mortality if the burn of the extent just described were full thickness in a 40 year-old patient?

   (A) 15%
   (B) 35%
   (C) 45%
   (D) 63%
   (E) 85%

945. If crystalloid and colloid are both employed for the support of a 70 kg patient with full thickness 45% body surface burn, what would be the net total volume required in the first 24 hours?

   (A) 3.0 liters
   (B) 5.0 liters
   (C) 6.5 liters
   (D) 8.0 liters
   (E) 10.0 liters

946. As remobilization of the sequestered extracellular fluid takes place, the volume requirements may decrease, but the energy requirements of healing have just begun. For a significant thermal injury as just described, the caloric requirement would approximate a daily total of

(A) 1000 kcal
(B) 2000 kcal
(C) 3000 kcal
(D) 4000 kcal
(E) 5000 kcal

947. If 3000 ml of fluid are being given one week post-burn and each contained 5% Dextrose solution, what is the calorie shortfall for the demand that must be made up?

(A) 600 kcal
(B) 1000 kcal
(C) 1500 kcal
(D) 2400 kcal
(E) 5000 kcal

948. A patient with closed head injury is not recovering cerebral function when it is discovered that the serum sodium is 88 mEq/L. The appropriate immediate initiation of therapy is

(A) push an intravenous bolus of 250 ml hypertonic saline solution
(B) 10% NaCl solution instilled via nasogastric catheter
(C) furosemide diuresis
(D) restrict water intake
(E) insufflate synthetic ADH as a snuff in the nasopharynx

949. Following prolonged aortic cross-clamping, the patient enters the intensive care unit and is found to have cardiac arrhythmia, decreased urine output and a serum potassium of 8.6 mEq/L. Each of the following treatments is appropriate **EXCEPT**:

(A) slow infusion of calcium gluceptate
(B) set ventilator for hypoventilation and increase respiratory dead space
(C) infuse 50% glucose with 10 units regular insulin
(D) 2 ampules of sodium bicarbonate infused in the arm opposite the calcium infusion
(E) potassium exchange resin (kayexalate) by retention enema

950. Eighteen hours post total thyroidectomy the patient is found in carpopedal spasm and complaining of tingling and shortness of breath. Each of the following maneuvers is appropriate **EXCEPT**:

(A) rebreathing into a bag
(B) infuse calcium gluceptate IV
(C) administer mithramycin
(D) give large amounts of oral calcium antacid tablets
(E) begin vitamin D treatment by mouth

ANSWERS AND TUTORIALS ON ITEMS 941-950

The answers are: **941-C; 942-C; 943-C; 944-E; 945-D; 946-C; 947-D; 948-D; 949-B; 950-C.**

941. The patient within a short period post burn is not likely to be loosing any appreciable quantity of the cellular component of whole blood. However, transudation of plasma and fluid is happening very rapidly following the burn injury, and hemoconcentration is taking place in the patient's circulation. On admission the hematocrit is likely to be rising to levels that are already too viscous for effective circulation, and packed red blood cells would further exacerbate this problem. The patient needs fluid and fast and in high quantities — the most readily available would be crystalloid, and it must be given to replace that which is lost. To maintain a longer period of circulating intravascular fluid, some colloid component of it may be important to sustain circulation, and plasma, albumin, and plasma expanders such as hydroxy-ethyl starch may serve this purpose. Packed red cells are contraindicated at this stage.

942. The major blood groupings identified the major red cell incompatibilities as based on one antigen or another, both or neither (A, B, AB, O); and to this was later added a minor, but significant incompatibility discovered through transplacental sensitization in succeeding pregnancies found to be present also in the rhesus primate (Rh +/-). This blood type demonstrates neither A nor B antigens with Rh being positive, yet this blood type is by no means universal in that it can be given to anyone. After major antigen typing, it is important to exclude a large number of minor incompatibilities that would lead to hemolysis with over a score known and probably an equal unknown number yet to be fully described, and that is done with a cross-match to rule out presensitization and the presence of preformed hemolytic antibody. That there is no reaction in cross-match might mean that it is worth the risk of Rh sensitization in the middle age man who needs blood, but that may not be the best policy for the young girl whose reproductive future may be compromised since we will not know until the event whether a future fetus might have received the genes that determine Rh positivity in it that will run into potential difficulty with Rh antibody induced by this transfusion sensitization. Major blood group typing, like tissue typing, attempts to minimize sensitization across compatibility differences in specificity, and the cross-match attempts to eliminate hemolytic reaction from preformed antibodies that the donor unit could encounter.

943. The classic "rule of 9's" states that the upper extremity is 9%, the front and back of the torso each 18%, and the lower extremity in entirety 18%, with 9% for the head and 1% for the genitalia. If the patient experienced a burn of half the body (18%), one complete upper extremity (add 9%) and one complete lower extremity (add 18%) the patient has a 45% body surface burn, if the head and genitalia are spared which together are 10% (with corresponding mirror image of the body given the additional 45%).

944. For a full thickness loss of this extent, the age and extent of burn sum to

325

approximate expected mortality. In this 45% full thickness burn in a 40 year-old sums to a high mortality risk of 85% all other factors not considered. If by reason of good health and meticulous surgical care, an extent of burn as described could show satisfactory improvement on those odds with a great deal of energy input.

945. Assuming the patient normally needs 2 liters of water for insensible losses as a daily fluid requirement without the burn, the injury requires the following additional fluid: one-half ml per kg times percent full thickness loss is in colloid (.5 x 70 x 45 = 1575 ml colloid) and three times that in crystalloid (1.5 ml x 70 kg x 45% burn = 4725 ml crystalloid). Adding 2000 ml of D5/W to the 1575 ml colloid and 4725 ml crystalloid sums to 8300 ml total fluid volume, which approximates 8 liters in his first 24 hours post burn.

946. In the absence of infection, just the energy requirement for this degree of thermal injury would be two to three times basal level even given bed-rest. Now that quantity of caloric energy will have to be supplied along with the fluids being given.

947. If the patient's requirements are 3000 kcal and the equivalent of 3000 ml D5/W are being given, the shortfall can be calculated by determining the caloric delivery presently. Since D5/W has 50 gm glucose in a liter, three liters gives 150 grams of glucose. Each gram of glucose supplies four kcal, so (150 x 4 = 600 kcal) are being delivered with a 2400 kcal shortfall. It is unlikely that this will be able to be adequately repleted with the same glucose concentration speeded up, since the volume requirements are no longer as high, so the glucose must be enriched or other

energy substrates added. Amino acids have the same value in terms of 4 kcal/gm, but they supply other nutrient needs. Adding some component of lipid doubles the kcal/gm of nutrient value. At one week post-burn, he may be able to take in enriched feedings by mouth. But the maintenance fluid should be shifted now for caloric enrichment whereas the primary requirement early in the post-burn course was for fluid volume and colloid. Over a prolonged period if no return to regular diet of mixed varieties of foods can take place, then trace metals and vitamins must be supplemented. All of this is assuming a normal recovery without intercurrent complication that force up demand and decrease utilization of energy fuels, such as sepsis, which is very likely in a burn of this extent).

948. This patient has severe hyponatremia and it may account for the encephalopathy that persists after his closed head injury. Administration of concentrated sodium by either IV or gastric route may be necessary as may diuresis be, but each is a second order treatment to attempt free water clearance. The simplest and earliest therapy should be to restrict water or any hypotonic fluid intake. In the syndrome of inappropriate ADH secretion (SIADH) the patient is retaining water and diluting the normal serum electrolytes, and the first objective is to keep this from getting worse by additional water intake. Since the ADH activity is excessive, exactly the wrong thing to do is to add additional ADH, which is a treatment for a problem opposite the one that is keeping this patient from waking up.

949. The emergency response is to decrease hyperkalemia. Then reduce excitability of neuromuscular conductivity and contractility. Calcium stabilizes cardiac membranes despite the continuing excess serum potassium, and the next steps are done to drop the high serum potassium by driving it into the intracellular space. Glucose with insulin crosses the membrane surface and expands intracellular space by glycogen deposits which expands the potassium rich intracellular space while the activation of the membrane pump creates a net flux of potassium into the cells. This is in competitive equilibrium with hydrogen ion, and that is the rationale for reducing hydrogen ion concentration to favor potassium transfer intracellularly. That is the therapeutic reason for the bicarbonate infusion, and it is the same reason that hypoventilation and increasing dead space would be contraindicated in this patient, since respiratory acidosis would counteract the effect of bicarbonate infusion, slow intracellular potassium transfer and worsen hyperkalemia.

950. It is the symptoms that are treated rather than the serum calcium numbers, but the patient complaint appears that support to the falling serum calcium will be necessary, so it should be begun until symptoms are relieved and then chronic support taken over by oral supplements. The vitamin D and calcium tablets accomplish the latter role after the IV calcium infusion. The immediate therapy of decreasing the alkalosis that is usually a part of hypocalcemia from the patient's excitement with the discomfort of tetany is effective in rapidly changing the quantity of ionized calcium in competitive equilibrium, since it is the ionized calcium that is the physiologically active component of the diminished total present in the circulation. Rebreathing causes CO_2

increase in the blood and a rise in the hydrogen ion concentration unbinding the calcium carried on serum albumin with competitive antagonism of rising hydrogen ion. The wrong answer is to prevent absorption of calcium into the blood stream, which is the action of mithramycin. This treatment is for hypercalcemia and has no role in the tetany of hypocalcemia.

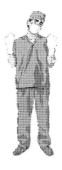

ANESTHESIA AND OPERATING ROOM

Items 951-960

951. With respect to hematocrit, at what level is oxygen flow to peripheral tissues optimal?

   (A)   15%
   (B)   25%
   (C)   35%
   (D)   45%
   (E)   55%

952. Which of the following blood products carries minimal risk of viral disease transmission?

   (A)   packed red cells
   (B)   serum albumin
   (C)   factor VIII
   (D)   fibrinogen
   (E)   platelet concentrate

953. A patient complains of very annoying pain in both shoulders and one side following laparotomy. Physical examination reveals a coin shaped burn over each deltoid area and lateral thigh. The most likely explanation is

(A) sterile abscess at injection sites
(B) electrocution entry and exit sites
(C) improper application of electrocautery grounding pad
(D) hypersensitivity reaction to adhesive tape
(E) nummular fixed eruption from medication hypersensitivity

954. During an open technique colonic anastomosis, pencil tip electrocautery activation produces an explosive noise accompanied by a flash of blue flame. Although the patient is not burned, the whole operating team is alarmed. The most likely source is

(A) alcohol used in the skin prep
(B) cyclopropane anesthesia
(C) a short circuit in the spark gap
(D) methane ignition
(E) improper grounding lead on the patient

955. A patient is intubated after anesthesia induction and the endotracheal tube fixed with a "bite block" and tape. The patient is then raised to semi-sitting position for skin preparation preceding thyroidectomy for a large right thyroid nodule. During the opening incision, the blood looks dark whereas adequate oximetry readings had been recorded during anesthesia induction. The most likely explanation is

(A) kinking of the endotracheal tube deviated by the right thyroid mass
(B) oxygen tank on anesthesia apparatus has run out and intake has not been switched over to auxiliary
(C) prolonged paralysis secondary to deficiency in acetylcholine metabolism
(D) advance of the endotracheal tube lumen into the right mainstem bronchus
(E) malignant hyperthermia

956. Patients with Graves' disease have a higher rate of which of the following complications attributable to anesthesia technique than patients generally?

(A) dental fractures
(B) corneal abrasions
(C) naso-alar cartilage necrosis
(D) hypotension
(E) aspiration

957. A 12 year-old boy with abdominal pain is brought to the operating room and anesthesia induced for laparotomy for suspected appendicitis. As the abdomen is scrubbed, the EKG monitor shows the heart is racing and the blood pressure dangerously high. A spot determination of plasma glucose with a chemical strip shows the blood glucose is elevated. A likely source for this crisis is

(A) ketoacidosis
(B) anesthetic reaction
(C) sickle cell crisis
(D) pheochromocytoma
(E) malignant hyperthermia

958. A patient has just undergone left pneumonectomy and is returned to the recovery room. Coughing vigorously on awakening, the patient is extubated, but continues to cough and abruptly produces large volumes of dilute blood-tinged sputum as he is gasping for breath. You should immediately

(A) reopen the incision
(B) compress the innominate artery against the sternum with a finger inserted through tracheostomy incision
(C) place the patient in Trendelenburg with the left side down
(D) sit the patient up in semi-Fowler's position
(E) perform bronchoscopic lavage

959. Patients with chronic obstructive lung disease have a higher incidence of each of the following intraoperative complications EXCEPT:

(A) bronchospasm
(B) pneumothorax
(C) atelectasis
(D) pulmonary embolism
(E) pneumonitis

960. A "street person" is admitted for debridement and irrigation with immobilization of an open fracture of the tibia and fibula that he cannot recall how it happened. The operation is performed under spinal anesthesia, and 48 hours postoperatively he becomes very agitated, incoherent, and bizarre in behavior. Immediate check of blood gases shows normal values without hypoxia. The likely diagnosis is

(A) pulmonary embolism
(B) acute schizophrenia with psychotic break
(C) drug dependance
(D) "ICU syndrome"
(E) ischemic heart disease

ANSWERS AND TUTORIALS ON ITEMS 951-960

The answers are: **951-C; 952-B; 953-C; 954-D; 955-D; 956-B; 957-D; 958-C; 959-D; 960-C.**

951. Hemoglobin is the chief oxygen carrier of blood. If there are no other rate limiting factors, the higher the hemoglobin, the greater the oxygen carriage capacity. However, hemoglobin is packaged in red cells, and the packed cell mass reflects not only the amount of hemoglobin if the red cells have the normal concentration within them, but also the rate at which blood can flow through capillaries. Many surgeons and more anesthesiologists might be concerned that a hematocrit of 35% was an indication for transfusion; however, the rheology of blood flow through capillaries is actually superior to that seen at the higher hematocrits which carry with them a higher viscosity resisting peripheral capillary perfusion. When hematocrit is very low, although the flow might marginally improve from that seen at hematocrit of 35%, the sacrifice of oxygen capacity means that oxygen delivery is decreased.

952. Human blood donor products carry with them risks of disease transmissibility from malaria through syphilis and hepatitis to HIV and other virions that may result in later development of communicable disease. Each of the subsequent fractionation steps in preparing blood or plasma constituents attempts to both screen and treat the product to minimize transmission risk. This risk is successively minimized but not reduced to zero in production of any of the listed products except albumin.

953. Electrocautery functions through the concentrated intensity at the narrow point of the cautery tip, with the grounding pad giving a much larger surface for that contact and decreased energy transmission for any unit of surface. If this grounding pad is inappropriately placed, has inadequate conductive lubricant applied, or dislodged, the other electrical conduction skinpoints serve as much more concen-

trated focal grounding points. The EKG leads used in monitoring the patient during this operation have served that capacity, and electrocautery has caused electrical burns at the sites of Einthoven's triangle. Hypersensitivity to tape, drugs, and other allergy would not have this peculiar distribution, and injection site reaction would be subcutaneous rather than a surface burn.

954. Explosive anesthetic agents have been nearly eliminated from contemporary operating rooms in the US, at least, but anesthetic agents are not the only the flammable gas. One agent often suspected but rarely proven is alcohol vapor. Alcohol flammability is much less than other fuels (which is why Indianapolis 500 race cars have eliminated gasoline and are powered by alcohol for the lower probability of ignition in collision) and there would be minimal to no alcohol residual at the time the colon anastomosis is being done late in the operation.

In the first instance, the alcohol applied to the skin would be minimal, and it would vaporize almost immediately after application and would have been long since gone or so dilute as to be even harder to ignite than it has just been noted to be in liquid form. Whether grounded or not, electrical energy is expected to be generated at the cautery tip, and improper setting can give rise to electrical burns, but does not account for the explosion. It is sometimes a surprise to recognize that microbes generate methane in the colon. The quantity of gas produced, particularly with endoscopic insufflation and vigorous bowel preparation prior to operation, can be decompressed when the colon is open and can be ignited by the spark from electrocautery.

955. When an airway is fixed in position when the patient is in a given posture, the alignment of that intubation must be checked again after the patient's position is changed. With flexion, the tube tip may have advanced since it is fixed at the teeth. The ventilation of both sides of the chest is routinely checked following intubation, but should also be checked following repositioning of the patient. "Running out of gas" is a conceivable but unlikely event, and most operating rooms don't run on bottled oxygen alone. Even room air ventilation would not produce desaturation unless the system were closed to ambient ventilation. Cholinesterase deficiency is a possible encounter, but the patient's ventilation is assisted immediately after paralysis is induced for intubation, and it is continued in the event spontaneous ventilation does not resume. Malignant hyperthermia would not give evidence of desaturation as obviously as other signs.

956. Many patients with Graves' disease have exophthalmus associated with this form of hyperthyroidism. Protection of the cornea from overhanging IV tubes, esophageal stethoscopes, electrical stimulators, and a host of electrical monitoring leads draped over the patient's head is the same as for patients being operated on for other causes, but most patients have the eyelids taped to protect the cornea with instillation of methyl-cellulose drops or antibiotic ointment. This may also be routinely done with patients with Graves' disease, but with less effectiveness if proptosis makes lid retraction and incomplete closure likely. The desiccation that may occur during the period of anesthesia or superficial contacts with the cornea in their protuberant position are more likely in Graves' disease

than in other patients. The other complications listed have no unique predisposing factors with Graves' disease, and some are less likely than for the median incidence for all patients in operating rooms.

957. Both anesthesia induction with or without transient hypotension from vasodilatation, and vigorous abdominal massage during abdominal preparation under anesthesia when the patient's abdominal guarding does not limit the rigor of manipulation, have triggered release of catecholamines from an unsuspected pheochromocytoma. The first encounter with an unknown pheochromocytoma in an operating room has high mortality even under contemporary monitoring and support measures, and the best defense is a low threshold for suspicion of this abnormality. It is further increased in likelihood in the combination of both blood glucose and blood pressure as physiologic effects of the catecholamine excess. It is unlikely that either diabetes or sickle cell anemia would be unknown at this age and in this setting, but neither would give this pattern, nor would hyperthermia. Only in the most general sense is this an anesthetic reaction, since it is more a reaction to the manipulation during this experience, and the physiologic effect of such anesthesia second order phenomena, e.g., vasodilation or hypotension, to which it is reactive.

958. What is described here is the rare but disastrous circumstance of blow-out of the bronchial stump soon after pneumo-nectomy. Saline is typically infused into the chest without chest tube drainage to replace the lung with fibrothorax in healing post pneumonectomy. In the course of coughing, the bronchial irritation from this disruption and leak of this pleural fluid is suggested and the coughing also accentuates the blow-out diameter. The patient is flooded with fluid from the open bronchus into the remaining functional lung, and this constitutes, in effect, acute salt water drowning. Accentuating this with further instillation of saline by broncho-scope is obviously not a good idea. A change in the patient's position can be life saving, with the left side down enlisting the help of gravity to slow fluid entry into the airway, and with the head down, drainage of the aspiration fluid is facilitated. The chest should be opened, but under the controlled circumstances of a return to the operating room, where assessment of the bronchial stump and securing it for both air and water tight seal can be reinforced.

959. Patients with structural derangement of lung structure such as emphysematous blebs or foci of inflammation have a higher rate of pneumonia following operation with typically lower resistance to inocula such as those that may come from intubation or aspiration. Bronchospasm is significantly higher in those patients with any degree of bronchitis, and atelectasis is the most common complication, each from the higher likelihood of inspissated secretions from the prior pulmonary inflammatory conditions. Pulmonary thromboembolism is related to the perfusion side of the lung, and associated with factors that are common to these patients and others of comparable age and disease distribution with no higher incidence in the chronic lung patient, although the consequences of thromboembolism may be more severe in these patients with compromised functional reserves.

960. The most probable event in a patient who is agitated postoperatively and the first obligation of the clinician is to assure that hypoxemia is not the cause, as it seems not to be in this instance. Both pulmonary embolism and myocardial infarction can give rise to anxiety and agitation in a patient, but they would not account for the timing and symptomatic state with apparently normal oxygen uptake and utilization. Mental illness is very prevalent among patients who are homeless, and this may or may not be characterized by intermittent psychotic episodes. The ICU syndrome is described as a combination of sleep deprivation and a barrage of stimuli in a very anxiety-provoking situation outside the patient's control. There is no evidence that this patient fits this description or that he is even in the ICU. What is worrisome is the circumstance of his original injury. If he were unaware of how it happened, either he was unconscious at the time of this severe injury or forgot it from some lapse immediately afterwards. "Lost" periods of time such as this are often associated with addiction to narcotics or serious bouts of alcoholism, and the patient's current status compatible with withdrawal.

It is also noteworthy in retrospect that there is some difficulty in the anesthetic course of the patient, but spinal anesthesia obviated some of the observations on "drug appetite" noted with induction of general anesthesia, but it may be noteworthy that the patient's post-operative pain would be less likely to be responsive to normal doses of some analgesic agents. The diagnosis could be proven by a challenge with some reversal agents such as nalorphine, but the patient's requirements at this point are to be comforted and treated for his significant local injury as well as his metabolic response to it. There are alternatives to infusions of alcohol or *ad libitum* narcotics, and others may be employed such as the use of minor or major tranquilizers and sedatives, but only while continuing to prove that his agitation is not due to hypoxemia.

An etiologic cause for agitation following an open fracture in any patient, not peculiar to the given clinical description of this patient, might be fat embolism, and this can be checked by examination of stained urine and other clinical evidence, but it is often reflected in respiratory problems and blood gas abnormalities later. Longer term management and rehabilitation for his orthopedic injury is more likely to be successful than for his addiction, but each must be addressed at this time during his hospitalization with precedence given to his addiction.

"Moderation in all things — above all else, in the practice of moderation."
Glenn W. Geelhoed

PART VI
SURGICAL SPECIALITY REVIEW ITEMS

DIRECTIONS: Each of the following numbered items or incomplete statements is followed by a list of answers or completions of the statement. Select the **ONE** best response from the lettered options that is the best completion or correct answer to the statement in the stem.

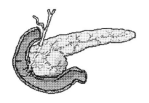

ENDOCRINE SURGERY

Items 961-970

961. The most important intra-operative monitoring device in a patient undergoing surgical exploration for pheochromocytoma is

   (A) central venous pressure line
   (B) urinary bladder catheter
   (C) intra-arterial pressure line
   (D) pulmonary artery catheter
   (E) esophageal stethoscope

962. Which of the following intra-operative maneuvers is contra-indicated during surgical exploration of a patient with metastatic carcinoid syndrome when hypotension results?

   (A) whole blood infusion
   (B) somatostatin analog injection
   (C) albumin concentrate infusion
   (D) epinephrine injection
   (E) β-adrenergic blockade

963. Which of the following imaging techniques is most closely associated with functional abnormality in pre-operative localization of hyper-functioning parathyroid tissue?

   (A) selective venous sampling
   (B) computerized tomography
   (C) real time ultrasonography
   (D) barium swallow esophography
   (E) magnetic resonance imaging

964. Which of the following statements best characterizes positive lymph node involvement with thyroid carcinoma for a patient with a 1.5 cm papillary thyroid cancer in the right thyroid lobe?

   (A) positive nodes change the Stage from I to II
   (B) positive nodes extend the thyroidectomy to radical neck dissection of the affected side
   (C) positive nodes require chemotherapy as adjunct to operation for cure
   (D) positive nodes change the Stage from II to III
   (E) positive nodes do not change the clinical staging

965. Hormones that regulate blood glucose by causing it to increase include all of the following **EXCEPT**:

(A) corticosteroids
(B) insulin
(C) growth hormone
(D) glucagon
(E) norepinephrine

966. Suppression tests in the diagnosis of insulinoma are generally considered safer than provocative testing. Which of the following pre-operative tests for insulinoma is a suppressive test?

(A) fasting
(B) tolbutamide
(C) glucagon
(D) diazoxide
(E) calcium

967. Endocrine hyperfunction of each of the following hormones can constitute a clinical crisis for a patient. Hypofunction can also cause critical illness in a deficiency or lack of response from all of these hormones **EXCEPT**:

(A) insulin
(B) thyroxine
(C) parathormone
(D) cortisol
(E) catecholamine

968. Which of the following patients is most likely to have a single hyper-functioning parathyroid adenoma found in one parathyroid gland?

(A) a hemodialysis patient following 10 years of chronic renal failure
(B) a 23 year-old woman with asymptomatic hypercalcemia
(C) a teenager from a family with hereditary multiple endocrine adenopathy
(D) a 60 year-old arthritic con-suming milk and alkali in large quantity for 25 years
(E) a young man with kidney stones whose family has had isolated primary hyperpara-thyroidism in several affected individuals

969. Each of the following clinical maneuvers is beneficial in the patient with hypercalcemic crisis **EXCEPT**:

(A) saline infusion
(B) magnesium administration
(C) furosemide diuresis
(D) calcitonin injection
(E) mithramycin administration

970. In Cushing's syndrome there are increases in the measurements of each of the following manifestations **EXCEPT**:

(A) blood sugar
(B) urinary corticosteroids
(C) bone density
(D) blood pressure
(E) waistline girth

ANSWERS AND TUTORIALS ON ITEMS 961-970

The answers are: **961-C; 962-D; 963-A; 964-E; 965-B; 966-D; 967-E; 968-B; 969-B; 970-C.**

961. Abrupt changes in blood pressure can be a critical feature of operation for pheochromocytoma. Manipulation of the tumor or excitation following infusion of its catecholamine content into the circulation may elevate the blood pressure to dangerously high levels requiring urgent pharmacologic intervention. Occlusion of the effluent through venous ligation is signaled by a decrease in the catecholamine-stimulated blood pressure elevation. This physiologic response can be helpful in locating ectopic or residual chromaffin tissue following completion of excision of the primary tumor or in search for bilateral disease, metastatic or second primary functioning tissue.

962. Injection of epinephrine or any analog of it or catecholamine-releasing agent causes a discharge of kinin, and a paradoxical fall in blood pressure results from injection of epinephrine or any of its congeners. This "bradykinin shock" is diagnostic of a carcinoid syndrome, and may also result in bronchoconstriction. One of the few therapies that results in pharmacologic reversal may be the administration of somatostatin analog; however, blood and fluid volume resuscitation is recommended for hypotension in any patient with carcinoid syndrome while catecholamine therapy is contraindicated.

963. Each of the radiographic imaging methods may detect mass lesion presence, but the venous sampling measures local secretion near the site of the catheter tip. This may help lateralize a source of parathyroid hyperfunction. Because C-terminal growth hormone fragments circulate for hours in the systemic circulation until cleared by the kidney, N-terminal parathyroid hormone assay may be helpful, since its serum half-life is measured in minutes, and it is more highly correlated with the end-point source of the secretion. Form/function correlation is critically important in pre-operative localization for endocrine surgery, since mass abnormality does not imply directly that the identified lump is the source of the patient's syndrome unless the intermediate secretion excess can be identified as originating from that mass.

964. Unlike the clinical staging for breast cancer or other more frequently encountered cancer, regional lymph node status does not change the staging of papillary thyroid cancer. Clinical staging is principally determined by the size of the primary lesion and presence or absence of distant metastatic manifestations, so the patient described would be Stage I with or without the positive nodes adjacent to the primary thyroid cancer.

965. Insulin is a regulatory hormone for blood glucose causing it to decrease, and the other hormones listed are "counter-regulatory hormones" that cause blood sugar to increase. Norepinephrine does that immediately by glycogenolysis. Glucocorticoids, growth hormone, and glucagon are involved in the process of gluconeogenesis to cause a sustained increase in blood sugar.

966. Each of the studies listed is a provocative test that causes the release of insulin and can further dangerously lower blood sugar in the hypoglycemic hyperinsulinemic patient except diazoxide. Diazoxide inhibits insulin release and can be used both diagnostically for insulinoma identification and therapeutically to sustain blood sugar in a patient with the metastatic malignant islet cell disease.

967. Hypofunction of insulin can give ketoacidosis, and insufficient thyroid hormone can lead to myxedematous coma. Parathormone insufficiency is manifest in tetany, and insufficient cortisol gives Addisonian crisis. Although hyperfunction from excess catecholamine can give hypertensive attack as seen with pheochromocytoma, there is no remarkable clinical syndrome of hypofunction associated with catecholamines, requiring replacement of the hormone.

968. In hereditary kindreds, all parathyroid cells inherit the same genetic defect. As a consequence, primary hyperplasia is the rule in both isolated hyperparathyroidism that is familial as well as multiple endocrine adenopathy. All secondary hyperparathyroidism has a stimulus that affects all available parathyroid tissue, so multiple gland disease is nearly invariable in such patients with, for instance, chronic renal failure. Ingestion of excess calcium may change the renal excretion, but should not affect hyperplasia or neoplasia in the parathyroid gland in humans. In sporadic primary hyperparathyroidism, such as that commonly seen in patients who present with asymptomatic hypercalcemia, over 90% will have single gland disease, manifest as a solitary hyperfunctioning parathyroid adenoma.

969. Diuresis with both saline and furosemide are important first steps in the hypercalcemic patient to get calcium clearance. Calcitonin may be helpful in decreasing serum calcium as mithramycin invariably is, but with higher toxicity associated with its use. Magnesium is another divalent cation which would exacerbate hypercalcemia and require many of the same overloaded systems in its clearance, and would be contraindicated in a hypercalcemic crisis.

970. Cushing's syndrome is manifest by truncal obesity, gluconeogenesis that is expressed in elevated blood sugar, and excess corticosteroid excretion in the urine. However, bone density is decreased, with calcium resorption and osteoporosis, sometimes to the point of pathologic fracture.

"I have taken all knowledge to be my province."
Sir Francis Bacon (1561-1626)

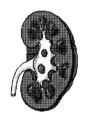

TRANSPLANTATION SURGERY

Items 971-980

971. A liver transplant performed in the right upper quadrant of an infant with biliary atresia using part of an adult cadaver donor liver is technically prescribed as

    (A)   an orthotopic autograft
    (B)   a heterotopic allograft
    (C)   an orthotopic isograft
    (D)   a heterotopic xenograft
    (E)   an orthotopic allograft

972. Causes of early kidney transplant dysfunction includes each of the following **EXCEPT**:

    (A)   minor histocompatibility antigen mismatch
    (B)   hyperacute rejection
    (C)   ureteral obstruction
    (D)   prolonged warm ischemia in donor organ
    (E)   venous obstruction and thrombosis

973. Which statement would apply to kidney transplantation from the flank of the donor to the iliac fossa of the recipient between identical twin siblings?

    (A)   a rejection episode can be anticipated within 14 days of transplant
    (B)   the operation is an orthotopic isograft
    (C)   immunosuppression should not be required for the recipient
    (D)   the donor is left with half renal function at 6 months postoperatively
    (E)   the recipient can be expected to have one half the donor's renal function at 6 months

974. Which of the patients listed in the ICU with certified cerebral death is a candidate for cadaver renal donation?

    (A)   an HIV-negative, hepatitis B positive drug addict
    (B)   a patient with Stage III Hodgkin's lymphoma
    (C)   a patient in cardiogenic shock on epinephrine support for 3 days following massive myocardial infarct
    (D)   a patient with intra-abdominal sepsis and gram-negative septicemia
    (E)   a patient with undifferentiated intracranial extensive glioblastoma multiforme

975. Which of the following conditions precludes transplantation from the donor for a recipient who is blood Type O-positive?

(A) a "zero antigen match" in histocompatibility
(B) a primary intracranial malignancy in the donor
(C) a creatinine of 1.2 mg/dl in the donor
(D) a positive cross-match
(E) a history of glomerulonephritis in the recipient

976. An ultrasound (US) scan shows a large, unilocular, fluid-filled space adjacent to a kidney transplanted in the iliac fossa which has been steadily growing since the transplant operation 2 weeks ago. The asymptomatic patient's BUN and creatinine are normal. The most likely diagnosis is

(A) urinoma from leaking urine
(B) ileus in adjacent bowel
(C) lymphocele
(D) organizing blood clot
(E) abscess

977. Six years postoperatively, a transplant recipient is noted to have progressive severe systolic hypertension. Renal function on maintenance immunosuppressive drug treatment is normal. The most likely cause is

(A) glomerulonephrosclerosis
(B) chronic rejection
(C) recurrent glomerulonephritis
(D) essential hypertension
(E) renovascular stenosis

978. Which of the following access procedures is preferable for the primary initiation of maintenance hemodialysis for a patient with end-stage renal disease?

(A) arteriovenous fistula (Breschner) in forearm
(B) Scribner shunt cannulation
(C) femoral venovenous (MacIntosh) catheterization
(D) bovine xenograft arteriovenous conduit in the thigh
(E) prosthetic vascular graft loop from brachial artery to cephalic vein AV fistula

979. Which statement is **NOT** true for diabetic patients for end-stage renal disease (Kimmelstiel-Wilson disease)?

(A) steroids in the immunosuppressive regimen would exacerbate the diabetes
(B) immunosuppressive corticosteroids may worsen vision through cataract formation
(C) diabetic foot ulcers may be more troublesome following immunosuppression
(D) diabetes is a contraindication to transplantation because of problems with immunosuppression complications
(E) hip replacement surgery may be necessary following increased bone resorption with immunosuppression drugs

980. Liver transplantation has exhibited its highest success rate in which group of patients?

(A) patients with alcoholic cirrhosis
(B) patients with massive primary hepatoma
(C) infants with biliary atresia
(D) young adults with tumor metastatic to the liver
(E) fulminant viral hepatitis

ANSWERS AND TUTORIALS ON ITEMS 971-980

The answers are: **971-E; 972-A; 973-C; 974-E; 975-D; 976-C; 977-E; 978-A; 979-D; 980-C**.

971. The first descriptor explains the location of the implanted graft, and the liver is placed anatomically where the prior liver had been before excision making it orthotopic. The second descriptor refers to the source of the donor organ, and it is from one individual to another within the same species but not genetically identical, making it an allograft.

972. The transplanted kidney may fail for reasons of vascular, ureteral, or parenchymal damage that stems from prolonged ischemia, or hyperacute rejection that stems from presensitization of the recipient to donor antigens. Minor histocompatibility antigens would not likely be a source of hyperacute rejection if the recipient had no prior experience with them, and minor mismatches are not a

contraindication to transplantation in a patient whose crossmatch is negative.

973. Transplantation between identical twins is an isograft, with the kidney placed in heterotopic position in the iliac fossa. Both donor and recipient could be expected to have renal hypertrophy restoring each to the full renal function of the donor within weeks postoperatively, a biologic "two for the price of one" result. Rejection would not be anticipated, since perfect histocompatibility obtains, therefore, no immunosuppression would be necessary for the recipient.

974. Blood-borne dissemination of viral, bacterial, malignant or other transmissible disease is a contraindication to transplantation as is prolonged ischemic changes that come from normothermic hypoperfusion. Metastasizing carcinoma or lymphoma may also contraindicate organ donation, but intracranial neoplasm, even if high-grade and undifferentiated rarely metastasizes outside the skull, and such patients may be considered donors.

975. Malignancies that may be metastatic and have access to the systemic circulation are generally contraindication to transplantation, but this does not include intracranial primary neoplasms. A history of glomerulonephritis may suggest that recurrent disease is possible, but not immediately and does not preclude transplantation. Histocompatibility matching attempts to minimize antigenic differences, but a zero antigen match is still possible for organ transplantation, whereas a positive crossmatch rules out the donor organ for this recipient. A creatinine of 1.2 mg/dl reflects adequate renal function for a patient who is being transplanted for chronic renal failure.

976. A perinephric abscess would not be asymptomatic, and leaking urine would be reflected in reabsorbed urea to distort renal function tests. The ileus is unlikely, since a graft is outside the peritoneal cavity, and an organizing blood clot is frequently heterogeneous on US scan. In the process of implanting the kidney, iliac lymphatics are disrupted, and may frequently leak a lymph collection around the kidney. These lymphoceles are often self-limited.

977. Recurrent primary renal disease or chronic rejection would not be likely with normal renal function, nor would parenchymal histologic changes of glomerulonephrosclerosis be compatible with normal renal function tests. Essential hypertension is very common; however, it would not be characterized by onset with this timing and severity. Intimal proliferation and atherosclerosis may take place around the area of the vascular suture line, and this stenosis at the site of a continuous scarring may cause renal vascular hypertension through the mechanisms of renin release. This differential diagnosis is important, since this condition may be reversible.

978. External devices that transfer through the skin such as the Scribner shunt or the MacIntosh catheter are useful for acute dialysis, but for chronic dialysis, all materials should be implanted beneath the skin with percutaneous puncture only at the time of dialysis. Conduits, of autologous, xenograft or prosthetic material may be useful when the veins *in situ* are no longer usable, but the forearm AV fistula has the best utility and longevity once matured for chronic hemodialysis.

979. All the complications listed are possible in patients with transplantation and more likely in the diabetic because of the end-vessel disease and decreased local immune response. Although diabetic patients have a higher complication rate than transplantation patients without prior diabetes, these increased risks do not contraindicate transplantation for diabetic end-stage renal disease.

980. Generally speaking, infants have fared better with liver transplantation than adults, and specifically those with congenital abnormalities without inflammatory or neoplastic disease have done better with an anatomic defect in the primary liver rather than with a secondary destruction of it by viral, malignant, or toxic insults.

"Rules are just to take up slack when the brains run out."

Popashvily (1945)

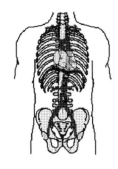

ARTERIAL VASCULAR SURGERY

Items 981-990

981. Which of the following statements regarding diabetic foot ulcer is **NOT** true?

   (A) infecting organisms are frequently anaerobic
   (B) one of the etiologic bases for diabetic ulcers is endarterial insufficiency
   (C) one of the etiologic bases for diabetic foot ulcers is neurotrophic injury
   (D) hyperbaric oxygen treatment is occasionally helpful in their treatment
   (E) major arterial reconstruction (aorto-iliac and femora-popliteal) remarkably improves blood flow to the site of the ulcer

982. The principle correctable component of peripheral ischemic disease is

   (A) atherosclerosis
   (B) elevated serum cholesterol
   (C) distal thrombosis
   (D) smoking
   (E) ergotism

983. Which of the following statements is true concerning "trash foot"?

   (A) it results from embolization of crumbled atherosclerotic debris and platelet aggregates from arterial atheromata
   (B) it can be prevented with platelet-aggregation inhibitors
   (C) amputation is most often avoidable with intact limb salvage by arterial reconstruction
   (D) heparinization is not necessary in its management
   (E) only a single end-artery is usually affected

984. A difficult operation is undertaken for a ruptured abdominal aortic aneurysm with the finding of extensive atherosclerotic disease extending beyond the iliac arteries necessitating graft extension to the femoral arteries bilaterally. After a protracted operation, back bleeding was poor at the distal anastomosis, and when aortic cross-clamping was released, the patient became hypotensive. Although blood pressure returned to normal, urine output did not. Intensive care unit management of this situation would include all of the following **EXCEPT**:

   (A) bicarbonate infusion
   (B) heparinization
   (C) warming the extremities with hyperthermia blanket
   (D) tourniquet amputation of the lower limbs
   (E) hyperventilation settings for the ventilator

985. A 72 year-old patient had prior elective aortic aneurysm resection but returned to a surgeon with the unusual complaint that both lower legs fell asleep when he had been kneeling on a church bench. Physical examination reveals tense pulsatile masses in the flexor space behind both knees. The most likely diagnosis is

(A) Baker's cysts
(B) popliteal aneurysms
(C) bursitis
(D) osteoarthritis
(E) lesser saphenous thrombophlebitis

986. A 23 year-old woman with past history of birth control pills as the only medicine she has taken comes in with severe hypertension and an abdominal bruit is heard. Her renin determination is very elevated and she is poorly responsive to blood pressure control medication. The most likely diagnosis is

(A) atherosclerotic aortorenal occlusive disease
(B) acute vasospasm
(C) fibromuscular hyperplasia
(D) focal embolic renal occlusion
(E) Paige kidney

987. A middle-aged man complains of an unusual giddiness and fainting when he has been engaged in vigorous activity using his upper extremities. It has never happened while he is jogging or at rest. A bruit is audible in the right subclavicular fossa along with other physical findings. This suggests the most likely diagnosis

(A) right proximal subclavian artery occlusion
(B) right carotid high-grade stenosis
(C) vertebral artery aneurysm
(D) expanding aortic arch aneurysm
(E) right brachial artery occlusion

988. The most valuable indication for carotid endarterectomy under local anesthesia is

(A) it is less expensive
(B) the patient is aware of what is taking place
(C) continuous evaluation of the patient's cerebral status is possible relative to inter-ruption of blood flow
(D) it prevents hyperpyrexia from general anesthesia malignant hyperthermia
(E) it takes less time

989. Which of the following findings is an indication for carotid endarterectomy?

(A) total carotid occlusion discovered on arteriography
(B) ulcerated atheroma at carotid bifurcation
(C) 30% narrowing of carotid arteries bilaterally
(D) acute stroke
(E) 50% bilateral common carotid stenoses

990. An endarterectomy is carried out at the site of prosthetic graft suture to a popliteal artery in a femoral-popliteal bypass, with good back flow and excellent high volume blood flow at the completion of the bypass procedure. Four hours later, there is total occlusion of the graft and popliteal artery. The most likely cause is

(A) a kink in the graft
(B) intimal flap
(C) hypercoagulability
(D) vasospasm
(E) retrograde propagation from distal arterial embolus

ANSWERS AND TUTORIALS ON ITEMS 981–990

The answers are: **981-E; 982-D; 983-A; 984-C; 985-B; 986-C; 987-A; 988-C; 989-B; 990-B.**

981. Diabetic foot ulcers are an arterial insufficiency, but of an end-organ vasculitis and occlusion rather than major arterial occlusive disorders. Therefore "replumbing" the main lower extremity vessels does not result in remarkably improved blood supply. For that, various pharmacologic therapy or sympathetic blockade appears more beneficial, at least temporarily. It is true that a large number of the organisms are anaerobic, which is responsible for the name "fetid foot", and hyperbaric treatment has some benefit while it continues. Neuropathy is one component of the diabetes, as well, and this neurotrophic component prevents injury avoidance (as it does in leprosy) and perpetuates injury. The principle vessels responsible for the vascular component of diabetic foot ulcers are beyond the reach of vascular reconstruction.

982. Intrinsic vascular disease such as atherosclerosis is highly unlikely to be reversible in a major way, but cholesterol control can slow its progression. The acral ischemia of ergotism is historically interesting but is clinically uncommon. The effect of nicotine on peripheral circulation is dramatic and may make a marginal difference between salvage from ischemia and extremity loss. The progression of vascular disease under various regimens of diabetic control is a subject of some debate; however, there appears to be some minimal unpreventable progressive vascular disease even in the most compulsive control regimens. Further extension of marginal therapeutic methods should not be undertaken in patients who persist in the single most correctable cause of peripheral ischemic disease.

983. A showering of atheromatous debris and aggregated blood thromboemboli plugs end-order vessels in the foot, often resulting in dry gangrene. The process nearly always leads to at least partial amputation, and it is not preventable by antiplatelet active drugs. Heparinization is a necessary component of treatment but not sufficient to reverse embolization from atheromata which do not dissolve with thrombolysis.

984. The syndrome described is compatible with severe lower extremity ischemia and rhabdomyolysis. The patient must be protected against the acidosis and hyperkalemia from the necrosing tissues of the ischemic lower extremities, and it may even be necessary to isolate them from the circulation by tourniquet amputation. The kidneys have shut down possibly from the hypotensive insult but compounded with rhabdomyolysis causing protein precipitation in the kidneys, particularly when acidosis was present. It is for that reason that alkalinization of the circulation through administration of bicarbonate and ventilator settings to blow off an excess CO_2 are appropriate treatments. The one maneuver that would be contraindicated would be to accelerate rhabdomyolysis and increase the oxygen demand in the ischemic tissues by increasing the temperature. Rather than a hyperthermia blanket, hypothermia would be more appropriate in this setting.

985. Vascular atherosclerosis is a generalized disease and reconstructive surgery is palliative. Following resection of an aneurysm in one area, the same propensity exists in others, and popliteal aneurysms are likely to be found in a patient who has multiple other sites of arterial disease. If the patient's cardiac status (remember that vascular disease is generalized, and this is the site of the biggest and most important of the diseased

blood vessels) is able to withstand another operation, elective repair of these additional aneurysms should be considered.

986. This is a classic setting in which renal vascular hypertension is due to a focal and fixable benign process. Aortorenal bypass beyond the segment of fibromuscular hyperplasia should result in a long-term cure of restored renal blood flow and normal blood pressure. She is too young to have extensive atherosclerotic disease absent any lipid disorders or family history, and there is no evidence to suggest embolus. Besides, if the kidney was totally occluded on the arterial side, there would be less renin production to raise the blood pressure. External compression of the kidney that might similarly raise the renin production ("Paige kidney" effect) is not evident here, it is not needed to explain the syndrome when the abdominal bruit suggests arterial turbulence through a high-grade stenosis from a significant renal arterial stenosis. Fibromuscular hyperplasia is the more usual etiology in this setting.

987. The syndrome described is compatible with subclavian steal syndrome. In this instance, there is a proximal subclavian occlusion, and with exertion of the upper extremities, the blood flow is reversed from the vertebrobasilar system. The flow reverses because of the lower resistance runoff with exercise of the right upper extremity, and dizziness results from the "stolen" blood flow from the cerebral and cerebellar distribution. This same reversal of flow would not occur with the occlusions listed in the other options, and vertebral aneurysm would not give the symptoms, although it might give rise to the bruit.

988. The patient's cerebral blood flow in its most important evaluable aspect — cerebral function — is possible to evaluate under local anesthesia whereas this is abolished by general anesthesia. The other options listed, though debatable, even if true, are not principle determinants of the selection of local anesthesia for carotid endarterectomy.

989. It would be dangerous to revascularize a patient who is in the acute phase following stroke, and there is no need for reconstruction of the carotid on the side of total occlusion that has been present for some indeterminate period. Neither 30% nor 50% narrowing is hemodynamically significant. However, the risk of distal embolic phenomena from the ulcerated surface of the atheroma plaque makes preventable neurologic damage a strong indication for endarterectomy for the patient with ulcerated atheroma.

990. In the course of tearing out atheroma, the endothelium is lifted, and if this is not appreciated by retrograde backflow, the full head of arterial systolic pressure may pick up the cut edge of the intima and dissect it forward with total occlusion resulting and secondary graft thrombosis. Anticoagulation is not likely to prevent this, and patient hypercoagulability is highly unlikely. There is no prior evidence of an arterial system thrombus that may embolize, and it is unlikely that the graft would kink postoperatively when excellent flow was maintained immediately postoperatively. Vasospasm does not give rise to this clinical pattern nor would it halt a bounding high flow arterial pulse. Attempts are made to prevent this complication by inspection of the cut edge of the intima and tacking down the upstream edge where dissection might lift the intima from the muscular tunics of the arterial wall.

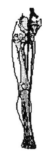

VENOUS VASCULAR SURGERY

Items 991-1000

991. Which of the following conditions is **NOT** a hemodynamic threat to life, but may be a harbinger of underlying malignancy?

(A) deep venous thrombosis
(B) migratory superficial thrombophlebitis
(C) pulmonary thromboembolism
(D) *phlegmasia cerulea dolens*
(E) splenic vein thrombosis

992. The association of risk factors with varicose veins strongly suggests an etiology linked to

(A) prolonged standing
(B) multiple pregnancies
(C) Western life style
(D) high-fiber diet
(E) tropical filariasis

993. Which of the following elements is **NOT** a component of venous thrombogenesis?

(A) incompetent valves in perforating veins
(B) venostasis
(C) Virchow's triad
(D) hypercoagulability
(E) disruption of endothelial intima

994. The single biggest disadvantage of venography in the diagnosis of deep venous thrombosis is

(A) inaccuracy
(B) causes thrombosis in some patients in whom it might not otherwise be present
(C) lack of sensitivity
(D) lack of specificity
(E) high cost

995. Which of the following statements about radiolabeled fibrinogen scanning is **NOT** true?

(A) it reliably demonstrates preformed clot
(B) a blood-borne viral disease transmission is possible
(C) it accumulates in post-operative wounds and hematomas
(D) it is not useful in pelvic vein assessment
(E) it gives a positive reading in wound infection which it cannot distinguish from thrombosis

996. Each of the following are true for operative indications for a patient with thromboembolism **EXCEPT**:

(A) deep venous thrombosis confirmed
(B) recurrent thromboembolism
(C) thromboembolism recurs while on full therapeutic heparinization
(D) angiographic confirmation of thromboembolism is secure
(E) patient's ability to withstand a repeated embolism is compromised

997. Which of the following statements about venous thrombosis is **NOT** true?

(A) Coumadin therapy is useful in prevention
(B) early ambulation reduces risk
(C) low dose subcutaneous heparin is appropriate therapeutic anticoagulation for treatment of established thrombosis
(D) platelet active agents such as salicylates are useful in prevention
(E) intermittent compression pumps may prevent venostasis during prolonged operations

998. Inappropriate therapy for chronic venous stasis ulcer would include

(A) Unna boot
(B) vein stripping
(C) femoral-popliteal bypass
(D) skin graft
(E) elevation while at rest

999. Following femoral-popliteal bypass a patient is returned to the ward where you have an interest in preventing stasis in blood flow. The correct positioning of the patient would be

(A) the legs elevated above the heart to gravity-assist venous return
(B) the legs straight and neutral on the level of the supine patient
(C) patient should be sitting up with hips and knees flexed
(D) compressive stockings should be applied up to mid-thigh
(E) semi-Fowler's position

1000. Which of the following statements relating to vena cava operations is **NOT** true?

(A) it is a treatment for pulmonary embolism retrieval
(B) caval clipping attempts to compartmentalize the inferior vena cava
(C) ligation of the inferior vena cava has hemodynamic consequences
(D) sieving procedures can still transmit smaller thrombo-emboli
(E) the venous interruption procedure may, itself, give rise to venous thrombosis

ANSWERS AND TUTORIALS ON ITEMS 991-1000

The answers are: **991-B; 992-C; 993-A; 994-B; 995-A; 996-A; 997-C; 998-C; 999-B; 1000-A.**

991. Each of the options that involve clots in the venous system pointed at the heart (deep venous thrombosis, *phlegmasia cerulea dolens*, pulmonary thrombo-embolism) is a hemodynamic threat to life, as is splenic vein thrombosis which could propagate to occlude the portal system. Migratory superficial thrombophlebitis has nuisance value in terms of febrile morbidity and tenderness, but is moreover a sentinel of underlying malignancy, perhaps based in hypercoagulability which occurs in some cancers.

992. The classic Western medical texts have it all wrong: they relate varicose veins to prolonged standing and multiple pregnancy, and heavy exertional effort. In the developing world the birth rate is higher, people are far less sedentary, and certainly they have to work harder without "labor-saving devices" in abundance. Men develop varicose veins as frequently as women in the Western world, without — clearly — at least the risk factor of multiple pregnancies. Since there is such a geographic disparity in varicose vein incidence, it must have something to do with Western life styles since the same high incidence is acquired by immigrants from low incidence areas to industrial environments. Fiber content in the diet is in the opposite direction, being more prevalent in the areas of lesser varicose vein incidence as are tropical filariasis conditions.

993. Incompetence of the valves in perforating veins is an etiologic agent in varicose veins, but not linked to thrombogenesis. Each of the other options listed is individually and collectively, as components known as Virchow's triad, the basis of venous thrombogenesis.

994. The gold standard for the determination of deep venous thrombosis was and remains venography. It is the most accurate clinical examination by which all others are judged in comparison to this standard, and has few false positives or false negatives creating admirable accuracy. It may be expensive, but it is comparable to other tests employed for far less accuracy in suggesting the diagnosis. However, the hyperosmotic contrast injected in the deep venous system may set up the third or missing link in Virchow's triad to initiate thrombogenesis by intimal disruption and endothelial inflammation, so that in approximately 5% of patients deep venous thrombosis is actually caused by the diagnostic test that would otherwise have proven negative.

995. Since fibrinogen, whether labeled or otherwise, can only find its way into a clot that hasn't yet been formed when it is converted into fibrin, this method has no role in detecting venous thrombus already present. It is not reliable in assessing pelvic veins, and furthermore, fibrin formation occurs in healing wounds, hematoma, and wound infection, all of which would be revealed as false positive tests. Since it is a serum derived donor product, transmission of hepatitis or HIV is a risk.

996. Thromboembolism and its potential is an indication for operation, if *angio-graphic* evidence is shown of *recurrent* pulmonary embolism on *adequate* heparinization or the presence of contraindications thereto. Each must be satisfied for operative intervention. Venous thrombosis is not an adequate indication for operation nor does it have to be confirmed when superseded by thromboembolism evidence and its recurrence confirmed.

997. Therapeutic heparinization requires partial thromboplastin time that is over 100 seconds. Low dose heparin is not therapy but prophylaxis, and in fact is not an anticoagulating dose. No deep venous thrombosis monitoring is required, since no anticoagulative effect is expected. For resolution of established deep venous thrombosis, full therapeutic heparin anticoagulation is required. Methods such as intermittent calf compression, early ambulation, antiplatelet active agents and low dose heparin may be helpful in deep venous thrombosis prevention, as is coumarin interference in prothrombin activity.

998. Chronic venous stasis ulcer is a very troublesome and limb-threatening condition. Often, it is a result of a very large incompetent perforating vein, and ligation of these nearby perforating veins with or without superficial vein stripping is a component of therapy. Putting the limb at rest to decrease venous pressure is appropriate therapy, and that would include elevation and Unna boot immobilization. However, new vascularization of arterial inflow would increase venous pressure rather that decrease it, and an arterial operation should not be performed for a chronic venous stasis ulcer.

999. It is wise to avoid venostasis, but not at the expense of raising resistance to arterial run-off following a fresh arterial by-pass. In addition, compression stockings brought up to mid-thigh would compress the newly implanted graft and would be contraindicated on arterial basis for whatever presumed benefit they might give to diminish venostasis. The ultimate in venostasis is arterial inflow occlusion. The neutral position is best, with the patient encouraged to ambulate periodically to achieve the pumping action of muscular contraction, but flexion at the knee whether in bed (semi-Fowler's) or in a chair (sitting up) should be discouraged.

1000. The intent of any venous interruption procedure is interception of the *next* embolus, and does nothing to retrieve the prior embolus, relying on thrombolytic systems and anticoagulation to prevent new clot formation. The clip has hemodynamic consequences, particularly if it becomes — in effect — a total caval ligation when the next thrombus migrates to it. It may also set up endothelial damage and the intimal portion of Virchow's triad, and be itself a source of venous thrombosis. The patient who has already had a pulmonary embolus has some hemodynamic compromise and right heart strain, and a sudden reduction in venous return may change that further. At the same time, large collateral venous pathways may take over the function of the cava, and then they, too, can carry the thromboembolic risk. It is for that reason that left ovarian vein drainage into the left renal vein is frequently ligated at the time of inferior vena cava compartmentalization. Whether from inside the cava (Mobin-Uddin umbrella, Greenfield filter) or from outside, (Mile's clip) or a combination of both (plication), these procedures are only halfway effective preventive measures in patients who still have the thrombogenic risk of Virchow's triad, and the intent of the venous interruption procedures is only to tide the patient through the period when their reserves have marginal tolerance for a repeat thromboembolism.

"Before undergoing a surgical operation, arrange your temporal affairs — you may live."

Reny de Gourmont (1858-1915)

351

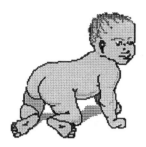

PEDIATRIC SURGERY

Items 1001-1010

1001. Which of the following statements is true regarding congenital diaphragmatic hernia?

(A) it is most common on the right side

(B) both lungs are normal when re-inflation can take place with reduction of the hernia

(C) severe respiratory insufficiency often follows surgical repair when the diaphragm is intact and the gut returns to the abdomen

(D) the peritoneal cavity is typically capacious and empty since much of the contents have migrated

(E) strangulation and infarction of the visceral components ectopic in the chest are frequent problems complicating repair

1002. The delivery room calls to report a newborn has been delivered with a protruding upper midline abdominal mass. You find that it is darkened, matted, stiff and dried without evidence of covering lining. The most likely diagnosis is

(A) exstrophy of the bladder
(B) omphalocele
(C) eventration
(D) gastroschisis
(E) prune belly

1003. Tracheoesophageal fistula is a congenital defect with several forms. The most common of these is

(A) atresia of the trachea with a proximal segment of the esophagus connected to the distal tracheal stump

(B) atresia of the esophagus with proximal and distal esophageal stumps adjacent to a normal trachea without fistula

(C) esophageal atresia with a blind proximal pouch and a distal esophageal stump fistula connection to the trachea

(D) atresia of the esophagus with both ends of the esophagus fistulized at different points to the trachea

(E) tracheoesophageal fistula without atresia of either esophagus or trachea (H-type)

1004. Which of the following statements is true regarding pyloric stenosis?

(A) genders are equally affected
(B) it is commoner in Cauacians than Blacks
(C) bilious projectile vomiting is characteristic
(D) metabolic acidosis is a complication
(E) its most common onset is 24 months of age

1005. Which of the following features of *pectus excavatum*, a pediatric chest wall deformity, is true with implications for management recommendations?

(A) it can be measured by filling the defect to overflow with water and measuring the aspirant that remains on the chest surface to quantify the defect
(B) it results from complete failure of sternal fusion
(C) the primary etiology is failure of rib growth with the gap between opposite sides represented in the anterior thoracic defect
(D) it is rarely functionally significant in terms of abnormal blood or air flow in the chest
(E) it becomes a greater cosmetic problem later in life for females than for males

1006. Wilms' tumor is a malignant renal tumor about which of the following statements only one is true?

(A) if the tumor extends through the capsule of the kidney, survival is less than 50% following therapy
(B) combination chemotherapy is a treatment recommended for nearly all patients as an adjunct to surgery
(C) bilateral renal involvement is incurable
(D) there are no recognized patterns of associated congenital anomalies
(E) the tumor is not radio-sensitive

1007. Which of the following statements is true for the infant with persistent jaundice?

(A) biliary atresia occurs before birth from intrauterine infection with hepatitis B
(B) Australia antigen is invariably present with variable results to tests or the antibody against it
(C) toxoplasmosis is frequently associated with intrahepatic biliary atresia
(D) ultrasonography is most helpful in distinguishing surgically correctable biliary atresia from other forms of persistent jaundice
(E) percutaneous external biliary drainage and refeeding bile into the upper GI tract through a tube is known as the Kasai procedure

1008. Which of the following statements about pediatric neuroblastoma is true?

    (A)   survival, compared stage for stage, is much better than for patients with Wilms' tumor

    (B)   the older the patient is at diagnosis, stage for stage, the better the prognosis

    (C)   patients with osseous metastases have a 50% complete response rate to combined radiation and chemotherapy

    (D)   remarkable improvements in treatment success rate for advanced stage disease have progressed rapidly in the past decade from poor prognosis to better than even chance of survival

    (E)   rarely it may be seen to mature with the growth of the infant, passing through neuroblastoma to ganglioneuroma.

1009. Trisomy-21 (Down's syndrome) is a combination of multiple congenital abnormalities that may include each of the following **EXCEPT**:

    (A)   duodenal atresia
    (B)   muscle hypotonia
    (C)   Brushfield spots
    (D)   neuroblastoma
    (E)   endocardial cushion defect

1010. Hirschsprung's disease is a colonic defect in children that results from

    (A)   a bowel atresia acquired following birth
    (B)   an infectious disease
    (C)   a segment of colon that cannot relax, constituting a functional bowel obstruction
    (D)   absence of parasympathetic innervation in the dilated megacolon
    (E)   a rectum that appears normal but is devoid of parasympathetic ganglion cells in the myenteric plexus on submucosal biopsy

ANSWERS AND TUTORIALS ON ITEMS 1001-1010

The answers are: **1001-C; 1002-D; 1003-C; 1004-B; 1005-D; 1006-B; 1007-D; 1008-E; 1009-D; 1010-E**.

1001. The diaphragmatic hernia that is most frequent is through the posterior lateral left hemidiaphragm (Bochdalek), since few visceral hernias pass the liver on the right side of the abdomen. A fundamental defect associated with diaphragmatic hernia is hypoplasia of the lung on the affected side, and it is frequently necessary to place these children on special respiratory support which may include extrapulmonary oxygenation with extracorporeal membrane oxygenation (ECMO). It is not easy to reduce the hernia when the abdomen is opened and the viscera retrieved from the chest, since the abdomen frequently cannot accommodate the viscera which have "lost domain". The distended abdominal viscera in the tense closure push up the repaired diaphragm further compromising pulmonary ventilation. The diaphragmatic defect is typically large, and the viscera are not usually compromised by strangulation, and infarction of the gut in the thorax is a very unusual complication.

1002. This is a serious congenital abnormality and the outcome is determined by the condition of the viscera protruding from the abdomen at the time of treatment. Both gastroschisis and omphalocele have a protrusion, the former above and the latter at the umbilicus; however, the omphalocele is covered with a peritoneal sac and the bowel is typically in better condition because it is not as exposed as the stomach and the other matted viscera typically are in gastroschisis. Prune belly is a disorder of the abdominal musculature, and exstrophy of the bladder is a mucosal extrusion above the pubis at the lower rather than the upper end of the abdominal midline. Eventration refers to a chronic condition of the diaphragm not used in the context of this newborn congenital anomaly.

The viscera must be returned to an abdomen that has not accommodated them, after care is exercised regarding the vitality of the bowel and blood supply to it. This usually involves creating a new extra-peritoneal environment for the bowel before gradually reducing it in steps into the abdominal cavity.

1003. Esophageal atresia with a proximal blind pouch and a distal tracheoesophageal fistula (TEF) connecting the trachea to the distal atretic end of the esophagus occurs in nearly 90% of instances. The much more readily envisioned and discussed H-type fistula between both nonatretic esophagus and trachea (analogous to the acquired tracheoesophageal fistula in adults) is only 5% of the total of TEFs. Atresia of the trachea would be hypothetical, since such an infant would not survive to diagnosis. It is the esophageal atresia with or without connection to the trachea that has survivability since breathing is not totally impaired.

1004. There is a peculiar age, gender, and race predilection to this disease with an etiology that is unknown but with some apparent mixture of hereditary and environmental factors. The majority of patients are Caucasian males, with the most common onset in infancy from two weeks to two months. Projectile vomiting is characteristic, but it is nonbilious because of the obstruction at the level of the pylorus. The vomiting, however, does give rise to a complication that is metabolic alkalosis rather than acidosis because of the vomiting of gastric acid.

1005. The principle concern about *pectus excavatum* is typically cosmetic. This depression in the area of the sternum does not result from any failure of lateral rib growth or sternal junction fusion failure. The volume of the depression can be approximated by the fluid volume that it can hold, but the presence of the defect is not the indication for its repair, and the best use of this information is to point out changes over time in progress through growth. Indications for surgical correction should rest on functional impact on normal activities or exertion as in sports. It is typically males who are more concerned about the cosmetic deformity later than females, since central cleavage accentuates other contours developing in the pubescent female. Functional indications for repair are the same in both genders.

1006. Wilms' tumor is one of the earliest examples which suggests adjunctive systemic chemotherapy and tumor reduction could be employed with successful outcome for even advanced disease. Even when metastases to liver and lungs are present or when the tumor is bilateral, patients still have better than 50% survival prognosis. A whole list of associated congenital anomalies have been described in association with Wilms' tumor. The tumor is radiosensitive, and advanced stages of the disease are treated with radiotherapy, but there is a high complication rate to this treatment when high doses are employed with children. Wilms' tumor appears to be an ideal arena for the multidisciplinary treatment of cancer with a successful outcome in the majority that would not be intuitively obvious given the extent of the disease in some instances that respond to combined treatment.

1007. Persistent jaundice must be differentiated in the newborn as in the adult from causes that are hepatocellular or those related to the collecting system. Toxoplasmosis may be a source of hepatitis as may hepatitis-B virus, but neither is invariably associated with biliary collecting abnormalities. In fact, biliary atresia and jaundice do not occur *in utero*, but are acquired after birth with no proven association with any one of a number of candidates for transmittable disease. The Kasai procedure is an internal drainage of a filleted liver porta into the upper GI tract, and does not involve percutaneous bile drainage. To distinguish surgically correctable biliary tract atresia from that which occurs too proximal in the liver or that which is due to hepatocellular disease (both of which would require replacement by means of liver transplantation) ultrasonography is most helpful, since dilated ducts and the presence or absence of a gall bladder may be visible for anatomic definition of the level of the atresia.

1008. Neuroblastoma is the most common solid tumor in newborns, and one that has yielded least to the combined assault of surgery, radiation, and chemotherapy. The classic neuroblastoma may rarely be seen to mature with the growth of the infant, passing through neuroblastoma to ganglioneuroma, a benign encapsulated tumor that can be excised and the patient cured despite earlier biopsy diagnosis of the same tumor at birth confirming undifferentiated neuroblastoma. There have been no remarkable improvements in survival, which is uniformly worse than that seen with Wilms' tumor and gets worse with advancing age of the patient at diagnosis. With the possible exception of massive chemotherapy and radiation that ablates both tumor and bone marrow with marrow transplant rescue as an experiment, treatment has been based in frustration with the failures of regimens that had worked so well with Wilms' tumor. A rare insight into tumor biology is the occasional evidence of tumor maturation under the influence of some factors not clearly understood but certainly not entirely due to the pressures of therapy. Neuroblastoma is a tumor awaiting an infusion of new information before it can be managed.

1009. Trisomy-21 has multiple manifestations, and some of the congenital findings are later associated with developmental defects such as those seen in the duodenum and cardiac abnormalities. Primary malignancy of the neuroblastoma variety is not among these associations.

1010. The megacolon of Hirschsprung's disease is an acquired phenomenon, but the congenital defect is an absence of parasympathetic ganglia in the myenteric and submucosal plexus of the nondilated component, usually the rectum. This is not an atresia, but does constitute a functional bowel obstruction, since it cannot propel. The dilated portion of the colon is hypertrophic, responding normally to normal innervation propelling against this functional obstruction. There are many associations, including Down's syndrome, enterocolitis, and an overwhelming predominance in male infants and those affected with strong family history. Although it mimics some abnormalities seen with Chagas' disease, this congenital Hirschsprung's disease is not infectious.

"Sometimes when a doctor gets too lazy to work, he becomes a politician."
J. Chalmers DaCosta (1863-1933)

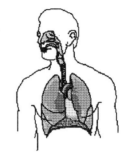

THORACIC SURGERY

Items 1011-1020

1011. Which of the following suggests unresectability of a left upper lobe lung cancer?

   (A)   hemoptysis
   (B)   pneumonia
   (C)   malignant pleural effusion
   (D)   a cough specimen with positive sputum cytology
   (E)   clubbing and blueness of fingers

1012. Management of pulmonary complications of tuberculosis refractory to antibiotic management include each of the following **EXCEPT**:

   (A)   decortication
   (B)   chest wall reconstruction
   (C)   hyperbaric oxygen therapy
   (D)   bronchoscopic brush biopsy and lavage
   (E)   lobectomy

1013. Which of the following associated conditions indicates dissemination of small cell carcinoma of the lung?

(A)   Cushing's syndrome
(B)   myasthenic (Eaton-Lambert) syndrome
(C)   superior sulcus syndrome
(D)   hypertrophic pulmonary osteoarthropathy
(E)   polycythemia

1014. Which of the following is **LEAST** likely as a diagnosis when a left upper lobe "coin lesion" is discovered on the chest X-ray screening of an asymptomatic 40 year-old white male?

(A)   sarcoidosis
(B)   hamartoma
(C)   adenocarcinoma
(D)   squamous cell carcinoma
(E)   tuberculosis

1015. *Pneumocystis carinii* pneumonia

(A)   occurs only in patients who are HIV-positive
(B)   begins as a perihilar infiltrate pattern on chest X-ray
(C)   responds to erythromycin
(D)   usually presents as a pro-ductive cough
(E)   only rarely causes severe hypoxia

1016. A 54 year-old man with a "barreled chest" undergoes mediastinoscopy for staging of lung cancer identified by a positive sputum cytology. Hilar lymph node biopsy has shown frozen section histology negative for tumor. Three hours following mediastinoscopy the patient is in dyspneic crisis with a cyanotic dusky complexion and fearful expression with neck veins distended. You should immediately

(A)   order chest X-ray
(B)   insert large bore needle in both sides of the chest
(C)   ventilate with ambulatory manual breathing unit (AMBU) bag
(D)   place a bag over patient's nose and mouth for re-breathing
(E)   perform tracheotomy

1017. Cyanosis is a prominent clinical feature of each of the following conditions **EXCEPT**:

(A)   *cor pulmonale*
(B)   tetralogy of Fallot
(C)   aortic stenosis
(D)   pulmonary atresia
(E)   tricuspid stenosis

1018. Pulmonary artery banding in children is indicated in which of the following conditions?

(A)   large ventricular septal defect
(B)   coarctation of the aorta
(C)   "pink" tetralogy of Fallot
(D)   distal pulmonary atresia
(E)   aortic stenosis

1019. The most frequently performed procedure for coronary insufficiency currently is

(A)   internal mammary artery bypass
(B)   coronary endarterectomy
(C)   coronary thrombectomy
(D)   aortocoronary bypass graft
(E)   percutaneous coronary angioplasty

1020. Satisfactory methods of treating mitral valve disease include each of the following **EXCEPT**:

(A)   mitral commissurotomy (Harken)
(B)   xenograft valve prosthesis (Carpentier-Edwards)
(C)   tilting disk mitral valve prosthesis (Bjork-Shiley)
(D)   ball valve prosthesis (Starr-Edwards)
(E)   aortic homograft prosthesis

ANSWERS AND TUTORIALS ON ITEMS 1011-1020

The answers are: **1011-C; 1012-C; 1013-C; 1014-A; 1015-B; 1016-B; 1017-C; 1018-A; 1019-D; 1020-C**.

1011. Pneumonia, hemoptysis and clubbing are all signs that may be related to benign pulmonary disease as well as resectable malignancy, and positive sputum cytology on cough specimen does not rule out resection for cure since it is presumed to originate from the cancer already identified in the left upper lobe. If the cytology were from a catheter trans-bronchial aspirant from the right lung, it would suggest bilateral disease making this patient with clubbing and pneumonia inoperable as well as suggesting a tumor that is nonresectable. The single contra-indication to operation planned for resection for cure is the positive finding of a malignant pleural effusion, since this indicates that the cancer has spread beyond the confines of the lobe and would not be cured even by left pneumonectomy.

1012. Tuberculosis can result in local destruction of affected lung with cavitation. If this cavitary destruction is large, if it is multiple in one lobe, and if it is not successfully drained intrabronchially through the assistance of bronchoscopic brush biopsy to enter the cavity and lavage, lobectomy may be advised. A thickened pleura is likely, particularly if a secondary bacterial infection and empyema result which may require thorough drainage of the pleural space and decortication of the encased lung in order to allow expansion. If that expansion is not possible with the lung coming up to the chest wall, the chest wall is actually collapsed down onto the lung, in a type of chest wall reconstruction called thoracoplasty. Each of these surgical methods has been used with success with management of complications of tuberculosis. Hyperbaric oxygen therapy is not successful in managing these complications.

1013. Small cell carcinoma of the lung is associated with several paraneoplastic syndromes. Myasthenia symptoms, like those of myasthenia gravis, are described in the Eaton-Lambert syndrome. ACTH-like endocrine responses can be seen with a Cushinoid appearance. Both poly-cythemia and an unusual form of osteoarthropathy involving sub-periosteal growth suggests messengers with erythropoietin-like or growth hormone-like activity. Each of these are secondary to physiologic responses, and polycythemia may be a response to chronic desaturation even without the presence of an excess peptide mediator postulated. However, superior sulcus syndrome is a phenomenon of malignant obstruction to the innominate venous return and superior sympathetic chain, and indicates metastatic disease outside the confines of the lung.

1014. Sarcoidosis is found in younger age groups predominately, and as a rule it does not present as a solitary "coin lesion". It is also higher in incidence in African-American than in Caucasian patients. Adenocarcinoma may present in this fashion in the lung, and is probably more likely to represent metastatic disease than primary pulmonary adenocarcinoma. The fortunate but rare benign tumor known as hamartoma presents as a "coin lesion", but unfortunately the more common "coin lesion" encountered radiographically, even on screening asymptomatic patients, is squamous cell carcinoma. Tuberculosis may present as a solitary lesion, before cavitation in the later stages when communication with the bronchus occurs in later stages of caseation. These lesions are all primary pulmonary lesions and sarcoidosis is more likely to be perihilar in position and involving mediastinal lymphatic structures as a rule.

1015. One of the earliest presentations for *Pneumocystis* is a nonproductive cough. Because of the interstitial location of the protozoa, sputum production is remarkably absent. In such patients rapid and severe hypoxia and desaturation occur early; and,

as the major morbid feature, out of proportion to clinical findings on auscultation. Chest X-ray early in such patients shows perihilar infiltrate in a "butterfly" pattern, progressive to later consolidation. The protozoan does not respond to erythromycin antibiotic as *Mycoplasma* or *Legionella* often do. *Pneumocystis* occurs in patients who have been immunocompromised. This includes, but is not limited to, patients infected with HIV . Earlier cases of *Pneumocystis* showed a predominance among premature malnourished infants, lymphoma patients under chemotherapy, or patients immuno-suppressed for transplantation.

1016. Mediastinoscopy is a valuable staging procedure for identifying potential spread from lung cancer. In a patient with chronic disease, the mediastinum may be displaced by intrapleural expansion. Both mediastinoscopy and node biopsy may result in entry into the pleura that can be unrecognized at the time of the procedure, and the ventilation of the patient during the operation can result in a ruptured emphyse-matous bleb. The patient's clinical con-dition is nearly instantly recognizable as tension pneumothorax. There is no time for chest X-ray, and especially not if the patient is sent away to a radiography suite for it, out of an environment of higher nursing intensity. The symptoms are not suggestive of upper airway obstruction, and if hematoma or other compression were obstructing the lower trachea or bronchi, tracheotomy would be above this obstruction and would serve no purpose in relief of it. AMBU bag ventilation is contraindicated, since this would serve to further insufflate air under tension higher than that which a patient is already experiencing from the intrapleural air accumulation through the ventilatory effort. Clinical exam which would consist of listening to each side of the chest might suggest which side to begin, but thoracostomy is urgently indicated. One of the safest and quickest ways to carry this out is with a large bore needle on a 50 ml syringe. Inserting this in the pleural space of each side of the chest, the side most suspicious by clinical examination first, causes the plunger to jump from the barrel of the syringe on the side with tension pneumothorax, simultaneously diagnosing and relieving the patient's inhalatory emergency until longer term management can proceed through placement of tube thoracostomy.

1017. Malformation of the tricuspid valve (Ebstein's deformity) causes reduction in right ventricular output, and, hence, cyanosis. The same is true for reduction in pulmonary flow in the shunting seen in the tetralogy of Fallot and pulmonary atresia. An increase in pulmonary vascular resistance as in *cor pulmonale* also constitutes a pulmonary arterial flow restriction, and each of these reductions in pulmonary arterial blood flow is associated with cyanosis. Aortic stenosis, however, should not affect hemodynamics or oxygen saturation in the right circulation, but is a problem in the perfusion of blood from the left side of the heart that has already been oxygenated, so cyanosis is absent.

1018. High volume left to right shunt can give refractory congestive failure in patients too ill or too small to undergo total surgical correction. Temporary palliation may be achieved by diminishing pulmonary artery pressure through a constriction of the pulmonary trunk. This would hardly be necessary in a patient who already had an atretic segment of pulmonary artery. The patient with pink tetralogy is manifesting compensation whereby congestive failure is not prominent from left to right shunt. In the classic operation for cyanotic tetralogy, pulmonary blood flow and pressure was actually increased to early systolic systemic levels by creating a fistula through the subclavian artery diversion (Blalock-Taussig) or aortopulmonary window anastomosis (Waterston). This is the reverse of the pressure dynamics attempted with a pulmonary banding procedure.

Both coarctation of the aorta and valve stenosis are, in effect, "banding" of the left ventricular outflow, causing some degree of left heart strain, and pulmonary banding would not address any therapeutic purpose in lowering a normal pulmonary arterial pressure besides creating additional right ventricular strain. Only the patient with significant congestive failure from refractory pulmonary hypertension that cannot undergo total anatomic correction should undergo this palliative procedure, and with improvements in both medical management of pulmonary hypertension and earlier definitive repair, the palliative pulmonary banding procedure is becoming much less commonly indicated.

1019. Thrombectomy for coronary artery thrombosis is as temporary as coronary endarterectomy, both of which do not improve blood flow long-term and, hence, myocardial performance. The Vineberg internal mammary artery bypass was useful when originally proposed and remains so for selected indications, but the majority of patients today undergo bypass grafting from aorta to coronary arteries through reversed saphenous veins or some other conduit than the internal mammary artery.

Percutaneous transcatheter coronary angioplasty might be applicable to patients with isolated lesions, but most coronary atherosclerosis is generalized with not just a single focal significant stenotic lesion, so even patients with coronary angioplasty procedure are standby candidates for coronary artery bypass graft from aorta, which is the most frequently performed operation.

1020. The repair of a stenotic valve in the mitral position can take the form of mitral commissurotomy to increase mobility of fused or stenotic mitral valve leaflets, although restenosis may be a long-term result. There is a dynamic tension between long-term recurrence of problems and low maintenance in adjunctive medication requirement with anticoagulation required for some prosthetic materials. Natural tissue seems to require less vigilance with respect to thrombotic problems which occur with less frequency with tissue, whether of xenograft or homograft origin, than with prosthetic synthetic materials. The ball valve design has been satisfactory if maintained with adequate anticoagulation, but the tilting disk has had an unacceptably high rate of dislocation, leading to embolization and sudden valvular insufficiency. For that reason, not only are those patients who require valve replacement not currently getting the option of tilting disk prosthesis, but there is a long-term recommendation for replacement of those already in place with a very low threshold for re-operation at the earliest sign of any symptoms.

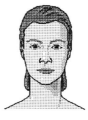

PLASTIC AND RECONSTRUCTIVE SURGERY

Items 1021-1030

1021. To cover a surface wound that the surgeon wishes to revise later by sequentially excising portions of it until only primary unwounded skin is closed for the end result, the graft selected would be

(A) full thickness free graft
(B) split thickness skin graft
(C) banked allograft skin
(D) xenograft
(E) microvascular composite graft

1022. Which of the following techniques would be most appropriate for an immediate release of scar contracture across joint surfaces?

(A) full thickness pedicle flap
(B) split thickness skin graft
(C) myocutaneous composite graft
(D) skeletal traction for constant tension on joint
(E) Z-plasty revision

1023. The purpose of "meshing" a split thickness skin graft includes each of the following **EXCEPT**:

(A)   it can be expanded to cover much more surface than the size of the original graft donor site

(B)   it allows oxygenation of the granulation bed

(C)   it conforms to the irregular shape of the recipient bed

(D)   it allows serum to ooze without lifting the graft from its attachment to the bed

(E)   it enhances further wound contracture

1024. What is the appropriate sequence for the repair of a cleft lip and palate diagnosed at birth for a young male newborn?

(A)   repair of both cleft lip and palate before baby is released from hospital after birth

(B)   repair of cleft lip at 10 weeks, and cleft palate one year later

(C)   repair of cleft palate at one month, and repair of cleft lip at one year

(D)   repair of nasal deformity as soon as possible after birth, cleft lip at one year and cleft palate at puberty

(E)   repair of cleft lip, palate and nasal deformities at one operation just before the child goes to school at age four

1025. A young man is seen in the emergency room after a head-on deceleration collision in which he passed through the steering wheel and struck his face against the windshield. The mandible appears intact, but there are fractures bilaterally and in the central compartment of the face whereby the lower face is "floating" in dysjunction from the cranium. This injury is known as

(A)   LeFort I
(B)   LeFort II
(C)   LeFort III
(D)   temporomandibular dysjunction
(E)   Caldwell-Luc maxillary sinus

1026. The management of decubitus ulcers ("pressure sores") involves each of the following components **EXCEPT**:

(A)   prevent compression of the ulcerated area by relief of weight-bearing from the site

(B)   maintenance antibiotic therapy

(C)   contouring of the skeletal protrusion by osteotomy

(D)   excision of the ulcer, devitalized facia and inflammation back to bleeding tissue

(E)   restoration of anatomic padding by transfer in of vascularized skin and subcutaneous tissue with or without muscle

363

1027. Each of the following techniques is currently available and recommended for breast reconstruction following mastectomy **EXCEPT**:

(A) myocutaneous flap using latissimus dorsi
(B) saline-filled prosthesis
(C) myocutaneous flap using transverse rectus abdominis (TRAM)
(D) silicone implant
(E) myocutaneous flap using gluteus maximus

1028. Which of the following factors is most important in minimization of scar formation in closure of an elective surgical incision?

(A) size of the suture
(B) number of throws on the suture knot
(C) dressing technique
(D) careful tissue handling
(E) antibiotic irrigation of the wound

1029. Intra-arterial injection of illicit drugs by addicts may give rise to serious problems in the hand. These include all of the following **EXCEPT**:

(A) Volkmann's ischemic contracture
(B) the "puffy hand syndrome"
(C) distal digital gangrene
(D) carpal tunnel syndrome
(E) gas gangrene of the deep palmar space

1030. Which of the following statements is true of a knife laceration of the wrist in a suicide attempt that has severed several tendons, nerves, and the ulnar artery?

(A) the severance of the flexor digitorum superficialis may be undetected if the profundus is intact
(B) the ulnar artery ends should be found and re-anastamosed as early as possible in the procedure
(C) the patient would likely die from exsanguination if not rescued and resuscitated
(D) if the nerve ends are not found and repaired at the time of acute injury, it will be too late to attempt to find and fix them at a later date
(E) the patient will be able to oppose the thumb if the median nerve is sectioned at this level

ANSWERS AND TUTORIALS ON ITEMS 1021-1030

The answers are: **1021-B; 1022-E; 1023-B; 1024-B; 1025-C; 1026-B; 1027-D; 1028-D; 1029-D; 1030-A.**

1021. One of the putative disadvantages of split thickness skin grafts is that there is an increased secondary contracture rate. That works to the advantage of the therapeutic intent here, in which there is an intent to consecutively decrease the wound size. A microvascular composite graft would in this instance be totally inappropriate, since imported blood supply along with accessory structures beyond surface epithelium is unnecessary and this process is far too complicated for the simple purposes of resurfacing. Full thickness skin graft would be limited in donor sites, and would not be expandable to cover the defect nor would it contract later in the course of progressive shrinkage which is the intent. Allograft "skin" would not take for a period long enough without immuno-suppression which is a very high price to pay for a wound closure and eventual elimination. Xenograft would not take at all, but would be used as a biologic dressing, often until a vascularizable graft can be obtained, and if that would be a split thickness skin graft, that could be used here from the start.

1022. Scar contracture across joint surfaces may require much more extensive resurfacing than the scar tissue excised, since *contracture* is the nature of the problem that has lost mobility in the joint. The simplest way to release the scar contracture bands that have caused the joint to be drawn up in flexion contracture is to release these scar bands and to reorient the scars so as to not impair motion of the joint. "Z-plasty" involves the geometric incision of the longitudinal contracting band with upper and lower incisions on apposite sides and at angles to the incised scar. The triangular flaps thus created are interposed, thus releasing the contracture.

If split thickness skin graft were used to resurface the scar excised over the contracted joint surface, the recontracture of this joint can be confidently predicted. Full thickness graft would result in less contracture, and myocutaneous flap still less, but each involves the movement of a considerable amount of tissue with a question about limited number of donor sites which would also require closure. Skeletal traction also results in immobility of the joint — in extension rather than flexion, but is unlikely to be successful if the contracting bands are already present, would be painful in their disruption if possible at all, and would not give immediate results. The best method for immediate scar contraction release to restore mobility would be Z-plasty revision; that is triangular flap interposition along the line of contracture.

1023. "Meshing" a split thickness skin graft on a grid allows an expansion of 4 to 1 or more surface area coverage than the original split thickness skin graft surface size. Transudation of serum can occur without lifting the graft, but there is little or no advantage in allowing air or enhanced oxygen directly through the interstices. It can be "accordioned" into conformability to irregular recipient beds and facilitates contracture of the surface wound. For these reasons, "meshed" split thickness skin grafts are highly useful for resurfacing burn wounds or other large granulating surfaces.

1024. The sequence of repairs in "cleft craft" begins with the cleft lip, and that is usually repaired by the "rule of tens": a child at ten weeks, ten pounds and ten grams hemoglobin undergoes repair of cleft lip, and one year later the cleft palate is repaired. After the lip and palate have already been repaired, plastic revision of nasal deformities, such as insufficient columella length, is postponed until puberty.

Clefts in lip and palate have not remarkably interfered with sucking response on the part of the child, and feeding such an infant is remarkably easier than most parents originally envision. Often spoon feeding is begun earlier than usual. In some underdeveloped areas of the world, adult patients with uncorrected clefts may be encountered. They can undergo cleft lip and palate repair, having fully accommodated appearance and speech defects in that interval, sometimes adjustment to the repaired palate and lip is difficult. Before self image has developed, the cleft lip would have been repaired, and just at the time when speech is becoming a very important issue, the palate cleft will be repaired. At the time of heavy concentration on body image in puberty, revisions of columella or vomer deficiency can be undertaken. This sequential repair in "cleft craft" gives the best functional as well as cosmetic results.

1025. In the classification of facial fractures, LeFort III fracture represents craniofacial dysjunction. In this instance, the bony skeleton of the face is separated from the rest of the skull and there is a floating dysjunction. LeFort I fracture separates alveolar ridge and palate from the zygoma and nose. LeFort II fractures the nasion so the central triangle of the face is movable. In LeFort III the entire upper jaw, cheek bones, and nose are movable by grasping the upper teeth while holding the skull, with elongation of the face by distraction. Caldwell-Luc is an opening made into the maxillary sinus, and temporomandibular dysjunction would not necessarily involve a fracture at all. LeFort III is the most severe form of facial fracture, involving separation of the suborbital face from the rest of the skull.

1026. Relief of pressure on the ulcerated area — the etiology of the pressure sores — is a method helpful in treatment and also prevention of recurrence. This may also involve relief of the pressure from the inside by rongeuring or excising bony prominences, especially when they may be affected by necrosis and osteomyelitis from the ulcer contamination. This means that excision of the devitalized tissue back to bleeding tissue would be an appropriate preparation for a recipient bed to have transferred in some vascularized soft tissue with skin, and most probably associated muscle because of its vascularity exceeding that of subcutaneous fat through some rotation of an anatomic well vascularized but expendable bit of autologous tissue. The pressure ulcer did not begin as a wound infection, and is usually not complicated by any systemic sepsis for which the antibiotics would be indicated. Circulating antibiotics would not be delivered through blood flow to an area of ischemia from pressure so that antibiotics would not be delivered to the site where they would be putatively useful. For that reason, maintenance antibiotics would not have a primary role and only infrequently an adjunctive role, being useful only in treatment of an infection complicating the primary problem of pressure ulceration.

1027. Yes, the gluteus maximus is used for this purpose, as are the other myocutaneous flaps from latissimus dorsi or "TRAM" flap using microvascular anastomotic techniques. Saline-filled prosthesis is appropriate, but with any prosthetic graft in this position a fibrous capsular contracture may often occur within an encased and hardened shell that is inappropriate as a breast replacement. Such concerns have reached the level of withdrawal from common use of the silicone prosthetic implant, both for reasons of this encapsulation and for alleged immunologic disorders, so this form of prosthetic breast replacement is not currently recommended.

1028. All full thickness incisions in skin heal by scar formation. Minimization of that scar formation is addressed by many factors, including the body position of the skin so wounded, the sharp versus blunt damage to the tissue, prolonged exposure and desiccation, contamination, foreign body presence, tension in proximation and motion of the incision site after closure and dressing. Of these, the single most important factor is careful tissue handling in closure.

The wound is immediately closed by a "plasma glue" which is a transudate and sometimes an exudate of the injured tissue when the integument is broken. It is true that fine suture has less reaction than suture of the smae type but larger caliber, but this factor is part of the technique of gentle tissue handling as are also other considerations such as tension of the closure, and suture technique. The dressing that is applied may involve immobilization as in a plaster splint or supracuticular tension such as adhesive tape "butterfly" closure. Irrigation of the wound is significant in removing foreign body and devitalized cells. The presence or absence of antibiotic is much less important, and can be a negative factor if the chemical reaction of the introduced drugs further damages tissue. Each of the other factors in consideration relate to minimization of further tissue damage as in the first rule of medicine or surgery *"primum non nocere"*.

1029. Addicts who have exhausted venous access, or for a special sensation known as the "flash" or "hand tripping", resort to intraarterial injection, since the artery can be located by its pulse when adjacent vessels are obliterated or scarred and impalpable. The excipients may embolize distally giving digital gangrene, and arterial occlusion can give rise to Volkmann's ischemic contracture. The material mixed is often quinine since it has comparable texture to the heroin it is used to dilute, and this sets up the redox potential for anaerobic growth so that gas gangrene is a possible deep palmar space infection that may be a risk to both life and limb.

Carpal tunnel syndrome is the entrapment of the median nerve from compression within the limited space at the volar surface of the wrist, often brought upon patients with prolonged amyloid deposit or repetitive manual stress. It would not be typically associated as a complication of narcotic addict angio-access.

1030. This is an unsuccessful method of suicide, as the patient is now aware, since exsanguination is unlikely, and the ulnar artery need not even be identified for anastomosis, since it is expendable, and there are many more time consuming priorities in the procedure that must follow in repair of this injury. It is true that the flexor superficialis tendon disruption will not be noticed if the profundus is intact, since the patient can still flex the fingers up to the distal phalanx with the action of the deep tendons, and flexor tendon injury in the superficialis system must be searched for to be detected. A very significant injury is the section of the median nerve, and it will receive the most meticulous attention in the repair. It is highly disabling, since the patient will not be able to oppose the thumb, because the recurrent nerve from the median innervation of the thumb comes off distal to the laceration. The repair of the median nerve can be accomplished acutely, or this procedure can be done on a delayed basis with results that will not be impaired by the delay. A great deal of the success of the result is dependant upon rehabilitation directed by the patient, and given the circumstances this may be less than ideal; however, the median nerve should take first priority in attention, the flexor tendons next with the profundus being the highest priority and superficial severed tendons the last options in repair while the ulnar artery is simply ligated.

"Some kinds of critical patients require operation even before resuscitation."
Glenn W. Geelhoed

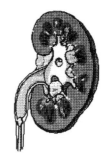

UROLOGIC SURGERY

Items 1031-1040

1031. Which of the following statements are **NOT** true regarding prostate carcinoma in a 95 year-old man?

   (A)   presence of prostate carcinoma is 95% likely in the prostate of any 95 year-old American man

   (B)   treatment should be designed to prevent the spread of the disease

   (C)   it is associated with an elevated prostate specific antigen

   (D)   it typically follows an indolent course

   (E)   management is by observation

1032. Which of the following processes involving the kidneys does **NOT** produce hypertension?

   (A)   polycystic kidney disease
   (B)   renovascular stenosis
   (C)   glomerulonephritis
   (D)   nephrectomy
   (E)   coarctation of the aorta

1033. An agitated 28 year-old man comes to the emergency room stating he is having another episode of ureteral colic, having previously passed urate stones on several occasions. He states he is allergic to intravenous pyelogram (IVP) contrast. He demands Demerol. His urinalysis is unremarkable. The most likely diagnosis is

(A) urate stones
(B) von Munchausen's syndrome
(C) narcotic addiction
(D) IVP contrast hypersensitivity
(E) a malpractice litigant baiting the clinician

1034. A 14 year-old boy enters the emergency room with bright red blood at the urethral meatus. He is not forthcoming with any history, and his midstream urinalysis is unremarkable as are other preliminary laboratory studies. A likely diagnosis might be

(A) prostatitis
(B) instrumentation
(C) epididymitis
(D) mumps
(E) syphilis

1035. A newborn male has bilateral flank masses and sonographically confirmed hydroureter. The most likely diagnosis is

(A) uretero-vesicle stenosis
(B) bilateral suppurative pyelonephritis
(C) primary hydronephrosis
(D) infantile prostatism
(E) urinary bladder atresia

1036. A patient with normal blood pressure, blood counts, and blood chemistry is noted to have an opaque calcium calculus in both kidneys incidently described on a routine chest X-ray. On an IVP, multiple diffuse cysts were seen in both kidneys. Repeat examination is again normal and the patient denies symptoms. A likely diagnosis is

(A) polycystic kidney disease
(B) von Hippel-Lindow syndrome
(C) medullary sponge kidney
(D) miliary biogenic renal metastases
(E) septic arterial emboli from infected cardiac valve vegetations

1037. Arteriography may be employed in the defining of the extent of the blood supply of hypernephroma but has what additional principal advantage?

(A) it would rule out operation by demonstration of hepatic metastases
(B) it would determine unresectability for cure by demonstration of renal venous tumor extension
(C) it can be used to facilitate operation by occluding the principal and collateral blood supply to the tumor
(D) it may involve demonstration of portal venous tumor invasion
(E) chemotherapeutic transcatheter infusion is delivered direct to the tumor

369

1038. Each of the following treatments is acceptable in managing benign prostatic hypertrophy **EXCEPT**:

(A) proscar (Fenastamide)
(B) transurethral resection
(C) suprapubic prostatectomy
(D) perineal prostatectomy with interstitial radiation therapy
(E) transrectal biopsy and observation

1039. A 56 year-old woman with chronic fatigue has mild anemia and eosinophilia on blood count, and occult microscopic hematuria on clean catheterized urinalysis. A sonogram ordered to check her pancreas suggests a left renal mass. A likely diagnosis is

(A) glomerulonephritis
(B) renal carbuncle
(C) hypernephroma
(D) squamous cell carcinoma of the renal pelvis
(E) staghorn calculus

1040. Newer techniques alternative to pyelolithotomy include all the following **EXCEPT**:

(A) basketing the stone for retrieval by ureteral catheter
(B) ECSW lithotripsy
(C) chemically dissolving calcium oxalate stones by infusion into the kidney
(D) pulverizing the stone by laser or shock energy introduced through ureteral catheterization
(E) laparoscopic minimally invasive nephrolithotomy

ANSWERS AND TUTORIALS ON ITEMS 1031-1040

The answers are: **1031-B; 1032-D; 1033-C; 1034-B; 1035-D; 1036-C; 1037-C; 1038-D; 1039-C; 1040-C**.

1031. It is inappropriate to do radical therapy to contain the threat of malignant spread in a tumor of almost any kind in a 95 year-old patient, particularly prostate cancer. Since it is very likely to be present, and it is less likely to be causing problems because of its indolent behavior, observation would be adequate to see if there were symptoms related to it. It there were, treatment would be related to those symptoms, such as relief of urinary tract obstruction or bleeding.

1032. Renovascular hypertension may occur with arterial stenosis or proximal narrowing as in coarctation, atherosclerosis or fibromuscular hyperplasia. Polycystic kidney and glomerulonephritis can also result in nephrogenic hypertension, since while the kidney is present it can give rise to renin which produces hypertension as an end result of its peptide activation sequence. If the kidney is absent, it not only does not excrete, it doesn't secrete either, so nephrectomy should not be associated with a hypertensive response.

1033. With a well practiced story, patients who request narcotic often get it when the story cannot be corroborated, and urate stones would not be radio-opaque, and could not be demonstrated if IVP contrast were contraindicated. The urinalysis does not suggest hematuria, and his agitated state might suggest either psychic problems (and the story a component of the von

Munchausen's syndrome) or narcotic withdrawal. IVP contrast hypersensitivity can be tested for, but not with results in the period of time during which he requires his alleged pain to be treated. Narcotics should be withheld until further confirmation of his alleged problem is corroborated. So as not to withhold information from him regarding your reasons for not complying, he should be told about the skepticism, not regarding his pain, but regarding his diagnosis which cannot be confirmed.

1034. There is no evidence for urinary tract pathology beyond the urethra, and the clinical context is that often seen with manipulation and fear of consequences. Mumps would have acute orchitis and the inflammatory conditions of epididymitis or prostatitis are not likely to give a negative physical exam and blood work. This is not the presentation of chancre, either, so the patient should be invited to talk about his fears to the limit that he is willing to do so over a follow-up observation.

1035. This syndrome is recognized to be a feature of newborn males, and it is embryologically derived in an obstructive uropathy also known as "posterior urethral valves." These paramesonephric (Müllerian) remnants give a high grade obstruction which causes reflux and hydronephrosis with massive megaureter. The syndrome should be reversible with relief of the urethral valves and decompression if the renal cortex has not been totally destroyed, but in the newborn there is a good deal of resiliency for recovery. It is likely that the hydroureter will require ureteral tapering and reimplantation at a later stage in the process. There is no early reason why any newborn should have

suppurative pyelonephritis or embryologic reasons why atresia or stenosis at other sites should develop, and that is why the particular anatomic point of obstruction has been termed infantile prostatism.

1036. Medullary sponge kidney is often a surprise finding on IVP in patients who are undertaking this test for some other indication. Sometimes the medullary cysts have calcific calculi, and that may indicate the study, but not usually for cause of ureteral colic, since the stones are not often released into the collecting system. The other options are not likely to be the underlying diagnosis in an asymptomatic patient, particularly those that deal with pyogenic inflammatory processes. Polycystic kidney has a different distribution of the cysts, which typically enlarge the kidneys much more and von Hippel-Lindow findings are associated with this syndrome beyond the presence of renal cysts, such as retinal findings and liver abnormalities.

1037. Hypernephroma is one tumor that is better managed surgically following radiographic devascularization. A spring coil with thrombogenic material can be placed in the feeding vessels and reduces tumor bulk and vascularity encountered in subsequent operation. This is also a method for stopping hemorrhage in tumor or palliating patient by tumor reduction in metastatic sites. Arteriography would not reach the portal venous system and would not be used for identifying hypernephroma extensions to it which would be unlikely. Both identification of hepatic metastases, or intravascular extension into the renal vein would not contraindicate operation, since patients respond to tumor reduction in the former instance, and the patient can still be cured even with demonstrated presence of intravascular venous invasion.

1038. Benign prostatic hypertrophy's management is principally designed to relieve urinary tract obstruction symptoms and also to rule out the presence of malignant prostate disease. If there is no obstruction, observation can be safely followed after biopsy confirmation in some age groups that no malignant prostate component is present. Open prostatectomy was the standard before wide-scale application of transurethral resection techniques, but now a new therapy has been made available in the form of an enzyme inhibitor that shrinks benign prostatic hypertrophy and may postpone or eliminate the requirement for operations designed to relieve obstruction. This tendency toward more benign and less invasive procedures for benign prostatic hypertrophy would preclude a radical perineal prostatectomy, and no interstitial radiation implant source would be required for the benign disease.

1039. A complex of microscopic hematuria, eosinophilia and a renal mass strongly indicate hypernephroma. The patient is not the right age for glomerulo-nephritis, and squamous cell carcinoma is typically found only after prolonged resident renal calculus which is not suggested by the sonogram. Metastasis to the kidney would be more unlikely than the primary origin of this tumor in the kidney given the triad of the findings.

1040. Although lesser invasive procedures have been developed for kidney stone removal, most have involved cystoscopic manipulation of ureteral catheters to retrieve stones or fragments or pulverizing

the stone through extracorporeal shock wave lithotripsy or direct contact with the stone through the ureteral approach. As yet, no available chemical dissolves the calcific stone without causing damage to the surrounding tissue that would preclude its use.

"The sickest patients tolerate the biggest operations, but only if they pay IMMEDIATE METABOLIC DIVIDENDS."
Francis D. Moore, 1968
Personal Communication

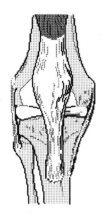

ORTHOPEDIC SURGERY

Items 1041-1050

1041. Each of the following maxims of management of extremity fractures is true **EXCEPT**:

(A)   avoid mobility in the upper extremity, preventing nonunion for a solid fusion

(B)   open fractures are contaminated wounds and treated as potential osteomyelitis

(C)   avoid conversion of any closed fracture to an open fracture by immobilization and splinting to minimize soft tissue damage

(D)   orthopedic management is a second order priority following shock resuscitation

(E)   avoid mobility in lower extremity fractures to prevent nonunion and achieve a solid fusion

1042. Which is the ultimate criterion of successful outcome from orthopedic management?

(A)   correct anatomic alignment on X-ray

(B)   no visible deformity on clinical exam

(C)   adequate function of the part post injury

(D)   primary healing without evidence of callus

(E)   the shortest possible duration of the treatment course

1043. Hematogenous osteomyelitis in patients with sickle cell anemia may uniquely be due to

(A)   *Staphylococcus aureus*

(B)   *E. coli*

(C)   *Hemophilus*

(D)   *Gonococcus*

(E)   *Salmonella*

1044. A 9 year-old girl falls from her bicycle on her outstretched arm and is seen in the emergency room complaining of pain about the shoulder. The most likely diagnosis is

(A)   impaction fracture of the proximal humerus

(B)   Colles' fracture

(C)   acromioclavicular ligament tear

(D)   clavicle fracture

(E)   fracture of the radial head

1045. "Clipping" in football is an illegal procedure incurring penalty on the part of the perpetrator. The injuries sustained by the one clipped resulting from force to the lateral aspect of the knee is likely to include each of the following **EXCEPT**:

(A) hemarthrosis
(B) tear of the medial collateral ligament
(C) inter-trochanteric fracture
(D) anterior cruciate ligament disruption
(E) torn lateral meniscus

1046. A middle-aged woman is knocked down and run over by a taxi, sustaining a crush of the right knee with open fracture with fragments of tibia protruding through the skin. Surgical management of this injury should include each of the following **EXCEPT**:

(A) arteriography
(B) open surgical debridement
(C) copious irrigation with saline solution
(D) prolonged systemic antibiotics
(E) emergency total knee replacement

1047. Which of the following fractures is **LEAST** clinically significant and can be treated without casting or immobilization?

(A) fracture of the medial malleolus and deltoid ligament disruption of the ankle
(B) fracture of the fibula at the lateral malleolus
(C) trimalleolear fracture
(D) fracture of the head of the fibula
(E) fracture of the calcaneus

1048. Which of the following statements regarding femur fractures in preschool children is true?

(A) if perfect alignment of fracture fragments with anatomic continuity seen on X-ray takes place in the treatment alignment, the fractured limb is likely to grow longer than the normal opposite side
(B) internal fixation is generally necessary
(C) an intramedullary rod accelerates recovery for earlier rehabilitation
(D) hip contracture is a significant problem with plaster spica immobilization
(E) management with traction is inappropriate in young children

1049. Which of the following statements is true for fractures that occur in children?

- (A) the epiphyseal growth plate and its junction are infrequently the site of fracture involvement since this area of the bone is more flexible than bone in mid-shaft which is where most fractures in children occur
- (B) a "greenstick" fracture is a transverse fracture breaking through the cortex on both sides of a long bone
- (C) in a fracture through the cortex on one side of a long bone in children with the opposite cortex intact, during fracture reduction of an angulated deformity the opposite cortex should actually be broken to complete the fracture
- (D) appropriate casting involves immobilizing the joint above, but not necessarily below the fracture site
- (E) because they are growing, children's bones knit more slowly than those of adults who do not have the more widespread demand on calcium deposition

1050. An elderly patient experiences a fall in circumstances not recalled by the patient or witnessed by others. The patient was brought by ambulance to the emergency room because he could not get up, when found by a daughter. Even with assistance, weight-bearing on the left is impossible. In the emergency room, raising the sheet to expose the feet you note that the left leg is shortened and externally rotated with the foot flat in bed on its lateral surface with the toes pointing to the patient's left. On X-ray you expect to find

- (A) an impacted spiral fracture of the mid-femoral shaft
- (B) an inter-trochanteric fracture
- (C) a fracture separation of the pelvic symphysis
- (D) impaction of the femoral head through the fractured acetabulum (arthrokatadysis)
- (E) a pathologic fracture

ANSWERS AND TUTORIALS ON ITEMS 1041-1050

The answers are: **1041-A; 1042-C; 1043-E; 1044-D; 1045-C; 1046-E; 1047-D; 1048-A; 1049-C; 1050-B.**

1041. The *mobility* of the upper extremity is crucial for normal funciton. Therefore, nonunion in fracture healing is preferable to a fused joint. The patient who cannot get his hand to his mouth or manipulate it in maneuvers of daily care cannot take care of himself, and is permanently disabled requiring attendants. If a fracture through a joint appears such that fusion is likely, the joint should be excised rather than to have it fused in a position of nonfunction. The *stability* of the lower extremities is functionally crucial. Here any mobility that might be a result of midshaft nonunion is a severe disability. Stable fusion is required for weight-bearing, and if that should require fusion of a joint, that is preferable to excess mobility that cannot be weight-bearing.

Open fractures are contaminated and potentially infected, and the handling of bony fractures should avoid further damage to soft tissue including conversion to an open fracture. So long as it achieves the desirable functional result, closed fixation is less of a risk than open fixation with the additional potential contamination.

1042. Anatomy is less important than physiology as a criterion of end results. If a hand looks very abnormal, but functions as a hand, it is preferable to a cosmetically pleasing but nonfunctional result. Radiographic alignment in perfect anatomic reduction is often not desirable to achieve long term optimum function, particularly in younger patients. Remodeling of bone will take the place of precise alignment so long as function is not impaired. All healing occurs by bone callus, so that minimum callus may not be preferable (e.g., in a femur fracture where a large callus is desirable for strength). A short course that achieves a dysfunctional result is almost never to be preferred over a protracted process with functional end result.

1043. Of all forms of hematogenous primary osteomyelitis to originate in the metaphysis of growing bones, *Staphylococcus aureus* is the most common cause. However, unique to sickle cell patients is an unusual osteomyelitis due to *Salmonella*. Young children with ear infections may have *Hemophilus* and sexually active patients may have arthritis based in *Gonococcus*. The most common etiologic organism in all patients would be *Staphylococcus* and the one unique to sickle cell anemia patients is *Salmonella*. This clinical fact is significant because treatment is different predicated upon these findings.

1044. Clavicle fractures are common in all age groups, but particularly in children, and result from the mechanism of injury as described. When the force of the fall is transmitted up the arm to the clavicle, that strut is the only connection of the upper extremity to the trunk, and can fracture with the stress. The clavicle is a membranous bone and heals very readily in nearly all instances when immobilized with a figure-of-eight immobilization. Colles' fracture and radial head fracture could both result from this trauma but neither would give rise to the discomfort around the shoulder. Acromio-clavicular (A-C) ligament injuries would not be likely in this age group, but this is a possible site of disruption in older patients, but not typically with this mechanism of stress from a fall on an outstretched arm as much as direct trauma to the shoulder.

1045. Ligamentous injury in the knee can be worse in outcome than fracture of bone. Remember that stability is an important function of the lower extremity, and ligamentous disruption can lead to excess mobility and a loss of stability. When force is applied to the lateral aspect of the knee, soft tissue stretching occurs on the medial side, and the medial collateral ligaments may be the first to go. With further deformity, the anterior cruciate ligament is frequently torn, and with it meniscus tears occur. This is know as the "terrible triad of O'Donaghue" and may end at least an athletic career if the knee cannot be relied upon for stability in being "planted" for forceful maneuver. Hemarthrosis is nearly inevitable with the tearing of ligaments and their blood supply. The force at the knee should not give rise to femoral fracture, at least not at the level of the hip where fracture site is so much more common in older patients who begin to demineralize.

1046. The crush injury sustained in a joint such as the knee has high likelihood of neurovascular injury as well. Physical exam is important, but arteriography can identify intimal disruption and partial separation of the artery even if minimal pulses are felt from collateral or other sources distally. Removal of the debris by sharp dissection and extensive irrigation are indicated as an emergency, and therapeutic levels of antibiotics are indicated. It is contraindicated to implant any foreign body in this degree of contamination, and it is uncertain whether the patient would need this form of pros-thesis later. If the long-term result is a healing in fusion of the knee, recall that stability is the main function of the lower extremity and this may be more appro-priate for the patient in terms of weight-bearing than an artificial knee would be, which would be very difficult to assess with the traumatic disruption of the joint early on after injury.

Any attempt at reconstruction with implantation of prosthesis soon after the injury would result in a nonunion at the traumatic bone disruption with a risk of osteomyelitis and potentially a pseud-arthrosis at the site of infection. It is

conceivable that the patient would have a fused knee and a functional pseudoarthrosis below the knee which might imitate in functional result that which could be achieved with a much later attempt at total knee replacement.

1047. The purpose of the fibula in the lower extremity is joint stabilization at the ankle and secure ligamentous connections. The fibula contributes very little to stability at the knee, and is not weight-bearing in its upper proximal extension. In fact, the head of the fibula can be excised and frequently is for either bone grafting or for relief of compartment syndromes, without functional consequence. Therefore, a patient who has a fracture of the proximal fibula may be treated with minor analgesics and could even be given some weight-bearing support so as to minimize discomfort at the fracture site, but will not be concerned with stability of the lower extremity, since weight-bearing is intact as it is aligned through the intact tibia. Each of the fractures at the ankle and foot are significant, since they disrupt the anchoring position of important ligaments that hold the ankle mortis. None of them are treated without fixation in plaster immobilization and some instances are treated with open fixation as well.

1048. The femoral fracture would not require internal fixation in children, and an intramedullary rod would be particularly inappropriate, since it would align the bone fragments anatomically with even greater length if there was some distance between the fragments in opposition.

The young child is going to be growing, and the later disposition of that hardware that will shrink relative to the size of the child is another consideration.

Rehabilitation is not speeded by open reduction or internal fixation, and children tolerate traction which is the preferred form of management. Some overlap is not only acceptable but desirable, since increased vascularity in the fractured limb is a response to injury that makes epiphyseal overgrowth on the involved side very likely, so that limb length would be discrepant with the injured limb being longer if perfect anatomic opposition were achieved by careful reduction. Limb length discrepancy would obviously lead to a limp or other consequences with spinal and pelvic alignment. Femur fractures in young children can be handled with traction or plaster spica immobilization, and in young children contracture at the hip is not a problem.

1049. Are you surprised by this response? It is not often that a clinician is ready to fracture a bone in order to set it, but in this instance, angulation may be accentuated on the side of the cortical fracture, with overgrowth at the fracture site deviating the alignment of the bone to the opposite side. By disrupting the bone across both sides, alignment can be maintained during healing, while perfect alignment at the time of reduction may be followed by angulation because of the healing. Because the growth plate in children's bones is weaker, a distressingly large number of children's fractures disrupt the growth plate with many associated problems in growth that cannot be completely predicted or ameliorated and add another dimension to expected functional result following treatment. Both the joint above and below the fracture is immobilized. It may be helpful to remember that "ortho pedics" means "straight child".

1050. Pathologic fracture is a fracture that occurs spontaneously or results from minimal trauma in a bone weakened by a metastatic or primary bone tumor. An elderly individual with osteoporosis already has the weakening, which is most remarkable for the significant public health problem for the elderly of hip fractures sustained in falls. The foreshortening and external rotation suggests inter-trochanteric hip fracture. A spiral fracture of the midshaft in the femur would be unlikely without extraordinary circumstances in the mechanism of injury, since the demin-eralized femoral neck would be a much weaker site for the stress to disrupt. The arthrokatadysis (Otto pelvis) is a highly unusual disorder that may arise from a number of circumstances besides the trauma that brought this patient to the emergency room, and it is likely that a blow sufficient to perforate the acetabulum would likely break the hip at the femoral head as well if not preferentially. A pelvic disruption is not a necessary component of the symptoms presented, and is much more uncommon than hip fracture. This scene is a very common clinical phenomenon happening nearly daily in many emergency rooms with the injury described being the most common among them.

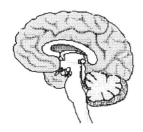

NEURO-SURGERY

Items 1051-1060

1051. Which of the following statements concerning papilledema is **NOT** true?

(A)   it results from intracranial obstruction of the retina's venous drainage
(B)   it is seen as a primary problem in diabetes mellitus
(C)   retinal hemorrhages and exudates are often associated
(D)   loss of venous pulsations is an early feature
(E)   increased intracranial pressure is the most frequent cause

1052. Which of the following studies is contraindicated in a drowsy patient with papilledema whom one suspects of having acute closed head trauma?

(A)   carotid arteriography
(B)   lumbar puncture
(C)   CT scan
(D)   MRI
(E)   echoencephalograph

1053. CT scan shows multiple solid 2 cm nodules in both cerebral hemispheres. This pattern is strongly suggestive of

(A)   glioblastoma multiforme
(B)   astrocytoma grade IV
(C)   multiple meningioma
(D)   metastases
(E)   pseudotumor

1054. A 40 year-old man has developed ptosis of the left eyelid with the left pupil dilated in an eye that deviates laterally. He has no complaints of headache, dizziness or drowsiness, and this new finding has gradually worsened in four weeks. An arteriogram is ordered for evaluation with the clinical information of the request suggesting

(A)   meningioma, left frontal sulcus
(B)   left occipital arteriovenous malformation
(C)   pontine tumor
(D)   cerebellar aneurysm of basilar artery
(E)   left internal carotid aneurysm

1055. Which of the following clinical signs is the most sensitive indicator of head injury from deceleration resulting in closed head trauma?

(A)   level of consciousness
(B)   blood pressure
(C)   pulse
(D)   cranial nerve function
(E)   deep tendon reflexes

1056. A young man waiting for a bus was stabbed in the back and the his parcels were snatched. He fell without seeing his assailant, since he could not support himself upright because his right leg was powerless. On emergency room examination you find that he has a stab wound on the right side of the spine, but he has lost sensation in his left lower extremity. Other physical findings you would anticipate would include each of the following **EXCEPT**:

(A) a loss of vibratory sensation on the right side
(B) he has lost proprioception on the right side
(C) he can distinguish heat from cold on the right side but not the left
(D) the left lower extremity is hyperreflexic
(E) pinprick sensation is absent at the groin and left lower quadrant of the abdomen

1057. Cervical collars are placed on patients before evaluation of multiple injury from deceleration to stabilize the neck because

(A) an open airway is maintained
(B) it avoids jugular compression in order to prevent cerebral edema
(C) it safeguards ventilation because of high cervical innervation of the diaphragm
(D) carotid sinus response is prevented
(E) it hyperextends the cervical vertebrae for radiographic evaluation

1058. Which of the following findings would be critically important information from skull X-rays or repeated examination and follow-up of the patient?

(A) linear temporal skull fracture line
(B) minimally depressed parietal skull fracture
(C) midline suture separation of 1 mm
(D) occipital linear skull fracture line
(E) opacified left frontal sinus

1059. Each of the following features of the Glasgow coma scale is true **EXCEPT**:

(A) a Glasgow coma scale for an adult less than 7 is a good prognostic indicator
(B) vocal response to the examiner at a measurement of 5 shows a well-oriented patient
(C) motor response score 3 shows flexion indicating decorticate response
(D) motor response at level of 2 shows extension indicating a decerebrate response
(E) eye opening in response to pain is a positive response of 2

1060. A 12 year-old boy was the catcher of a baseball game when he was struck in the lateral side of the head by the batter. He was knocked out, but revived a few minutes later and was comfortable, although complaining of a headache and scalp bruise in the emergency room, where he later became nauseated and drowsy. Appropriate management at this stage would be

(A) cerebral arteriogram
(B) discharge home in the care of his mother with a follow-up appointment in 72 hours
(C) hospitalization for observation following skull X-ray
(D) lumbar puncture
(E) outpatient CT scan scheduled for the following morning

ANSWERS AND TUTORIALS ON ITEMS 1051-1060

The answers are: **1051-B; 1052-B; 1053-D; 1054-E; 1055-A; 1056-D; 1057-C; 1058-A; 1059-A; 1060-C**.

1051. Increased intracranial pressure causes obstruction of venous return which first eliminates venous pulsations, leading to venous engorgement and papilledema which can then progress to hemorrhage and exudates in the retina. This process is an early sign of primary intracranial problems, and a patient with diabetes with these problems should have investigation of an intracranial pressure increase, since it is not associated primarily with diabetes.

1052. A patient with an increased intracranial pressure as evidenced by papilledema has risk from lumbar puncture that can decompress the cerebrospinal fluid lower in the lumbar thecal space, and this may bring about a shift of the intracranial contents downward to cause herniation of the brain and compression of the medullary respiratory control centers. Consequently, no CSF should be withdrawn, nor should any loss be risked by leaking at a lumbar puncture site in a patient suspected of having acute intracranial pressure increase. Echoencephalography, CT and MRI scanning are imaging techniques that allow determinations of any shift in midline structures or identification of space occupying defects or swelling that may account for the intracranial pressure increase. Arteriography can show distortion of the vasculature which would allow an inference of the same information. Of the options, the lesser invasive studies would be preferred and lumbar puncture would be contraindicated.

1053. Primary intracranial neoplasms may be invasive, and can become quite extensive, but are rarely multiple. That is true for both the lower grade neoplasms such as meningioma as well as high grade glioblastoma and astrocytoma. Pseudotumor is a clinical reflection of a variety of unrelated conditions that give rise to intracranial pressure increase from brain swelling, and would not show tumors, multiple or otherwise. The presence of multiple tumors in the substance of the cerebrum distributed bilaterally suggests metastatic cancer from an origin typically outside the head, most often spread by the hematogenous route.

1054. Over half of the internal carotid aneurysms present with oculomotor nerve palsy, because of the adjacent structures' proximity. Without symptoms of increased intracranial pressure or dizziness, tumors, whether in the frontal sulcus or pons, would not be likely and do not explain the III nerve palsy, and the pontine tumor would be far more morbid in presentation. Vascular abnormalities in the occiput might give visual disturbances, more likely than cranial nerve dysfunction. Basilar artery aneurysms are rare, but in this instance would give symptoms of dizziness or imbalance. The internal carotid artery aneurysm on the left is the diagnosis strongly suggested.

1055. In acute head injury, examination of the patient takes place after assessing the level of consciousness, since a conscious patient does not have disruption of the very sensitive indicator of cerebral function. Cushing response can be determined in a comatose patient by blood pressure and pulse, and tendon reflexes may help lateralize damage as might cranial nerve examination in a patient who does not have cerebral function. The level of consciousness is rather rapidly and readily assessed also making it a highly valuable indicator.

1056. This patient has suffered a Brown-Séquard syndrome. Brown-Séquard described the clinical findings of this lesion which involve loss of motor innervation on the same side, and loss of sensation to pinprick and temperature on the opposite side of hemisection of the spinal cord. Both vibratory and proprioception sensation are also lost on the same side as the motor loss, since they are in the posterior column which is not crossed,

similar to the motor innervation. The Brown-Séquard syndrome results from either a complete hemisection of the cord — in this case the right thoracic spine — or in compression of it or interference with its blood supply. There should be no change in motor reflexes in the left lower extremity which has intact motor innervation. (This clinical vignette, as are most of the others encountered in this book, is unfortunately not imaginary, but is a real story with recent history.)

1057. Cervical fracture can give spinal injury with sequelae of paralysis or loss of sensation. However, a high cervical fracture gives an additional risk of immediate threat to life from suffocation, since cervical spine innervation of the phrenic nerve would be interrupted from dysfunction high in the cervical spine, and patients with transverse myelitis at C-2 level cannot breathe. There is no likelihood of carotid compression without a displacement that would have to be greater than arterial pressure, and jugular compression may raise venous pressure but would not result in cerebral edema under most circumstances. The cervical collar must be removed in order to get appropriate radiographs of the cervical spine, and hyperextension at scene of injury is not for this purpose. A patent airway is the first priority in the management of the trauma victim, but the cervical collar does not accomplish that, and that must be achieved and assured before a collar is applied.

1058. Skull X-rays would be a low priority in the evaluation of patients with closed head trauma were it not for one critical area in which the skull fracture makes a clinical difference of urgent significance. Fractures in most areas of the skull would not be significant except in confirming the evidence of a severe blow to the head, and if not depressed considerably or displaced, no further surgical treatment of the fracture itself is indicated. That includes the parietal depressed skull fracture, and the very minimal suture line separation, and the occipital linear fracture. An opacified frontal sinus without antecedent history of sinusitis might suggest blood in the frontal sinus, but its presence there is not life threatening nor an indication of collateral critical injury. However, a linear fracture through the temporal bone runs a risk of disruption of the entrapped middle meningeal artery. Laceration of this artery would allow hemorrhage into the cranium under arterial blood pressure giving rise to an epidural hematoma which is an urgent threat to life. Subdural hematoma is under venous pressure, and accumulates more slowly and is frequently accommodated by patients over time, whereas epidural hematoma from the arterial hemorrhage that can be induced by this position of a linear skull fracture is life threatening.

1059. The Glasgow coma scale is almost universally used for head injury patient evaluation. The three measured responses are to eye opening, motor response, and vocal response, with a score of 15 being an uninjured patient who is not ill. If six hours following injury, an adult has a Glasgow coma score less than 7, prognostic outlook is very poor. It is slightly better for such a low score in the pediatric age group.

1060. Mechanism of injury in this patient in the clinical scenario are a worrisome combination suggesting a very significant head injury. What is described is a classic "lucid interval" whereby the patient suffers an immediate concussion and loss of consciousness, but recovers completely from that, only to begin deteriorating within a short period of time under observation. These findings suggest a rapid increase in intracranial pressure and that is often indicative of blood loss into the head. The position of the blow to the head could suggest a temporal or parietal location of the blow, and skull fracture that might have lacerated the entrapped middle meningeal artery, which can give rise to an epidural hematoma. The rapid accumulation of blood under arterial pressure often gives rise to the sequence of events described by this patient. Any option that would suggest discharge home, even under observation, would be inappropriate. The patient should have hospitalization for continuous observation as well as skull X-ray to evaluate the possibility of a linear fracture through the lateral skull. With increasing intracranial pressure, lumbar puncture is contra-indicated, and CT scan might be appropriate, but certainly not as an outpatient and not the following day. Cerebral arteriography might be diagnostic, but there would be less invasive and more sensitive and specific studies with better reliability that could be achieved sooner. This patient has a serious problem that requires rapid evaluation and the probability of early intervention.

PART VII

HOW TO USE
THE STUDY OF SURGERY

Within the covers of this book are 1060 chances for you to commit yourself using your knowledge of surgery in practical clinical application. This is an excellent practice for taking the National Board of Medical Examiners examinations. Moreover, it is an excellent way to review salient topics in the broad field of surgery. Test items and tutorials offer the opportunity for review of the principles behind decisions. This book is also a directed review that should have most of the clinically important features of surgical discipline succinctly organized for a review that could be completed rapidly in study for the examinations.

Each clinical item offers a decision point that is an opportunity for you to make the right choice, in the estimation of the author, while the tutorial allows you the opportunity to prove him wrong, given changing surgical practice.

The context for typical clinical presentation is that of United States urban medical practice in 1995, unless otherwise noted, recognizing that the world is a fluid place with respect to disease and with respect to standards of medical practice designed to meet essential human needs in a variety of settings.

To review the terminology and mechanics of the NBME type examinations, this introduction will take you through the terms and their use in tests you may have encountered before. You may use the terms and design features of the test to help you in making the correct response *after* you recognize the right information and then pattern the response to what the examination is asking. The SUBJECT matter of this examination review book is SURGERY. The TEST ITEMS are designed to score your proficiency in management of surgically relevant information. Such items are categorized by DISCIPLINE; in this book that would be either ANATOMIC or SPECIALTY divisions within this discipline, and items are related to the discipline by CATEGORY with SUB-CATEGORIES. For example, in Part VI of the one-best-response items, the anatomic (first) division is:

GASTRO-
   INTESTINAL   category

       PANCREAS   subcategory

       EXOCRINE   sub-subcategory

The test items are SCORABLE UNITS in ITEM SETS. The item set usually begins with an incomplete HEADER, followed by TRAILERS. In an A-TYPE item ("One-best-response" — see below) the header is followed by 5 trailers; one of these is the ANSWER and 4 are called DISTRACTORS, plausible but false options in the combined judgement of the author of the item and the TEST COM-MITTEE who have to agree upon a one best response. If the answer is judged to be controversial, tricky, or called into question by any member of the committee, it is reworked or discarded. If the committee requires more than one *minute* to read or understand the wording of the header and trailers, the item is discarded. The examination is not a reading test, nor is it designed to be tricky. It is designed to be a valid exercise of your comprehension. The test should not be a test of rote memory recall, but a test of second order thinking in how this information can be processed and applied, rather than simply stored.

TEST ITEM LIBRARY (TIL)

The TIL consists of several basic ITEM TYPES which are basically multiple-choice items (MCQ) scorable by a machine from a coded response sheet.

A-TYPE items are the most frequent types of MCQ test items. In this type a header is followed by 5 trailers, one of which is the *best* response. The four distractors do not have to be *wrong,* but they must be inferior in the unanimous judgement of the experts on the reviewing test committee, or the item would not be included on the examination.

Random guess (or consistently marking one response trailer — "C", say — would give you a 20% correct score. Those odds can be raised by mentally blotting out the distractors that are clearly wrong, often narrowing to two plausible options (raising you already from 20% odds to 50%). If you genuinely don't know the preferred *better* of the two responses, choose by being first safe, and then practical.

MATCHING items may take the form of B-TYPE test items. In this type of

"set", up to 10 or more items are listed (such as diagnoses, techniques, micro-organisms, drugs, etc.) and a more limited list of trailers follow this list. The object here is to select the one heading item most closely associated with the numbered trailer. The test will tell you that each lettered heading may be used once, more than once, or not at all. It is better to learn this with this book open before you without time pressure than to use up test-taking time to study test-taking technique.

Now, what is the savvy way of approaching the B-type test item without becoming befuddled by it as an incoherent reading list or confused test of short-term memory of disjointed headings with no apparent (or, worse, misleading) pattern? Just read by *scanning,* not by *studying,* the listed headings. Then concentrate on the numbered trailers — remember — where the *scorable unit* lies. Often, the answer as to what close association there may be with the trailer is readily apparent, and would come to mind even without the suggestibility of the heading list. Locate the answers you know in the heading list, and mark those responses first. Next, return to items you were unsure of and look through the options to evaluate them for association with remaining unanswered items. To run through the optional headings evaluating each individually for every one of the trailers not only takes too much time, but the suggestibility of this method could get you to change answers that you would have answered correctly reflexly.

Do not be misled by the same word appearing in both heading and trailer as a cue to the correct response. Such a "cheap shot" should be edited out by the test committee. For example, if the term "nevus" appears in both heading and trailer, it is likely to be there as part of a term, and not as a word that should cue the correct response. Also beware of terms that sound like they should be categorized differently from that which the name implies; for example, intuitively, "cystosarcoma phylloides" should not be appearing in a list of benign lesions, nor "mycosis fungoides" in a list of malignancies.

When you are through with this matching set (or, for that matter, the examination as a whole), you should check it for *form*, but not *content*. Make sure you have completed each section, and that you have left no answers blank. If you are satisfied that you have completed all parts of the test, *leave*! Second-guessing and changing your answers has a high probability of your falsifying correct responses. Remember, it was the design of the test to see how you could manage information you know, not stumping you through devious trickery into unlearning something through cleverly presented distractors.

SETS — THE C-TYPE test item could be considered "comparison multiple true-false". This item type has a pair of headings with a second pair of options added — both, or neither. The responses are 4 possibilities to 4 test item trailers (in each set in this book).

> A. only A
> B. only B
> C. both A and B
> D. neither A nor B

In approach to the C-type set, the first two headers are important to compare and contrast; the second two headers will *always be the same*, and need not even be read, which would slow down consideration of the two first important items. Remember, the test item types are clustered together, and there will not be a random scatter of A-types among C-types, for example. This is *not* a test of ability to read instructions, or to pay attention to quick switches!

Begin evaluating a C-type test item by considering it as a 2 option heading. How do these options relate? How are they different? How are they similar? Then, drop down to the first trailer. Now there is a third point of perspective, since the 2 headings have to be true together or false together to the degree of their comparative *similarities* with respect to the trailer, or they *contrast* with each other now in the light of the trailer item. All that remains is to consider their sign, +/-, and align them to the 4 options — which are *always* the *same* in all C-types.

G-SETS are another test of pattern recognition. Here a short clinical scenario may be provided. (This may be one of the few parts of the exam where you can expect to encounter multi-sentence headings, sometimes even up to a short paragraph. Do not make a reading test of this! Scan it as you would the list of options in the headings of extended matching sets, and then drop immediately to the test item trailer. Here is the place for graphics — an X-Ray, clinical photograph, microscopic slide, pathology specimen (called in test committee argot PIX). The item you will *not* likely be expected to encounter is: "What is this?" More likely it will be, "What would you do about this?" Again, this is not a memory test to see if you have "banked" this pattern in a recallable mode, but a test of *judgement* about how you would *use* this information.

So, do not "come to cloture" too soon on PIX! The "flash of recognition" that happens when you think, "Ahah! I know what that is!" has not yet come to the point of the item which will ask you something beyond "what is it you are seeing here?" If it were not obvious, the PIX would have been tossed out by committee editing. If this were a vision test, it would not be limited to medical students! So, wait for the item before the satisfaction of knowing what is being asked.

K-TYPE items are phased out of the new NBME exams, so none are included in this book. The author has written them for many years, and they continue to be used in other examinations, so for future reference in the event that you encounter K-types in such tests as specialty board certification or licensure examinations, these will be explained and a suggestion offered as to how to approach them.

K-types are "multiple true false" items. This type gets a lot of testable information into a list of 5 trailers *each* of which needs to be evaluated. If an A-type item has one quick and easy answer found among 5 trailers, one doesn't need to know anything about how true or false the other 4 distractors might have been — they could have been written in another language and they contain no testable information unless one didn't recognize the answer among them.

K-type items were designed for value added to these distractors over A-types. That is an advantage; they can be tricky, and evaluate testmanship and fund of information more than action taken on it. That may be why they have been phased out of the NBME examinations after so many years of use. If that testmanship is a feature of the K-type, you and I together will turn that to your advantage (below).

After the heading, this clumsy instruction list follows:

A only 1, 2, and 3 are correct
B only 1 and 3 are correct
C only 2 and 4 are correct
D only 4 is correct
E all are correct

TESTMANSHIP MADE EASY

Now, how can you turn this cumbersome K-type answer key to work *for* you? If there were only *one* best response, this item would be written as an A-type; the K-type *allows*, no, *requires*, more than one correct response (unless D is correct!). So, what if you are unsure of several of the list of options? Here are your clues to beating the odds:

K-TYPE ANSWERING SEQUENCE: In a K-type item, always look at "4" *first*. If false, then C, D and E are excluded. (You are already up to 50-50 odds knowing only *one* option!) *Next*, look at "2". If "2" is also false, only "1" and "3" are left, and "1" and "3" are always right or wrong together.

Now, if that isn't test-taking skill perfection enough to get you to pass examinations for which you are thoroughly unprepared, here are several more hints!

MCQ TEST TAKING SKILLS: In the "one best response" A-type item, if you know the answer from the stem, scan the responses to find the closest approximation to what you *know* to be correct. Do *not* be prompted by the distractors to reconsider or change your answer! Those other options are there to mislead you as plausibly as possible, so if you are confident of the answer, don't become suggestible by a list that is 80% wrong! If you genuinely don't know, then scan the options for those you can surely exclude, giving a shorter list of possible correct options, increasing your chances of a correct selection even if it is a guess. But, it should be an educated guess, and use whatever information base you have — even if incomplete. Remember, this is just like it will continually be in clinical practice! To be less random and more rational, use what you know.

LOOK FOR EXCLUSIONS: For example, in a two item set, items on the greater, (lesser), bigger, better, etc., comparisons, "both" and "neither" are nonstarters, so your odds are 50-50 even before you add any of your information base to "tilt" in favor of a choice. If in doubt, tilt toward clinical practical applicability and patient safety. Do not be in a hurry to exenterate or radiate, or do radical chemotherapy with bone marrow rescue unless you know the condition is desperate, yet might yield to aggressive treatment for cure. Do *not* stand by and watch tension pneumothorax strangle a patient, even if you are inclined toward a psychiatry residency. Remember, you have to get there first!

TUTORIALS: One of the useful components of the tutorials is to recognize that the art of surgery advanced a great deal as a means of helping people solve human problems. There are, despite these advances, very painful limits on what can be accomplished, particularly for some forms of cancer, multiple organ failures, and degenerative disease. It is a humbling but very maturing honest recognition that there exists no surgically curative treatment for quite a number of altogether too common diseases. At the same time, there are diseases that can be successfully managed, but only with timely application of extraordinary surgical technique. These patients should not be denied what surgery *can* accomplish.

WRONG ANSWERS: There may be several cues to *wrong* responses. They are any option with one of the following terms in it: "always", "never", "all", "absolutely", since medicine is the sometimes unpredictable application of biologic science which is full of surprises anyway. Most medical messages are followed by many qualifiers. A good test committee that is vigilant should screen out these absolute items. But using the reverse of this principle to advantage, in an essay-type stem (patient presentation, for example), the longest response (with the most qualifiers) is often correct.

Mutually inclusive and mutually exclusive distractors will always be linked and will have to be true or false together in the first instance and opposite in the second. Mutually exclusive distractors *are* permitted in the A-type format. When they are, one of the two is almost always the answer, and all one need know at that point is the clinical value of the +/- sign.

Easy items to write are A-types that state in the heading, "Each of the following is correct **EXCEPT**...". These items are generally discouraged, since they require the examinee to switch from positive to negative thinking. However that is the objective in identification of a contra-indication, adverse reaction, excluded possibility — each clues that can limit the options that need to be known to be answered. Beware, however, of negatives in the heading stem: they can create a double negative, switching the answer if there is at least one trailing option with a negative within it.

HOW TO USE THE TESTS AND TUTORIALS

How did this author come to be qualified to write not just surgery texts, but a surgery examination book? It was not just by taking lots of tests or failing none of them or having excelled in them, but from having written them for over two decades. The "supply side" is at least as challenging, and teaches not only information but how this vital information can be successfully taught with evaluation of both student and the teacher. The author has written examinations and sat through multiple NBME test committees for allied health, medical students, surgical residents, and other certifying agencies for surgical technologists, recertifying surgeons and subspecialty sections in the last 15 years, voluntarily withdrawing from NBME test committees more recently to prevent conflict of interest within these pages. He hopes that you may be able to turn this experience to your benefit in this examination book, using some of the ideas that go into how the new NBME exams are written to help in taking them. The offer was once made to the students and residents that this experience and advice on improving test-taking performance would be shared with all or none, but not with a few who sought advantage over others. This book is written to make good on the offer to all.

Use this text to teach — not just test-taking (which should be brought to an even playing pitch for all students) but to sharpen clinical judgement. You may disagree with the "answer" given with the tutorial, and over time some of these answers will change with advances in the art (as has happened so rapidly with development of less invasive procedures). But having selected the *right* answer for the *wrong* reason is a failure for the opportunity missed — since a wrong answer is an opportunity to learn through that memorable incentive — particularly in this test book rather than on taking the exam for "all the marbles".

SUMMARY:

USING THIS TEXT AND THE NBME TEST AS A BRIDGE TO A LIFELONG HABIT OF EVALUATION

The intent of the NBME examination, this book, and a medical education, is less the cataloging of an encyclopedia of medical information than in evaluating how well you can use clinically important information in improved patient outcome. The stratification of the candidates' performance on the examination is not to identify the overall excellence of the superstar, but to test the cumulative adequacy of marginal candidates' responses, to assure — to the degree that a written examination is capable of contributing to this goal — that the practicing clinician would be safe and effective in guiding patient health problems toward a successful result.

If biologic information is clearly testable with right and wrong answers to well-designed items, but that information is less important in determining practical clinical choices, it is irrelevant for the purposes of this examination or for medical practice. Such applied information management is a skill that develops over time with changing technology, disease pattern or generation of significant new information. Some of the correct answers as written today will be provably wrong in only five years when you answer the same items differently on board specialty examination. I only wish I knew now which item responses will be proven incorrect in the future!

The purpose of continuing medical education is continuous quality improvement in both the physician and the performance of medical and surgical service. The author hopes that this book will assist you in this process by identifying areas of weakness and their correction through the life-long habit of assisted self-study,

392